MRCP PACES

180 Clinical Cases

Kevin O'Gallagher MBBS BA (Hons) MRCP (UK)
Specialty Registrar in Cardiology, London Deanery, London, UK

Daniel Knight MBBS BSc (Hons) MRCP (UK)
Specialty Registrar in Cardiology, London Deanery, London, UK

Michael O'Gallagher MBBCh BAO
Specialty Registrar in Ophthalmology, Belfast, UK

Eirini Merika MBBS BSc (Hons) MRCP (UK)
Specialty Registrar in Dermatology, London Deanery, London, UK

Omar Malik MBBS BSc PhD FRCP
Consultant Neurologist, Charing Cross Hospital, London, UK

Editors

Peter TK Milton MBBS BSc (Hons) MRCP (UK)
Specialty Registrar in General Practice, London Deanery, London, UK

Nick Oliver MBBS BSc (Hons) FRCP
Consultant Physician and Endocrinologist, Charing Cross Hospital,
London, UK

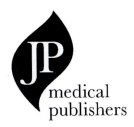

JP
medical
publishers

London • Philadelphia • Panama City • New Delhi

© 2015 JP Medical Ltd.
Published by JP Medical Ltd
83 Victoria Street, London, SW1H 0HW, UK
Tel: +44 (0)20 3170 8910   Fax: +44 (0)20 3008 6180
Email: info@jpmedpub.com   Web: www.jpmedpub.com

ISBN: 978-1-907816-52-9

British Library Cataloguing in Publication Data
A catalogue record for this book is available from the British Library

Library of Congress Cataloging in Publication Data
A catalog record for this book is available from the Library of Congress

Commissioning Editor: Steffan Clements
Editorial Assistant: Sophie Woolven
Design: Designers Collective Ltd

Typeset, printed and bound in India.

Preface

Representing the culmination of the membership examination process, PACES is widely recognised as an exceptionally difficult challenge. Demanding the incorporation of both clinical acumen and applied knowledge in a time-pressured environment, it is considered a rite of passage for the aspiring physician. Candidates can therefore be forgiven for approaching their preparation with trepidation.

This book aims to encourage an early, targeted approach for each component of the exam. It serves to guide readers through their preparation by providing a summary of clinical cases likely to be tested, and offers insight from candidates with recent experience of the current format, including the new station 5. It helps to remove the mystery from PACES, improving performance and maximising the chances of success through the development of a structured framework for the presentation of clinical findings.

The framework for successful presentation need not be complicated, as demonstrated in this book. Each clinical case is broken down to transform simple concepts and fundamental knowledge into an impressive display of clinical acumen. The successful candidate should adopt this framework, in order to display the necessary skills to be a safe, knowledgeable and insightful doctor suitable for admission to the Royal College of Physicians.

The book guides the reader through the carousel of the exam chapter by chapter. The introduction highlights the differences between the stations, the approach required for each, and defines the overall framework. It is therefore paramount for readers to familiarise themselves with the concepts defined in the introduction before moving on to the remainder of the text.

The format lends itself to both individual study and to group role-play, which will stimulate dialogue around the themes introduced. Exploring the themes and topics presented in each of the cases, structured in accordance with the framework, will equip candidates with the necessary skills to negotiate the PACES process.

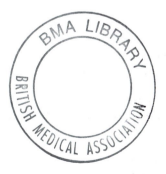

Kevin O'Gallagher
Daniel Knight
Michael O'Gallagher
Eirini Merika
Omar Malik
Peter Milton
Nick Oliver
October 2014

Contents

Contents

Contents

Contents

Contributors

Jamal Hayat BSc MBBS MRCP
Chapter 4
Specialty Registrar in Gastroenterology and General Internal Medicine
St George's Hospital, University of London, London, UK

Shruthi Konda BSc MBBS MRCP AICSM
Chapter 3
Specialty Registrar in Respiratory and General Internal Medicine
London Deanery, London, UK

Peter TK Milton MBBS BSc (Hons) MRCP (UK)
Chapters 2, 4, 6
Specialty Registrar in General Practice
London Deanery, London, UK

Bejal Pandya MBBS MRCP
Chapter 1
Consultant in Congenital Heart Disease
The Heart Hospital, University College London NHS Foundation Trust, London, UK

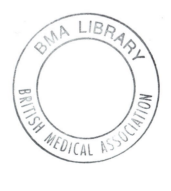

Glossary

ABPA	Allergic bronchopulmonary aspergillosis	BRCA	Breast cancer gene
ABPI	Ankle-brachial pressure index	BTS	British Thoracic Society
ACEi	ACE inhibitors	CABG	Coronary artery bypass graft
ACHD	Adult congenital heart disease	CAG	Coronary angiography
AChR	Acetylcholine receptor	CEA	Carcinoembryonic antigen
ACTH	Adrenocorticotropic hormone	CHADS-VASC	**C**ongestive heart failure – **H**ypertension – **A**ge ≥75 years – **D**iabetes – Prior **s**troke – **V**ascular disease – **A**ge 65–74 years – **S**ex **c**ategory
ADH	Antidiuretic hormone		
AF	Atrial fibrillation		
AHA	American Heart Association		
AIDP	Acute inflammatory demyelinating polyneuropathy	CIDP	Chronic inflammatory demyelinating polyneuropathy
AKI	Acute kidney injury	CNS	Central nervous system
ALS	Advanced life support/amyotrophic lateral sclerosis	CML	Chronic myelocytic leukaemia
		CMV	Cytomeglovirus
ALT	Alanine aminotransferase	COMT	Catechol-*O*-methyl transferase
ALS	Amyotrophic lateral sclerosis	COPD	Chronic obstructive pulmonary disease
AMTS	Abbreviated mental test score		
ANA	Antinuclear antibody	CRC	Colorectal cancer
ANCA	Antineutrophil cytoplasmic antibodies	CRP	C-reactive protein
		CRT-D	Cardiac resynchronisation therapy with biventricular pacemaker and defibrillator
APKD	Autosomal dominant polycystic kidney disease		
ARB	Angiotensin receptor blocker	CRT-P	Cardiac resynchronisation therapy with biventricular pacing only
ARVD	Arrhythmogenic right ventricular cardiomyopathy		
		CSF	Cerebrospinal fluid
ASAS	American Society of Abdominal Surgeons	CTPA	Computed tomographic pulmonary angiography
ASD	Atrial septal defect	CVA	Cardiovascular accident
ASO	Antistreptolysin O	CXR	Chest X-ray
AST	Aspartate aminotransferase	DC	Direct current
ATN	Acute tubular necrosis	DIP	Distal interpharengeal joints
AVNRT	Atrio-ventricular node re-entry tachycardia	DLE	Discoid lupus erythematosis
		DMARD	Disease-modifying anti-rheumatic drugs
AZA	Azathioprine		
BASAI	Bath ankylosing spondylitis activity index	DMPK	Myotonic dystrophy protein kinase
		DPLD	Diffuse parenchymal lung disease
BCG	Bacille Calmette-Guérin	dsDNA	Double-stranded DNA
BMI	Body mass index	DVLA	Driver and Vehicle Licensing Agency
BNP	B-type natriuretic peptide	EBV	Epstein Barr virus
BOS	Bronchiolitis obliterans syndrome	ECG	Echocardiogram

EHRA	Electronic health record architecture
EMG	Electromyogram
ESC	European Society of Cardiology
ESCKD	End-stage chronic kidney disease
ESR	Erythrocyte sedimentation rate
FBC	Full blood count
FFA	Fundus fluorescein angiography
FNA	Fine needle aspiration
FSH	Follicle stimulating hormone
FVC	Forced vital capacity
GBS	Guillain-Barré syndrome
GGT	Gamma-GT
GI	Gastrointestinal
GMC	General medical council
GORD	Gastro-oesophageal reflux disease
GP	General practitioner
GTN	Glyceryl trinitrate
GUCH	Grown up congenital heart (disease)
GUM	Genito-urinary medicine
HACEK	Haemophilus actinobacillus cardiobacterium einkella and kingella
HAS-BLED	**H**ypertension (systolic BP > 160 mmHg) – **A**bnormal renal function – Abnormal liver function – Previous **s**troke – Prior major **B**leeding or predisposition – **L**abile INR (<60% of time in therapeutic range) – Age >65 (**e**lderly) – **D**rugs predisposing to bleeding (antiplatelet agents, NSAIDs) – Alcohol use (>8 drinks/week)
HbA1c	Glycosylated haemoglobin
HCC	Hepatocellular carcinoma
HDL	High density lipoprotein
HDU	High dependency unit
HepA/B/C	Hepatitis A/B/C
HHS	Hyperglycaemic hyperosmolar syndrome
HIV	Human immunodeficiency virus
HLA	Human leukocyte antigen
HNPCC	Hereditary non polyposis colorectal cancer
HOCM	Hypertrophic obstructive cardiomyopathy
HRCT	High resolution computed tomography
HSMN	Hereditary sensory motor neuropathy
HSP	Henoch-Schönlein pupura
HTLV-1	Human T-lymphotropic virus type 1
HTT	Hungtingtin gene
IBD	Inflammatory bowel disease
ICD	Implantable cardiac defibrillator
ICP	Intracranial pressure
ILD	Interstitial lung disease
INO	Internuclear ophthalmoplegia
INR	internal normalised ratio
IPF	Idiopathic pulmonary fibrosis
	idiopathic pulmonary fibrosis
ISMN	Isosorbide mononitrate
ITU	Intensive therapy unit
IVIG	Intravenous immunoglobulin
JVP	Jugular venous pressure
LABA	Long acting β-agonist
LAMA	Long acting muscarinic anticholinergic
LBT	Blastic transformation of lymphocytes
LDH	Lactate dehydrogenase
LFTs	Liver function tests
LH	Luteinising hormone
LTOT	Long term oxygen therapy
LV	Left ventricle
LVOT	Left ventricular outflow tract
MAO	Monoamine oxidase
MAZE	The Maze procedure – open heart procedure requiring cardiopulmonary bypass
MDT	Multi-disciplinary team
MELD	Model end-stage liver disease
MEN2	Multiple, endocrine neoplasia, type 2
MI	Myocardial infarction
MND	Motor neurone disease
MR	Mitral regurgitation
MRA	Magnetic resonance angiography

MRC	Medical Research Council	PUVA	Photochemotherapy
MRCP	Membership of the Royal College of Physicians	RA	Rheumatoid arthritis
		RAPD	Relative afferent pupillary defect
MRI	Magnetic resonance imaging	REM	Rapid eye movement
MS	Mitral stenosis	RNIB	Royal National Institute for the Blind
MTP	Metatarsophalangeal	RNS	Repetitive nerve stimulation
MusK	Muscle specific kinase	RSR	Regular sinus rhythm
NASH	Non-alcoholic-induced steatohepatitis	RUQ	Right upper quadrant
		RV	Right ventricle
NCS	Nerve conduction studies	SAAG	Serum ascetic albumin gradient
NHS	National Health Service	SBP	Spontaneous bacterial peritonitis
NICE	National Institute for Health and Care Excellence	SCC	Squamous cell carcinoma
		SCLC	Small cell lung cancer
NIV	Non-invasive ventilation	SCUBA	Sub-millimetre common user bolometer array
NMJ	Neuromuscular junction		
NO	Nitric oxide	SHBG	Sex hormone binding globulin
NOAC	Novel oral anticoagulant	SHO	Senior house officer
NSAIDs	Non-steroidal anti-inflammatory drugs	SIADH	Syndrome of inappropriate antidiuretic hormone
NYHA	New York Heart Association	SLE	Systemic lupus erythematosus
OA	Oesophageal atresia	SPECT	Single-photon emission computerized tomography
OCP	Octacalcium phosphate		
OCT	Optical coherence tomography	SSRI	Selective serotonin reuptake inhibitor
OGD	Oesophago-gastro-duodenoscopy		
OGTT	Glucose tolerance test	SVC	Superior vena cava
PALS	Patient Advice and Liaison Service	TAVI	Transcatheter aortic valve implantation
PAN	Polyarteritis nodosa		
PANTHER	Prednisolone, azathioprine and N-acetylcysteine: a study that evaluates response in idiopathic pulmonary fibrosis	TB ELISPOT	Tuberculosis enzyme-linked immunosorbent spot test
		TBNA	Transbronchial needle aspiration
		TEDS	Thrombo-embolic deterrent stocking
PAS	Periodic acid-Schiff	TIA	Transient ischaemic attack
PBC	Primary biliary cirrhosis	TIPS	Transjugular intrahepatic portosystemic shunt placement
PCP	Pneumocystis carinii pneumonia		
PCR	Polymerase chain reaction	TLCO	Carbon monoxide transfer factor
PDA	Patent ductus arteriosus	TNF	Tumour necrosis factor
PEG	Percutaneous endoscopic gastrostomy	TPMT	Thiopurine methyltransferase
		TR	Tricuspid regurgitation
PEP	Post-exposure prophylaxis	TSH	Thyroid stimulating hormone
PMHx	Past medical history	TTA	Transglutaminase antibodies
PND	Paroxysmal nocturnal dyspnea	TTE	Transthoracic echocardiogram
PSC	Pancreatic stellate cells	UC	Ulcerative colitis
PTH	Parathyroid hormone	UDCA	Ursodeoxycholic acid
PUO	Pyrexia of unknown origin	US	Ultrasound

Glossary

UTI	Urinary tract infection	VT	Ventricular tachycardia
VDRL	Venereal disease research laboratory	VZV	Varicella zoster virus
VF	Ventricular fibrillation	WCC	White cell count
V/Q	Ventilation/perfusion		
VSDs	Ventricular septal defects		

Introduction: preparation for the exam

The MRCP PACES carousel

The PACES carousel consists of five stations, each lasting 20 minutes, through which candidates progress to encounter a variety of clinical scenarios. In the first instance, the need to distinguish between the types of stations, and the nature of their challenges, is paramount to success. Each station requires different skills and demands a tailored approach to demonstrate competency.

Stations 1–5

Candidates can expect to spend 20 minutes at each station.

Station 1 (Chapters 3 & 4)
Respiratory system examination: 10 minutes
Abdominal system examination: 10 minutes

Station 2 (Chapter 6)
History taking skills: 20 minutes

Station 3 (Chapters 1&2)
Cardiovascular system examination: 10 minutes
Nervous system examination: 10 minutes

Station 4 (Chapter 7)
Communication skills and ethics: 20 minutes

Station 5 (Chapter 5)
Integrated clinical assessment
Two brief clinical consultations: 10 minutes each

In broad terms the carousel can be broken down into three categories of station:

- The physical examination – stations 1 and 3
- Communications skills, ethical situations and history taking – stations 2 and 4
- The integrated clinical assessment – station 5

Skills examined

Having successfully negotiated the initial stages of membership, combined with experience in clinical practice, proficiency in the key areas under scrutiny is assumed in candidates embarking upon PACES. The key to success lies predominantly in mastering the ability to demonstrate the necessary skills under exam conditions. It is essential, therefore, to familiarise yourself with the seven areas being examined.

1. Physical examination requires a practised and polished approach. Importantly, the instruction to the candidate at each station will clearly set out what is required and this should be adhered to as closely as possible. Demonstrating this skill relies upon executing the appropriate examination in a way that identifies clinical signs while putting the patient at ease and maintaining patient welfare (see below)
2. Identifying clinical signs demands accurate interpretation of examination findings based on the foundation of clinical experience and targeted exam preparation
3. Clinical communication requires articulate, succinct and skilled use of consultation skills to engage in discussion with patients and examiners alike. The importance of good communication skills cannot be emphasised enough and forms the foundation of the framework upon which this book is based
4. Constructing a differential diagnosis is paramount to demonstrating core knowledge. Appreciating the need to highlight the logic behind the progression from physical examination to key clinical signs, upon which a list a differential diagnoses can be based, is crucial
5. Clinical judgement places an emphasis on clinical prioritisation and the ability to formulate management plans, negotiating with the patient where necessary, rationalising the need for investigation and/or treatment
6. Managing patient concerns looking to identify key issues, maintaining an awareness as to the possibility of sub-plots within a patient narrative, picking up on verbal and non-verbal cues alluding to fears and apprehensions
7. Maintaining patient welfare ensuring a patient centred approach where possible, maintaining respect and dignity throughout

In considering each of the three categories of station it is possible to appreciate the emphasis placed on each of the skills being examined at varying points in the exam.

> Check the most up-to-date guidance from the Royal College prior to sitting the examination.

Stations 1 and 3: presenting clinical cases in the physical examination stations

Clinical examination demands a structured approach, developed throughout undergraduate medical training and subsequently adopted in clinical practice, systematically working from general inspection in a stepwise progression through the hands and peripheral signs towards the target system of interest. Such standardisation of the examination seems intuitive, not least as it lends itself to eliciting clinical signs in an organised fashion, applicable to any patient regardless of pathology. Similarly, in considering viva questioning, it has long been accepted that the structured and organised answer, categorising where appropriate, best demonstrates a candidate's knowledge and encourages the examiner to look more favourably upon them. Thus, in considering the presentation of clinical findings, we would argue that the strong candidate would do well to develop a standardised, logical approach, developing a framework that best demonstrates their knowledge. Such a framework complements the structured approach of clinical examination and aids a confident and natural progression towards viva questioning, leading the examiner to develop a discussion rather than an interrogation.

The framework for successful presentation need not be complicated. In adopting the following structure you can transform simple concepts and fundamental knowledge into an impressive display of clinical acumen.

On completion of the physical examination in stations 1 and 3, take time to conclude the encounter with the patient and make the examiner aware of any further bedsides tests you would ordinarily perform at this stage in clinical practice. Thereafter:

1. Begin with a summary of the pertinent positive findings

The examiner expects a narrative on completion of your examination of the patient. That is not to say that what is required is a running commentary of each percussion, palpation and auscultation. Prioritise the clinical signs elicited and lead with the predominant finding. Naturally it takes practice to develop the ability both to elicit the clinical signs and to decide upon their relative importance. However, with some consideration of the likely pathologies to be encountered within each station and by studying relevant chapters in this book, it will become readily apparent as to how to proceed.

2. Follow with relevant negatives

In deciding upon a predominant positive finding, it is important to be aware that this will likely lend itself towards a predominant diagnosis. Indeed, the task thereafter is two fold. First establish how all other positive findings fit with the likely diagnosis or caveat towards the possible differential diagnoses. And secondly, and with equal importance, establish the relevant negative findings, which both support the diagnosis and rule out concomitant, often related, pathology. Negative findings are clinical signs that you would expect to find to support any given diagnosis, or signs that would be expected if a common complication of a diagnosis were present.

3. State the most likely diagnosis on the basis of both positive and negative findings

Decide upon, and state clearly, your likely diagnosis. To reiterate – in adopting this approach and commenting first on both the positive findings and relevant negatives, the likely diagnosis is one which should already have been described in all but name. It is important to understand that patterns of positive and negative findings are highly indicative of specific pathologies and so you should be sure that, in establishing a diagnosis on examination, your presentation reflects aspects that support and refute such a diagnosis and lead the examiner to a shared understanding in a logical manner. A useful phrase at this point is 'In summary, this patient has signs consistent with a diagnosis of X'.

4. Always proceed to offer relevant differential diagnoses

The differential diagnosis is one of the most valuable resources in PACES. While it is imperative that you should be sufficiently confident in the clinical signs elicited so as to commit to a diagnosis, thus demonstrating an aptitude for clinical medicine, it is equally important to recognise the potential for alternative answers to the problem posed. In everyday practice clinicians proceed with a working diagnosis and sensible list of differentials when encountering a new clinical scenario, relying thereafter on the results of investigations in the context of a full history to decide upon a firm diagnosis and subsequent management. To assume differently within the examination scenario would somewhat miss the point. The differential diagnosis serves both to demonstrate an understanding of the potential diagnoses of any given symptom, and in the context of the exam, to ensure that marks are gained for considering the pathology for which the patient has been selected for examination. Moreover, regardless of whether the actual diagnosis forms your working or your differential option, the importance is placed upon considering and investigating the possibility, thereby ensuring safe practice as a clinician.

Decide upon a short, sensible list of alternative diagnoses, starting with the most and ending in the least likely, from which the subsequent history and investigations will differentiate between. It will help to place the list of differential diagnoses in context, for example 'The differential diagnoses of a systolic murmur would include...' or 'The differential diagnosis for upper motor neuron weakness is...'.

5. Make reference to the importance of clinical context – a brief history

Briefly list the questions on history that would most benefit you in determining your diagnosis, establishing an underlying cause, gauging the severity of disease, or determining the need for medical management or intervention. While history should not form a large part of any given presentation, it offers the potential to demonstrate understanding and develop context, gaining valuable marks.

Moreover, the accomplished candidate will aim to demonstrate a holistic approach and include:

- Depression screening in chronic conditions
- Seeking to determine the impact of any given condition on the patient's quality of life
- Smoking cessation advice in conditions where smoking is a prominent modifiable risk factor

While on first glance such a list seems cumbersome, rest assured that with practice all can be covered swiftly and succinctly.

6. Demonstrate an understanding of the value and role of appropriate further investigation

As a general rule, an investigation should be referred to using the full and unabbreviated

name, alluding thereafter to the expected finding or result. Thus, where aortic stenosis forms the working diagnosis, 'I would request an ECG' becomes 'I would request a 12-lead electrocardiogram which I would expect to show sinus rhythm, demonstrating left ventricular hypertrophy as evidenced by enlarged QRS complexes within the anterolateral leads, and a strain pattern'.

At this stage it is important to appreciate the benefits of the framework upon which you are building. Where there is doubt as to the underlying pathology suggested by the examination findings, you should aim to commit to a working diagnosis, whilst incorporating all other reasonable possibilities as a list of differentials. In considering investigations, it is then possible to establish how you would arrive at a confirmed diagnosis and allows you to caveat your working diagnosis. For example, where the predominant finding of a systolic murmur has resulted in a working diagnosis of aortic stenosis, 'An echocardiogram would prove diagnostic in demonstrating a narrowed valve area with increased pressure and a stenotic jet across the aortic valve, while assessing the mitral valve to rule out evidence of regurgitation'.

7. Always proceed to offer a management plan

Having successfully navigated from examination findings, through diagnoses and the rationale of investigations the process reaches a crux. At this point, it is common for candidates to falter and not proceed to expand upon the diagnosis, and management thereof, due to concern as to whether they have arrived at the 'correct' answer. The strength of this framework lies in the fact that by discussing differential diagnoses and investigation first, the examiner should be content that in clinical practice such behavior would confirm or refute the working diagnosis and provide a platform on which to base your management. While you are not afforded the results of your chosen investigations, it is safe to assume that you can go on to discuss management of a single condition, regardless of whether the actual diagnosis was correct or lay within one of your differentials.

In discussing management, it is useful to consider the distinctions between conservative, medical and surgical intervention. While such categorisations complement the approach to management in surgical exams, they can be somewhat cumbersome in the medical context.

That said, they are a useful starting point in all but name. Conservative management should be considered as modifiable risk factors that require lifestyle change such as dietary advice and smoking cessation. Thereafter, risk factors that require medical treatment such as blood pressure can be discussed leading the discussion logically on to pharmacological management. It is important to note that conservative management is also often seen as a 'watch and wait' option, which has a certain implication of 'doing nothing' when really 'close monitoring' better reflects the rationale.

Most medical specialties have interventional management options such as percutaneous coronary intervention (PCI) in cardiology, transjugular intrahepatic portosystemic shunting (TIPS) in gastroenterology, coiling of subarachnoid haemorrhages in neurology. These procedures are considered minimally invasive procedures and are held in the realm of medical management. Confusion as to whether to consider them medical or surgical is unnecessary; the importance lies in understanding their indications for use and where applicable their role as either first line treatment or as options only where pharmacological therapy as failed.

In summary

You should aim to present the salient positive examination findings, avoiding a long list of normal findings, but including important negatives. With sufficient preparation and practice it will become easier to establish a working diagnosis that will form the basis of a differential list. Thereafter, appropriate investigation should reinforce the likely diagnosis upon which to form a management plan. You should then proceed to give a brief and fact-laden précis of the most likely diagnosis, and suggest initial management.

This framework encourages a logical progression for discussion of any patient within the examination setting. The proposed structure, expanded upon in this book, offers a framework that makes it possible to talk for several minutes in an authoritative and insightful manner. It is likely that any subsequent viva questioning will either be directed towards clarification of points of interest from your discussion or the examiner may choose to push the boundaries of your knowledge on any given topic. Regardless, this approach allows you to determine, in large part, the content of the discussion.

Station 2: history taking

Chapter 6 lays out commonly encountered themes in station 2. The detail included is not intended to serve as a reference text, rather to highlight the important principles of each case and offer insight as to the type of discussion and narrative required to communicate the salient points.

Prior to entering the room

The candidate information provides details of the scenario upon which the station is based, often setting the scene with simple patient details, the problem or presenting complaint, your role and the environment in which the encounter takes place. Comparatively, station 2 offers the most detail in the candidate information with which to prepare prior to entering the room. Thus, in each example we offer various approaches to utilise the time afforded to prepare for commonly encountered scenarios. Formulating a plan will prove invaluable in steering a logical and organised discussion from the outset and it can be useful to attempt working through potential lines of enquiry in your mind to preempt potentially difficult areas. Doubtless the patient will introduce the occasional theme or topic that will not fit with the best-laid plans but this stresses the importance of avoiding assumptions and remaining open to the patient's narrative as the station progresses.

It is worth taking the time to consider your individual approach to station 2. Some candidates choose to make use of paper and pen, which is provided, to jot down important phrases from the scenario, possible differential diagnoses, or pertinent questions to use as a prompt when faced with the patient. This can be useful but if you do not normally write your history as you talk with patients then don't suddenly start on the day of the exam! Be aware of the risk of failing to establish a rapport with the patient at the cost of focusing on your penmanship. Indeed, where you intend to use notes ask the patient if it is acceptable to write as you talk and thereafter be sure not to use it as a crutch. Focus on maintaining eye contact, keep notes short and try to avoid reading off them verbatim when dealing with the examiner.

On entering the room, begin with open questioning

The encounter with the patient is allotted 14 minutes, with a 2-minute warning from the examiner at 12 minutes. Thereafter, you may choose to take time to reflect upon the information gathered and organise their thoughts before engaging in a discussion with the examiner to conclude the station. The importance of stressing the timings of the station at this point is to highlight the considerable amount of time made available to interact with the patient.

On entering the room, introduce yourself to the patient and reaffirm your role to them as outlined in the scenario. Thereafter, begin with an open question and allow the patient to respond, uninterrupted, without directing the patient's response. Avoid interrogating with closed questioning from the outset, instead focus on establishing a rapport and employ attentive listening. Your aim is to make the patient feel at ease, and facilitate the passage of information with reassuring gestures, echoing important statements, gentle steering and repeated open questioning, underpinned with displays of empathy and sensitivity in response to appropriate cues. The initial stages should be used to allow the patient to unburden him or herself of information and get a feel for the agenda and themes of the station.

Choosing when to draw a line under open questioning will depend upon the nature of the information and readiness to proceed along a particular line of enquiry, the willingness of the patient to continue to talk openly without the need for continual encouragement, or where the information becomes seemingly tangential. The transition to closed questioning is often best achieved by interjecting with a summary of what the patient has said. Reiterating the key points, as you understand them, allows the patient to clarify or add further information as necessary. It also serves as a signpost to the examiner that you are shifting the emphasis of the consultation.

Proceed to closed questioning

Closed questioning should be used to confirm key aspects in the history relating to such areas as:

- Disease severity and/or classification
- Risk factors
- Recognised complications
- Relevant past medical history and family history
- Review of medication
- Consideration of quality of life and social history

Explore ideas, concerns and expectations

Actively determining and appropriately exploring ideas, concerns, and expectations is central to reaffirming the patient's agenda and uncovering other themes requiring discussion.

Often patients will have preconceptions as to the cause of their symptoms, or have a diagnosis at the forefront of their mind. Understanding the ideas or beliefs upon which these preconceptions are based is vital to achieving a shared understanding of the problems encountered. Often, exploring ideas will involve unpicking a web of information from previous consultations, family members, or research from search engines and internet sites.

Patient concerns or worries often relate to the impact of symptoms or a particular diagnosis on quality of life, ability to work, or relationships with loved ones or family members. It is important in this respect to attempt to gain an understanding of the impact of each problem from the patient's perspective. The stigma surrounding any given diagnosis is also a commonly encountered cause for concern.

Finally, having spent time gathering the relevant history, establishing a patient's expectations can be useful in transitioning to a management plan. Incorporating their expectations from the consultation, goals in relation to treatment, or envisaged outcomes, forms the basis of shared forward planning.

What to tell the patient

Summarise the case as you understand it and formalise a plan considering the need for:

- Immediate treatment for symptom relief
- The need for further investigation
- The need for a period of trial intervention/treatment before review
- The need for future consultation to explore the problem in more depth, with more time, after research
- The need for specialty referral

It is not uncommon to be confronted by areas of medicine in which you are not well versed, or lack knowledge. In such a situation it is not unreasonable to admit to the fact and suggest a plan in which the information is obtained or confirmed with a senior colleague and relayed to the patient at a later date. The premise is that in clinical practice this would be a reasonable course of action and places the importance on patient safety and the provision of accurate information. It should be stressed that this is not advocated as an acceptable approach to disguise failings in core medical knowledge!

The overall content and detail of the discussion with the patient should focus upon ensuring core understanding of the most important take home messages, using layman terminology and avoiding medical jargon. This is a key skill in of itself, vital to a patient-centred approach, which is increasingly favoured in these scenarios. Indeed, negotiating a management plan, with the patient at the centre of the decision making process, should be prioritised over an in depth discussion of the battery of available investigations and treatments.

What to tell the examiner

Impressing upon the examiner an appreciation of the pertinent points from the encounter upon which the investigation and management plans have been built, will lay the foundations for discussion of relevant themes. Be prepared to expand upon the details of specific issues touched upon in the history, including wider aspects such as prognosis and relevant follow up or specialist input.

Station 4: applied communication skills and ethical scenarios

To successfully navigate this station requires a fundamental appreciation of the core principles involved for any given scenario. Chapter 7 aims to provide you with a précis of those principles for commonly encountered situations. The exact nature of the station will depend upon the context of the encounter and the interaction with the patient. Preparing for a range of patient 'types' by role-playing with peers, is a useful exercise in the lead up to the exam. Practising applied communication skills through role-play should aim to explore ways of explaining the same information in different ways. Attempting to predict the reaction of the angry versus the withdrawn, depressed, patient or similar dichotomies in personalities or behaviours.

Station 5: integrated clinical assessment

Station 5 represents a global assessment of applied clinical skills, centred upon commonly encountered problems in daily practice on the wards or acute medical admissions. The 'brief clinical consultation' format challenges candidates to demonstrate a combination of both problem solving and communication skills, underpinned by sound clinical judgment. Indeed, it is the only station in which all seven areas of the marking scheme are assessed at one time. As such a significant proportion of the total marks available in the exam are attributed to station 5. It is important, however, not to over-prepare for this station simply because of the allocation of marks. The foundation of a strong performance in station 5 stems from thorough preparation for all other stations and relies upon successfully adapting the approach to demonstrate an amalgamation of the skills inherent to each.

In covering station 5, Chapter 5 focuses upon scenarios drawn from rheumatology and musculoskeletal medicine, endocrinology, ophthalmology and dermatology reflecting the areas of medicine previously examined prior to the introduction of the new format of station 5. However, the nature of the station is such that conceivably any area of medicine could be incorporated. Thus we encourage you to be mindful not only of the content presented but also the approach adopted in each scenario. Developing a systematic framework upon which to approach this station will equip you to face themes from any area of medicine.

Performing a focused history and examination

The history and examination should not be considered as separate entities and a stepwise approach, taking the history followed by an examination, should be avoided if at all possible. Instead, begin the dialogue with an open question that establishes the main area of concern allowing the early initiation of a relevant examination. Thereafter, the consultation can continue with an integrative approach, taking the history and examining the patient in parallel. With the identification of physical signs, targeted questioning should be employed to develop context and confirm or refute working diagnoses. Alternatively, the history may suggest additional areas or systems worth examining. It is through appropriate questioning and choice of relevant examination(s), with the potential need to prioritise breadth of interrogation at the expense of depth that forms the basis of an assessment of clinical judgment.

What to tell the patient

Summarising the case, clearly explaining any examination findings and relating them to a patient's symptoms where possible, is important in the first instance. Thereafter be sure to check the patient's understanding and answer any questions that arise. The discussion with the patient should resemble the conclusion of the history station and focus upon agreeing a management plan.

What to tell the examiner

The discussion with the examiner is likely to revolve around:

- Exploring the history and examination findings and how they correlate to diagnosis/ differential diagnosis offered
- Evaluating patient understanding and efficacy of your interaction – particularly in answering questions, allaying fears or dealing with areas of concern
- Justifying the need for further investigation and appropriate use of follow up arrangements
- Exploring management strategies

As such, succinctly presenting the examination findings in the context of the history is fundamental and requires practice to whittle the case down to the pertinent points.

Chapter 1

Cardiovascular system (station 3)

Case 1: Aortic stenosis

Instruction to the candidate

This 70-year-old man has been complaining of worsening shortness of breath on exertion. Please examine his cardiovascular system and present your findings to the examiner including a discussion of your proposed management.

Begin with a summary of positive findings

The auscultatory features leading to a working diagnosis of aortic stenosis include:

- A crescendo-decrescendo ejection systolic murmur, beginning after S1, peaking in mid-late systole, and ending before S2 (grade the loudness, **Table 1.1**)
- Most prominent in the right second intercostal space loudest in end-expiration with the patient sitting forward
- Equal radiation to the carotids
- The murmur can radiate to the apex (termed the Gallavardin phenomenon: high frequency components of the ejection systolic murmur radiating to the apex, falsely suggesting mitral regurgitation). This demonstrates that while the character and timing of the murmur with respect to the cardiac cycle are consistent, anatomical characteristics, such as the radiation, can vary and hence are not always reliable
- An ejection click after S1 indicates a pliable bicuspid valve

The following auscultatory features are consistent with severe aortic stenosis and should be commented upon where detected:

- Soft or absent S2
- Narrow or reverse split S2 (as A2 is increasingly delayed)
- Timing of the ejection systolic murmur: peak of the murmur is delayed with increasing severity. Importantly, the intensity of the murmur does not correlate with severity
- Presence of S4

Peripheral signs may include:

- Slow-rising pulse ('parvus et tardus': a diminished volume, delayed carotid upstroke)
- Narrow pulse pressure: not detectable by palpation, but should be requested from the examiner when commenting on blood pressure measurement. A narrow pulse pressure is a sign of severe aortic stenosis
- Aortic thrill
- Sustained, heaving undisplaced apex beat. In severe disease the left ventricle may become dilated and thus the apex beat will become displaced and harder to palpate with a weaker dispersed impulse

Follow with a summary of relevant negative findings

A common statement used in the cardiology station is 'the patient did not display signs of cardiac failure'. Such a statement relies upon an assessment of fluid status as evidenced by auscultation of the lung fields, height of the jugular venous pressure (JVP), and presence/absence of peripheral oedema. If a patient with valvular pathology has signs of cardiac failure this potentially relates to the inability of the

Table 1.1 The grading of murmurs	
Grade	**Description**
1	Faintest murmur, only heard after special effort
2	Soft but readily detected murmur
3	Moderately loud murmur with no thrill
4	Loud murmur with an accompanying thrill
5	Very loud murmur heard with just the rim of the stethoscope held against the patient's chest
6	Loudest murmur heard with the stethoscope held just away from the chest wall

heart to compensate for the valvular pathology – thus referred to as decompensation.

'There was no suggestion of associated valvular pathology'. In this case remember to comment on mitral regurgitation or, where there is the suspicion of a bicuspid valve (see below), aortic regurgitation.

Whenever valvular pathology is suspected the need to comment on any peripheral stigmata consistent with infective endocarditis is necessary, commenting on common sources including dentition and indwelling intravenous access.

State the most likely diagnosis on the basis of these findings

'This patient has signs consistent with severe aortic stenosis, likely secondary to calcific degeneration. He is clinically euvolaemic, displaying no features of decompensated disease. He does not have any features of infective endocarditis.'

Offer relevant differential diagnoses

The differential diagnosis can be considered in relation to the clinical sign, that of an ejection systolic murmur, and relating to the aetiology of aortic stenosis itself.

Differential of an ejection systolic murmur:

- Aortic stenosis
- Pulmonary stenosis
- Aortic sclerosis (calcified valve, with no stenosis or impediment to flow hence no radiation to the carotids nor impact upon pulse pressure)
- Subvalvular (hypertrophic cardiomyopathy with left ventricular outflow tract obstruction, subaortic membrane) or supravalvular (William's syndrome) lesions
- Flow murmur
  Aortic stenosis is the most common valve lesion in Europe and North America with calcific degenerative disease that occurs with advancing age (prevalence of 2–7% of individuals over 65 years of age) the leading cause. Congenital valvulopathy (bicuspid or extremely rarely unicuspid) which presents in younger individuals is the second most common aetiology. Thus, the age of the patient may provide a clue to the underlying pathology. Alternatively, consider the aetiology as congenital or acquired:

Congenital:

- Valvular: Bicuspid aortic valve (found in 2% of the population). Mention looking

for associated bicuspid aortopathy, namely dilatation, dissection, aneurysm formation and coarctation. The murmur of coarctation is best heard on the back in the interscapular area. 30% of patients with Turner's syndrome will have a bicuspid aortic valve
- Subvalvular: Subaortic membrane
- Supravalvular: Williams syndrome: both aortic and pulmonary stenoses are associated with this syndrome. Patients also have transient hypercalcaemia, elfin-like facies and learning difficulties with overly sociable persona

Acquired:

- Degenerative (the commonest cause in Western countries)
- Calcific, accelerated by:
  - Chronic kidney disease
  - Severe Paget's disease (in patients with more than 15% skeletal involvement, high output state from bony arteriovenous connections causes increased transvalvular turbulence and accelerated valvular calcification)
  - Hyperparathyroidism (aortic valve inflammation and calcification)
- Rheumatic fever (often with associated mitral involvement)
- Homozygous familial hypercholesterolaemia

Demonstrate the importance of clinical context – suggest relevant questions that would be taken in a patient history

Seek to elicit the cardinal symptoms that relate to survival and suggest severe disease:

- Asymptomatic: sudden death < 1%/year
- Dyspnoea secondary to heart failure: up to 2 years survival
- Syncope: average 3 years survival
- Angina: average 5 years survival

Establish exercise tolerance. It can be useful to make reference to the vignette, which may describe symptoms as in this case with shortness of breath on exertion. Beware of asymptomatic patients who may be limiting their activities to avoid symptoms.

Demonstrate an understanding of the value of further investigation

The three investigations to prioritise and discuss first are the electrocardiogram (ECG), plain chest radiograph (CXR) and transthoracic echocardiogram (TTE).

ECG: Left ventricular hypertrophy with or without accompanying strain pattern, i.e. ST depression and T wave inversion in the lateral leads.

CXR: Look for aortic calcification, which in severe diffuse cases is termed a porcelain aorta. This precludes cannulation or clamping of the ascending aorta during cardiothoracic surgery.

TTE: The gold-standard diagnostic investigation demonstrating:

- Transvalvular gradients and aortic valve area (**Table 1.2**)
- Degree of calcification, and tricuspid versus bicuspid valves
- Left ventricular wall thickness, systolic and diastolic function
- Aortic root dimensions and associated aortic pathology (especially important in the context of bicuspid valves)

Stress testing: Asymptomatic severe aortic stenosis can be further evaluated with a medically supervised exercise test, watching closely for symptoms, and abnormal haemodynamic response to exercise or arrhythmia. Discrepancies between transvalvular gradients and aortic valve area do occur and require further specialist investigation. For example, low dose dobutamine stress echocardiography is used in cases of severely stenotic aortic valve area with low transvalvular gradients in the presence of left ventricular dysfunction. Dobutamine increases myocardial contractility, revealing either a falsely low resting aortic valve area due to left ventricular impairment (with increasing valve area on stress) or increasing gradients (but static valve area) on stress due to true aortic stenosis.

Cardiac catheterisation: for investigation of concomitant coronary artery disease in pre-operative patients.

CT aorta and CT coronary angiography: A non-invasive assessment of coronary anatomy and suitability for peripheral arterial cannulation in patients in whom TAVI is being considered.

Transcatheter aortic valve implantation (TAVI)

TAVI is becoming a widely utilised interventional procedure in patients with severe aortic stenosis who are either declined conventional surgical aortic valve replacement during patient selection or are considered high risk. It has been demonstrated to provide both survival and quality of life benefits versus conservative management in inoperable patients with severe AS. Patient selection is key, and a multidisciplinary approach amongst non-invasive and invasive cardiologists and cardiothoracic surgeons is essential. It should also be remembered that TAVI is still an invasive procedure requiring a general anaesthetic, large bore vascular access and temporary cardiac pacing. Stroke is a major complication. Other complications include vascular injury, coronary embolisation, device embolisation, paravalvular leak and death.

Always offer a management plan

Symptomatic, severe AS requires aortic valve replacement. Aortic valve replacement is also indicated in moderate AS in the context of surgical coronary revascularisation or other concomitant cardiovascular surgery.

Asymptomatic mild to moderate aortic stenosis should receive outpatient follow-up to monitor the natural history of the condition.

In patients with severe aortic stenosis avoid medications that reduce preload (such as ACE inhibitors or nitrates), thereby reducing venous return and exacerbating transvalvular gradients.

Asymptomatic severe aortic stenosis:

- Truly asymptomatic patients should be closely followed-up, with the caveat that symptom onset should lead to surgical intervention being expedited
- Asymptomatic patients with an abnormal supervised exercise test (e.g. positive for

Table 1.2 Echocardiographic findings in aortic stenosis			
	Mild	Moderate	Severe
Valve area (cm^2)	1.5–2.0	1.0–1.4	<1.0
Peak gradient (mmHg)	<36	36–64	>64
Mean gradient (mmHg)	<25	25–40	>40

symptoms or a fall in blood pressure) require aortic valve replacement

- Aortic valve replacement is also indicated in asymptomatic patients with evidence of impaired left ventricular systolic function (due to the severe AS) or a rapid rate of progression of severity of AS (defined by increasing peak velocities ≥ 0.3 m/s per year)

Further reading

Vahanian A, Baumgartner H, Bax J, et al. Guidelines on the management of valvular heart disease: the task force on the management of valvular heart disease of the European Society of Cardiology. Eur Heart J 2007; 28:230–268.

Case 2: Mitral regurgitation

Instruction to the candidate

This 35-year-old man presents with dyspnoea. Please examine his cardiovascular system.

Begin with a summary of positive findings

Peripheral signs in mitral regurgitation includes:

- The pulse may be irregular, suggestive of atrial fibrillation
- Palpate at the apex for a displaced (clearly refer to anatomical landmarks), thrusting (volume-loaded) apex beat, which may be associated with a systolic thrill
- Auscultatory features include:
  - A pan-systolic murmur heard loudest at the apex in expiration in the left lateral position, radiating to the axilla
  - S3 gallop

  Signs of severity include:

- Left ventricular dilatation indicated by a displaced apex beat
- Signs of left ventricular failure
- A wide split S2 (an early A2 indicating premature aortic valve closure due to a large regurgitant volume across the mitral valve)

Mitral valve prolapse

Mitral valve prolapse is most commonly due to myxomatous degeneration, but also occurs with inherited connective tissue diseases including Marfan syndrome, Ehlers–Danlos syndrome, pseudoxanthoma elasticum and osteogenesis imperfecta. The auscultatory features of mitral valve prolapse include:

- A mid-systolic ejection click followed by a mid- to late-systolic murmur
- The click results from sudden tensing of the mitral valve apparatus bowing back into the left atrium
- Certain manoeuvres can alter the auscultatory characteristics of mitral valve prolapse:
  - The murmur is prolonged by reducing venous return (e.g. standing or Valsalva), thereby reducing left ventricular filling and thus increasing chordal laxity causing earlier prolapse and an earlier click (with a longer subsequent murmur)
  - Squatting increases venous return, ultimately delaying the click and reducing the duration of the murmur

Follow with a summary of relevant negative findings

The presence or absence of the following findings should be mentioned to the examiner:

- An irregular pulse suggestive of atrial fibrillation. Comment on the rate, embolic complications and any peripheral stigmata of anticoagulation that may be present
- Peripheral stigmata of infective endocarditis. Ask the examiner for the temperature and a urine dip (looking for microscopic haematuria), and comment on dental hygiene and the presence or absence of indwelling intravenous access
- Signs of cardiac failure, including pulmonary oedema, peripheral oedema, raised JVP and S3 gallop, which if present would indicate cardiac decompensation

State the most likely diagnosis on the basis of these findings

'The most likely diagnosis in this patient, who has a pan-systolic murmur and is in atrial fibrillation, is mitral regurgitation.'

Offer relevant differential diagnoses

The differential diagnoses of a pansystolic murmur include:

- Mitral regurgitation
- Ventricular septal defect
- Tricuspid regurgitation

Aortic stenosis can be mistaken for mitral regurgitation, especially when it radiates to the apex (termed the Gallavardin phenomenon).

The mitral valve consists of 2 leaflets (3 scallops each) contained within an annulus, anchored by chordae tendinae to papillary muscles that originate from the myocardium. The differential diagnosis of the underlying cause of mitral regurgitation can therefore be considered in terms of disorders of these various parts of the valve apparatus. Clues suggesting such aetiology can be identified during the clinical examination (**Table 1.3**).

Demonstrate the importance of clinical context – suggest relevant questions that would be taken in a patient history

As with any valve pathology, it is important to identify symptoms of heart failure. These include breathlessness, orthopnoea, paroxysmal nocturnal dyspnoea, and pedal oedema. Any history of palpitations should also be elicited, specifically considering the increased likelihood of AF.

Demonstrate an understanding of the value of further investigation

The most important investigations and their relevant findings include:

- A 12-lead electrocardiogram (ECG):
  - P mitrale (broad, bifid P waves) of left atrial dilatation
  - Atrial fibrillation
  - Look for ischaemic changes as a possible aetiology of mitral regurgitation
- A plain chest radiograph (CXR):
  - Cardiomegaly due to left ventricular dilatation
  - Evidence of left atrial dilatation
  - Pulmonary oedema
- Echocardiography: both transthoracic and transoesophageal echocardiography are important. They will demonstrate:
  - The severity of the valve lesion: determined by colour Doppler, regurgitant orifice area, regurgitant volumes and fractions, and by jet width
  - Clues which point towards the mechanism of the valve dysfunction: looking at all structures that make up the mitral valve apparatus
  - The physiological consequences of the valve lesion, namely regarding left ventricular cavity size and systolic

	Acute	Chronic
Leaflets	Endocarditis: review dentition, intravenous access, peripheral stigmata	Degenerative (the most common cause) Valvotomy for previous MS: check for scars MV prolapse: check for mid systolic click and movement with manoeuvres Rheumatic fever: check for concomitant MS Connective tissue diseases: such as rheumatoid arthritis, check the joints Anorectic drugs (fenfluramine, phentermine)
Annulus		LV dilatation
Subvalvular apparatus (chordae/ papillary muscles)	Ruptured papillary muscle during an acute ischaemic event Flail chordae	Flail chordae
Left ventricular posterior wall		Chronic ischaemia (circumflex territory causing lateral wall hypokinesis and hence posterior mitral valve leaflet tethering)

Table 1.3 Aetiology of mitral regurgitation and associated clinical signs

MS, mitral stenosis.

function. Systolic function should be 'hyperdynamic' if considered normal in severe MR, as the left ventricle offloads into both the aorta and the left atrium. Left atrial dimensions and pulmonary artery systolic pressure are also evaluated
  – To guide the nature of surgical intervention and the feasibility of repair versus replacement
• Cardiac catheterisation acts to investigate concomitant coronary artery disease in pre-operative patients, or to investigate a suspected ischaemic aetiology of mitral regurgitation

Always offer a management plan

The management of mitral regurgitation can be considered with regard to the medical and surgical options:

When discussing medical management the indications for specific therapies should be considered:

• Antibiotic prophylaxis: (see *Infective endocarditis*, p.40)
• In acute severe MR, nitrates, diuretics, and inotropes (to optimise prior to surgery) may be used
• In chronic severe MR with evidence of left ventricular dysfunction: ACE inhibitors, beta-blockers and potassium-sparing diuretics in accordance with conventional cardiac failure management
• Patients with AF should receive anticoagulation and rate control. Pursuit of sinus rhythm following AF in severe MR is unlikely to be successful in the long-term without correction of the underlying valvular lesion

> ### Mitral regurgitation and its various presentations
>
> Remember that MR can be acute, chronic and compensated, or chronic and decompensated. In PACES you will see the latter two presentations, but remember to mention during your present that cases of acute MR present as a medical emergency with pulmonary oedema.

The indications for surgery (preferably repair, otherwise replacement) in mitral regurgitation vary depending on whether the patient is symptomatic or asymptomatic:

• Symptomatic severe MR: surgery is indicated. In cases of significant left ventricular dysfunction (ejection fraction $\leq 30\%$, end-systolic diameter > 5.5 cm), response to medical therapy, likelihood of valve repair, and comorbid burden are all considered prior to a making a decision for surgical intervention
• Asymptomatic severe MR: asymptomatic patients with severe MR and normal left ventricular size and function can be followed up, but certain cases should be considered individually, e.g. females of child-bearing age with severe MR who want to consider pregnancy (and thus expose the cardiovascular system to increased circulating volume). Otherwise, in asymptomatic MR, surgery is indicated in the following circumstances:
  – Resting left ventricular ejection fraction $\leq 60\%$
  – Left ventricular dilatation (end-systolic diameter > 4.5 cm)
  – Patients with AF
  – Patients with resultant pulmonary hypertension
  – Patients undergoing other concomitant cardiovascular surgery, such as coronary artery bypass grafting (CABG) or other valve surgery
• In selected cases depending upon anatomical suitability and patient profile, there are percutaneous options for the treatment of severe MR. These would be considered following specialist referral, and include the Mitraclip and Cardioband devices.

Further reading

Vahanian A, Baumgartner H, Bax J, et al. Guidelines on the management of valvular heart disease: the task force on the management of valvular heart disease of the European Society of Cardiology. Eur Heart J 2007; 28:230–268.

Case 3: Ventricular septal defect

Instruction to the candidate

This 35-year-old woman feels well and is under cardiology follow-up. Please examine her cardiovascular system.

> **Clinical context of ventricular septal defects (VSDs)**
>
> VSDs are the second most commonly encountered congenital cardiac lesion after bicuspid aortic valves.

Begin with a summary of positive findings

The positive clinical findings in a patient with a VSD include:

Peripheral signs

- The morphologic features of known disease associations:
  - Down's syndrome.
  - Turner's syndrome
- The finding of a thoracic scar can be indicative of a childhood surgical closure
- A systolic precordial thrill may be felt on palpation

Auscultatory features

A pansystolic murmur loudest at the left sternal edge between the 3rd and 4th intercostal spaces. Note that the loudness of the murmur is not indicative of shunt size but rather of the pressure gradient.

To provide further clinical context, consider the various ways in which an adult can present with a chronic VSD:

- Surgically repaired without residual shunt
- With residual shunt, which can then lead to the following groups:
  - A well, young adult with a likely haemodynamically insignificant muscular VSD, with a large pressure gradient, and hence a loud murmur. ('Maladie de Roger')
  - An adult patient with varying degrees of pulmonary arterial hypertension and/or left ventricular volume overload
  - A cyanotic adult patient who has developed Eisenmenger's physiology

Follow with a summary of relevant negative findings

The following represent clinical complications of a VSD and it is, therefore, important to comment on the absence of the relevant clinical findings:

- Infective endocarditis: comment on the absence of peripheral stigmata, dental hygiene and the presence or absence of indwelling intravenous access
- Arrhythmia: either tachyarrhythmias, or bradyarrhythmias from complete atrioventricular block
- Signs of pulmonary hypertension
- Signs of left ventricular failure
- Cerebral (paradoxical) embolism due to the right and left heart communication
- Concomitant AR due to prolapse of the right coronary cusp can occur particularly in perimembranous VSDs

It is also important to comment on associated intracardiac lesions such as patent ductus arteriosus, tetralogy of Fallot, and aortic coarctation.

State the most likely diagnosis on the basis of these findings

The following is an example presentation to the examiner, relating to a patient with a haemodynamically insignificant and uncomplicated VSD:

'This patient has signs consistent with a ventricular septal defect, likely a small, haemodynamically insignificant left-to-right shunt ('Maladie de Roger'). She has no evidence of pulmonary hypertension, left ventricular failure or infective endocarditis. I would like to take a full history to establish her symptomatic status, and my investigation of choice would be an echocardiogram in the first instance to confirm the diagnosis, to quantitate the degree of shunting and to estimate left ventricular function and pulmonary arterial pressures.'

Offer relevant differential diagnoses

The differential diagnosis of a VSD can be considered either in relation to the underlying causes of VSDs, or to their anatomical classification.

The causes of a VSD include:

- A cardiac lesion as part of an underlying syndrome (Down's or Turner's syndrome)
- A congenital lesion, either alone or associated with other lesions (such as in tetralogy of Fallot)
- Ischaemic (acquired) VSDs, which typically occur approximately 5 days following a full-thickness septal myocardial infarction

Anatomically, VSDs are divided as follows:

- Perimembranous (80%)
- Muscular (15–20%)
- Outlet (5%)
- Inlet (<1%)

Demonstrate the importance of clinical context – suggest relevant questions that would be taken in a patient history

When informing the examiner of relevant questions to ask in a history, include those that would identify symptoms of heart failure and pulmonary hypertension. Also remark on questions that would shed light on the aetiology and previous management of the patient's VSD.

Demonstrate an understanding of the value of further investigation

The following list should be mentioned to the examiner as relevant investigations in the evaluation of patients with a VSD:

- An ECG may demonstrate electrocardiographic findings of left, right, or combined ventricular hypertrophy, depending on the size and direction of the shunt. If the VSD is small, a normal ECG can be expected
- A CXR may demonstrate the following radiographic findings:
  - Cardiomegaly due to left ventricular dilatation
  - Evidence of left atrial dilatation
  - An enlarged main pulmonary artery, with reduced peripheral vascular markings in patients with pulmonary hypertension
- Echocardiography, the gold-standard diagnostic investigation, will demonstrate:

  - The location and dimensions of the shunt
  - Quantification and direction of the shunt ratio, and the pressure gradient between the ventricles
  - An estimation of pulmonary arterial systolic pressure
  - Indices of left and right ventricular size and function
  - Any associated lesions, such as aortic regurgitation, which can be present with perimembranous VSDs
- Cardiac catheterisation is not routinely required, but can be used to determine pulmonary vascular resistance if pulmonary arterial pressure is suggested to be raised on echocardiography, and for shunt quantitation
- Cardiac MRI can be used for further evaluation of ventricular volumes, function and shunt quantification where echocardiography has not been diagnostic

Always offer a management plan

Patients with congenital lesions should be referred to a specialist adult congenital heart disease (ACHD) centre for follow-up. Additionally, consider advice on antibiotic prophylaxis (see *Infective endocarditis*, p.40).

The definitive management is a VSD closure if there is evidence of LV dilatation and/or failure. Surgical closure is the method of choice, but the procedure can also be carried out in a percutaneous fashion if the patient is considered too high-risk or unsuitable for surgical, or in the case of an anatomically suitable muscular VSD.

Patients with symptoms, left ventricular volume overload, mild pulmonary hypertension, or a history of recurrent (more than three episodes) infective endocarditis should all be considered for closure.

Closure is contraindicated at the extremes of the symptomatology spectrum, such as patients who have developed Eisenmenger's syndrome, or asymptomatic patients with small, haemodynamically insignificant lesions with no evidence of left ventricular volume overload. Severe pulmonary hypertension is also a contraindication to closure.

Further reading

Deanfield J, Thaulow E, Warnes C, et al. Management of grown up congenital heart disease. Eur Heart J 2003; 24:1035–1084.

Case 4: Hypertrophic obstructive cardiomyopathy

Instruction to the candidate

This 32-year-old man complains of palpitations and exertional dyspnoea. Please examine his cardiovascular system.

Begin with a summary of positive findings

The peripheral signs of hypertrophic cardiomyopathy include:

- A bifid (double) carotid pulse. This physical finding represents flow acceleration in early systole, followed by a second impulse in late systole
- The jugular venous pressure will be raised if the patient is in cardiac failure, with prominent 'a' waves, which indicate right atrial systole against a reduced compliance right ventricle due to the impact of the hypertrophied interventricular septum
- Precordial palpation may reveal a double apical impulse, represented by a heaving (pressure-loaded) apex beat with a palpable S4 due to forceful atrial systole against a non-compliant left ventricle

Auscultatory features of hypertrophic cardiomyopathy include:

- An ejection systolic murmur at the left sternal edge in mid to late systole with no radiation to the carotids
- A pansystolic murmur of mitral regurgitation due to systolic anterior movement of the anterior mitral valve leaflet
- A fourth heart sound (S4)

Auscultation in a HOCM case

The left ventricular outflow tract (LVOT) gradient and thus the loudness of the ejection systolic murmur vary directly with preload and afterload:

- Increasing preload by squatting or afterload by the handgrip manoeuvre reduces the gradient, with a consequently softer murmur
- Reducing preload by the Valsalva manoeuvre, standing from sitting, or use of diuretic or nitrate medications, or reducing afterload by administration of vasodilators will exacerbate the gradient across the LVOT, resulting in a louder murmur

Valsalva can be performed in the context of diagnostic studies for these purposes, but should not be performed as part of the clinical examination in PACES given the potential for symptomatic consequences.

Follow with a summary of relevant negative findings

The absence of the following clinical signs should be mentioned in cases of hypertrophic cardiomyopathy:

- Signs suggestive of cardiac failure. Cardiac failure may be due to diastolic dysfunction, or in the later stages of the natural history of the disease, due to systolic dysfunction
- The finding of an irregular pulse, suggestive of atrial fibrillation, is a marker of poorer prognosis
- Infective endocarditis: comment on the absence of peripheral stigmata, dental hygiene and the presence or absence of indwelling intravenous access

State the most likely diagnosis on the basis of these findings

The following quotation relates to a standard case of hypertrophic cardiomyopathy:

'This patient has signs consistent with hypertrophic obstructive cardiomyopathy. The ejection systolic murmur suggests a left ventricular outflow tract gradient, and the apical pansystolic murmur indicates mitral regurgitation secondary to systolic anterior motion of the anterior mitral valve leaflet. I would like to take a full history to establish his symptomatic status, a family history to establish pedigree of the disease, and my initial investigation of choice would be an echocardiogram.'

Offer relevant differential diagnoses

A suitable differential diagnosis that can be given to the examiner is that of an ejection systolic murmur as given in *Aortic stenosis* (p. 2).

Demonstrate the importance of clinical context – suggest relevant questions that would be taken in a patient history

Relevant history questions to mention to the examiner include direct questioning to elicit the following important symptoms:

- Palpitations
- Pre-syncope or syncope
- Exertional dyspnoea
- Chest pain

A family history of unexplained syncope or sudden, unexplained premature death should be sought. Many mutations responsible for hypertrophic cardiomyopathy are of autosomal dominant inheritance, so siblings and children have a 50% likelihood of being affected. A clear family pedigree is important with respect to establishing the diagnosis and the investigation and treatment of relatives.

The patient's job and driving status need to be sought in order to establish adherence to vehicle licensing regulations.

Demonstrate an understanding of the value of further investigation

The following investigations yield important diagnostic and prognostic information in hypertrophic cardiomyopathy:

- An ECG will show various combinations of the following electrocardiographic features:
  - Left ventricular hypertrophy
  - ST segment or T wave abnormalities suggesting abnormal repolarisation
  - Axis deviation
  - Left atrial or biatrial enlargement
  - Atrial tachyarrhythmia: atrial tachycardia, flutter or fibrillation.
- On CXR, abnormal findings are variable, and may include cardiomegaly due to left ventricular dilatation or evidence of left atrial dilatation
- Echocardiography is the gold-standard diagnostic modality demonstrating:
  - Different patterns of left ventricular hypertrophy, e.g. asymmetric (septal or apical) or concentric
  - A left ventricular cavity that is small in size
  - Atrial dilatation
  - Diastolic dysfunction, and systolic dysfunction in the later stages of the disease

- The presence and quantitation of LVOT obstruction
- The presence and quantitation of mitral regurgitation due to systolic anterior motion of the anterior mitral valve leaflet
- The absence of other conditions that might give rise to left ventricular hypertrophy, such as aortic stenosis or cardiac amyloid

- Holter monitoring can show the following findings:
  - Atrial and/or ventricular ectopy
  - Atrial fibrillation
  - Non-sustained ventricular tachycardia
- On supervised treadmill exercise testing, an attenuated or hypotensive response is indicative of haemodynamic instability and a risk factor for sudden death
- Cardiac MRI can be used for diagnosis and assessment of hypertrophic cardiomyopathy, especially when echocardiography has been inconclusive (particularly in cases of apical hypertrophy). It is also useful in the differentiation of alternative causes of myocardial hypertrophy. MRI can also be used to quantify fibrosis burden
- First degree relatives should be screened with an ECG and echocardiogram. Negative results in adult relatives should be reevaluated at 5 yearly intervals. Adolescent relatives require annual screening. Genotyping has been used in the research setting and also to establish family pedigrees

---

Risk stratification in hypertrophic cardiomyopathy

Following a clinical history, examination and investigations, the following risk factors for sudden death in hypertrophic cardiomyopathy can be used to guide management:

- A personal history of syncope or previous cardiac arrest
- A family history of unexplained premature sudden death
- Abnormal haemodynamic response to exercise on supervised treadmill testing
- Non-sustained VT on 24 hours Holter monitoring, or an episode of spontaneous sustained VT
- The presence of LVOT gradient on echocardiography (≥ 30 mmHg)
- Severe left ventricular hypertrophy (≥ 3 cm)

Always offer a management plan

It is important to consider the advice to give a patient who has a diagnosis of hypertrophic cardiomyopathy. This will include family screening, which is discussed in the investigation section of this case. With regard to driving, heavy goods vehicle or passenger-carrying vehicle driving licence holders will not be allowed to continue to hold this licence and need to inform the DVLA. Patients with an ICD need to inform the DVLA and adhere to this set of guidelines (see *The infraclavicular mass*, p. 33).

Additional points to advise patients about include telling them what they must avoid. Dehydration may exacerbate LVOT gradients. Patients should also avoid intense sports, particularly involving rapid bursts of exertion or simulating Valsalva (e.g. weightlifting).

Medical therapy in hypertrophic cardiomyopathy includes:

- Beta-blockers, rate-limiting calcium channel blockers and disopyramide are used for symptomatic LVOT obstruction
- Amiodarone should be considered for atrial or ventricular arrhythmia suppression
- A low threshold for anticoagulation exists for AF in hypertrophic cardiomyopathy due to the high risk of embolic stroke.

The management of AF may require specialist input from cardiomyopathy and electrophysiology subspecialties

Interventional options for patients with symptomatic LVOT obstruction include surgical septal myectomy, which remains the gold standard for this problem. Percutaneous alcohol septal ablation is an alternative approach.

Implantable cardiac defibrillators (ICDs) are considered according to risk stratification of the patient. Risk stratification should be performed on an annual basis with echocardiography, 24 hour Holter monitoring and supervised exercise treadmill testing.

Further reading

Maron BJ, McKenna WJ, Danielson GK, et al. American College of Cardiology/European Society of Cardiology Clinical Expert Consensus Document on Hypertrophic Cardiomyopathy. A report of the American College of Cardiology Foundation Task Force on clinical expert consensus documents and the European Society of Cardiology Committee for practice guidelines. Eur Heart J 2003; 24:1965–1991.

Case 5: Tricuspid regurgitation

Instruction to the candidate

This 55-year-old woman presents with flushing and dyspnoea. Please examine her cardiovascular system.

Begin with a summary of positive findings

The positive findings in tricuspid regurgitation include a combination of peripheral findings and auscultatory features.

The key peripheral signs to elicit and mention to the examiner are:

- The presence of giant 'v' waves on examination of the JVP
- Pulsatile hepatomegaly due to reflux of tricuspid regurgitation via the inferior vena cava

The auscultatory feature of tricuspid regurgitation is a pansystolic murmur heard loudest at the lower left sternal edge in inspiration ('Carvallo's sign').

Follow with a summary of relevant negative findings

The absence of signs of right heart failure (S3, peripheral oedema and ascites) and signs of pulmonary hypertension (a left parasternal heave, a palpable and loud P2) should be noted.

As with other valvulopathies, comment on the absence of peripheral stigmata of endocarditis, remembering however that right-sided lesions such as tricuspid regurgitation usually cause pulmonary septic emboli rather than peripheral embolic phenomena. Carefully inspect for risk factors for endocarditis such as poor dental hygiene and indwelling intravenous access. Importantly in right-sided lesion, comment on any signs of intravenous drug use.

State the most likely diagnosis on the basis of these findings

'This patient has signs consistent with severe tricuspid regurgitation. The 'Instruction to the candidate' mentions flushing and dyspnoea, which could be suggestive of carcinoid heart disease resulting from carcinoid syndrome. She has clinical features of right heart failure, but does not have any features of infective endocarditis.'

Offer relevant differential diagnoses

Offer to the examiner the differential diagnosis of a systolic murmur, as discussed in previous cases.

The anatomical structure of the tricuspid valve should be considered when discussing the underlying causes of tricuspid regurgitation. The tricuspid valve consists of three leaflets contained within an annulus, anchored by chordae tendinae to papillary muscles that originate from the myocardium. Disorders of any

of these structures can lead to TR (**Table 1.4**).

Remember that, just like MR, TR can be acute, chronic and compensated, or chronic and decompensated. In PACES you will see the latter two presentations, but remember to mention during your presentation that cases of acute TR can present, for example, in the setting of either RV infarction, or sepsis in the case of infective endocarditis.

Demonstrate the importance of clinical context – suggest relevant questions that would be taken in a patient history

Potential history questions to mention to the examiner would include those eliciting symptomatology as a result of the valve lesion, such as dyspnoea and peripheral oedema. Additionally, the clinical history can elicit features suggesting the aetiology of the valve lesion:

- Infective endocarditis: intravenous drug abuse or long-term indwelling venous access, fevers or rigors, and recent dental procedures
- Carcinoid syndrome: flushing, diarrhoea, weight loss and wheeze
- Rheumatic heart disease: history of childhood rheumatic fever

Table 1.4 Aetiology of tricuspid regurgitation and associated clinical signs

	Acute	Chronic
Leaflets	Endocarditis (review for signs of intravenous drug abuse, intravenous access (especially in patients receiving renal replacement therapy), peripheral stigmata)	Rheumatic fever (check for concomitant mitral stenosis)) Carcinoid syndrome (check for concomitant pulmonary valve and less commonly left-sided valve lesions, and flushed appearance) Leaflet malcoaptation or trauma due to RV pacing lead Anorectic drugs (e.g. fenfluramine and phentermine, also referred to as fen-phen)
Functional (annular dilatation)		Pulmonary hypertension Congestive cardiac failure
Subvalvular apparatus (chordae/papillary muscles)	Right ventricular myocardial infarction: ruptured papillary muscle (acute ischaemic event) Blunt trauma causing flail chordae	Leaflet prolapse
Miscellaneous		Ebstein's anomaly Dysplastic tricuspid valve Endomyocardial fibrosis

Demonstrate an understanding of the value of further investigation

The following cardiac investigations offer a complete assessment of tricuspid regurgitation:

- 12 lead electrocardiogram: If the ECG demonstrates widening of the QRS complex with RSR morphology in the right ventricular leads, this might be reflective of dilatation of this chamber. There may be delta waves suggesting pre-excitation in Ebstein's anomaly
- Echocardiography:
  - The severity of TR is assessed by colour Doppler and by jet width (vena contracta)
  - The mechanism and underlying cause of TR is elucidated by looking at all structures that make up the tricuspid valve apparatus
  - The impact of TR upon right ventricular cavity size and systolic function and right atrial dimensions must be assessed
- Cardiac MRI is currently the gold standard tool for determination of right ventricular size and systolic function
- Cardiac catheterisation is performed in cases of suspected pulmonary arterial hypertension

Always offer a management plan

Medical management of tricuspid regurgitation is limited to diuretics for relief of symptoms and treatment directed at the underlying cause. Atrial arrhythmias, particularly atrial flutter, are common and require management of both the rhythm itself (especially if poorly tolerated due to underlying congenital heart disease or pulmonary hypertension, for example) and anticoagulation where appropriate. Accessory pathways are also recognised in Ebstein's anomaly (for which the contemporary treatment is a Cone repair), and hence ablation should be sought to prevent conduction of atrial tachyarrhythmias via the accessory pathway.

Antibiotic prophylaxis should be taken as indicated (see *Infective endocarditis*, p. 40).

The definitive management of tricuspid regurgitation is surgery. Indications for surgery (which include plication, annuloplasty, or replacement) are:

- Symptomatic severe TR (without severe RV dysfunction) despite optimal medical treatment
- At least moderate TR in patients undergoing left-sided valve surgery

Evaluation of patient co-morbid status, right ventricular dysfunction, presence of pulmonary hypertension and previous cardiothoracic surgery are all considerations prior to deciding upon surgical intervention.

Significant TR may or may not resolve following surgical correction of mitral valve lesions, and predicting this post-operative course is imprecise. Furthermore, redo surgery for persistent TR following correction of left-sided valvular lesions carries a higher risk. Therefore severe TR secondary to mitral valve disease should be fully evaluated and concomitantly intervened upon in patients undergoing left-sided valve surgery.

The following features increase the mortality risk of surgical intervention for symptomatic severe TR:

- Poor functional class
- Left or right heart failure
- Pulmonary hypertension
- Previous valvular intervention (typically mitral valve repair or replacement) with unresolved TR

Further reading

Vahanian A, Baumgartner H, Bax J, et al. Guidelines on the management of valvular heart disease: The Task Force on the Management of Valvular Heart Disease of the European Society of Cardiology. Eur Heart J 2007; 28:230–268.

Case 6: Pulmonary stenosis

Instruction to the candidate

This 20-year-old woman presents with dyspnoea. Please examine her cardiovascular system.

Begin with a summary of positive findings

Peripheral signs of pulmonary stenosis include:

- JVP may be elevated indicating raised right atrial pressure, with giant 'a' waves indicating right atrial hypertrophy
- Parasternal heave indicative of right ventricular hypertrophy
- A thrill over the pulmonary valve area
- Presystolic hepatic pulsation

Auscultatory features of pulmonary stenosis include:

- An ejection systolic murmur heard loudest in the pulmonary area on inspiration. This can radiate to the left shoulder and the left lung field posteriorly
- An ejection click may be present with thin, pliable valves, followed by a soft P2
- S4

On identifying the positive findings of pulmonary stenosis, consider clinical signs which would point towards severe pulmonary stenosis:

- The peak of the ejection systolic murmur is delayed with increasing severity
- Absence of an ejection click (unless the stenosis is located at the infundibulum)
- Findings suggestive of right heart failure
- Presence of right ventricular S4

Follow with a summary of relevant negative findings

In addition to commenting on the absence of stigmata of infective endocarditis and on the absence of signs of right heart failure (including peripheral oedema and ascites), comment on features of tetralogy of Fallot and congenital cyanotic heart disease such as central cyanosis and clubbing.

State the most likely diagnosis on the basis of these findings

'This patient has signs consistent with pulmonary stenosis likely due to congenital heart disease. She has clinical features of right heart failure, but does not have any features of infective endocarditis. I would like to take a full history to establish her symptomatic status, and my investigation of choice would be an echocardiogram to confirm the diagnosis.'

Offer relevant differential diagnoses

Pulmonary stenosis is either congenital (for example, on its own or due to congenital rubella syndrome), with or without other associated lesions (tetralogy of Fallot, for example. See page 50), or acquired (for example, secondary to carcinoid heart disease).

Congenital pulmonary stenosis may feature as part of an eponymous syndrome:

- Noonan's syndrome: features include (amongst others) short stature, typical facies (webbed neck, hypertelorism, ptosis, flat nasal bridge), pectus excavatum, learning difficulties
- Watson's syndrome: affected individuals demonstrate dermatological features of neurofibromatosis type 1
- Williams' syndrome: features include transient hypercalcaemia, elfin-like facies and learning difficulties with an overly sociable persona. Aortic and pulmonary stenoses are associated with this syndrome

Demonstrate the importance of clinical context – suggest relevant questions that would be taken in a patient history

Relevant questions in any history of pulmonary stenosis would include:

- Exertional dyspnoea, chest pain and/or syncope
- Peripheral oedema

- Features suggesting aetiology, e.g. a history of maternal rubella

Demonstrate an understanding of the value of further investigation

Relevant investigations include:

- Pulse oximetry: if peripheral oxygen saturations are low, check a full blood count for secondary erythrocytosis and an iron profile
- Functional data such as 6-minute walk test or cardiopulmonary exercise testing (CPEX) can be informative both prognostically and to help guide management
- 12 lead electrocardiogram: whilst an ECG may be normal, it may show right ventricular hypertrophy (with or without strain) and right atrial enlargement
- CXR to look for dilated pulmonary arteries and reduced lung markings.
- Echocardiography will allow the following:
  - Doppler flow assessment of severity
  - Anatomical aetiology of pulmonary stenosis: valvular, subvalvular

(infundibular and subinfundibular) or supravalvular
  - Pathophysiological consequences of pulmonary stenosis: right ventricular wall thickness, cavity size and systolic function, and right atrial dimensions
  - To exclude other coexisting congenital cardiac lesions
- Cardiac MRI: For accurate quantitation of pulmonary flow, RV size and function assessment, and cardiac morphology +/- associated lesions

Always offer a management plan

Medical management of pulmonary stenosis is limited to diuretics for symptomatic relief. Antibiotic prophylaxis should also be considered (see *Infective endocarditis*, p. 40).

Interventional options include balloon valvuloplasty, which in anatomically suitable cases of severe symptomatic pulmonary stenosis offers excellent long term outcomes, and valve replacement (either surgical or percutaneous).

Case 7: Mitral stenosis

Instruction to the candidate

This 35-year-old woman presents with exertional dyspnoea. Please examine her cardiovascular system.

Begin with a summary of positive findings

Consider the patient demographics given in the candidate information. The patient is female (rheumatic mitral stenosis has a 2:1 prevalence of female:male) and she is 35 (symptoms usually present in the 3rd to 4th decade of life).

Peripheral signs of mitral stenosis include:

- Mitral facies: The malar flush of pink and purple patches on the cheeks
- Pulse: presence or absence of AF, and rate
- Palpate at the non-displaced apex for a tapping apex beat (palpable first heart

sound). A tapping apex beat and an opening snap are both clinical indicators of a pliable mitral valve, which would be more suitable to percutaneous balloon mitral valvuloplasty

Auscultatory features of mitral stenosis include:

- A loud first heart sound and opening snap after S2: both indicate pliable (rather than calcified) mitral valve leaflets
- A low pitch, rumbling mid-diastolic murmur, best heard at the apex with the bell of the stethoscope on expiration in the left lateral position
- If the patient is in sinus rhythm, a presystolic murmur (termed presystolic accentuation) will be heard as left atrial contraction forces blood across the stenosed mitral valve

Signs of severity in mitral stenosis include:

- The interval between S2 and the opening snap (and thus the duration of the diastolic murmur) is the auscultatory feature of severity in mitral stenosis. This is reflective of the degree of left atrial pressure. Higher left atrial pressure causes earlier mitral valve opening, and hence an earlier opening snap. Thus, the time between S2 and the opening snap is reduced with higher left atrial pressures, indicating more severe MS. In such cases the diastolic murmur is therefore longer
- The presence of pulmonary hypertension is also a feature of severe MS. The Graham Steell murmur is a rare early diastolic murmur of PR in the pulmonary region secondary to marked pulmonary hypertension

Follow with a summary of relevant negative findings

Important relevant negative findings which, if absent, are important to note, include:

- Arrhythmia (atrial fibrillation): comment on the rate, embolic complications and peripheral stigmata of anticoagulation
- Stigmata of infective endocarditis
- Pulmonary oedema (due to raised left atrial pressure)
- Signs of pulmonary hypertension, including:
  - Raised JVP
  - Left parasternal heave (pressure-loaded right ventricle)
  - Loud P2
  - Graham Steell murmur (rare)

State the most likely diagnosis on the basis of these findings

'This young woman has signs consistent with severe mitral stenosis with a pliable mitral valve, likely secondary to rheumatic fever. She is clinically euvolaemic, but is in atrial fibrillation with signs of pulmonary hypertension. I would like to take a full history to establish her symptomatic status and previous history of rheumatic fever, and my investigation of choice would be an echocardiogram to confirm the diagnosis.'

Offer relevant differential diagnoses

Any list of the differential diagnosis of mitral stenosis should start with rheumatic fever, which is by far the commonest cause. Less common causes include:

- Connective tissue disease (most commonly systemic lupus erythematosus or rheumatoid arthritis)
- Carcinoid heart disease
- Drugs: methysergide
- Mucopolysaccharidoses

Anatomic lesions that mimic mitral stenosis arise above the left ventricle and therefore also reflect raised pressures back to the pulmonary venous system. All of these conditions can manifest as pulmonary oedema and pulmonary hypertension, but the auscultatory features will differ from those described in mitral stenosis.

- Cortriatriatum: a congenital abnormality in which the left (or right) atrium is divided by a membrane, thus separating the pulmonary veins from the mitral valve and creating a triatrial heart
- Left atrial myxoma
- Pulmonary vein stenosis (this was reported more frequently following early experiences of pulmonary vein isolation in AF ablation)

Demonstrate the importance of clinical context – suggest relevant questions that would be taken in a patient history

Mitral stenosis tends to present in the 3rd to 4th decade of life with a stepwise decline in exercise tolerance. The chronology of symptoms tends to be revealing of the natural history of the condition. Pregnancy may unmask less severe mitral stenosis due to the increase in circulating volume during the second trimester. Symptoms to directly ascertain include:

- Exertional dyspnoea
- Palpitations (low index of suspicion of AF)
- Peripheral oedema
- Childhood history of rheumatic fever, country of birth and childhood
- History of cerebral embolic events
- More rarely, haemoptysis has been described.
- Hoarse voice secondary to left atrial dilatation compressing the recurrent laryngeal nerve has also been described in the setting of mitral stenosis, termed Ortner's syndrome
- Dysphagia can also manifest from oesophageal compression by a dilated left atrium

Demonstrate an understanding of the value of further investigation

An investigative work-up in a case of mitral stenosis would include the following:

Table 1.5 Echocardiographic features of mitral stenosis and their relationship to severity

	Mild	Moderate	Severe
Valve area (cm²)	1.6–2.0	1.0–1.5	<1.0
Mean gradient (mmHg)	<5	5–10	>10

- 12-lead electrocardiogram:
  - P mitral (broad, bifid P waves) of left atrial dilatation
  - Atrial fibrillation
- Plain chest radiograph:
  - Evidence of left atrial dilatation
  - Pulmonary oedema
  - Prominent pulmonary artery in patients with pulmonary hypertension
  - Splayed carina
- Echocardiography: the gold-standard diagnostic investigation. This demonstrates:
  - Severity: mitral valve area can be measured by Doppler flow and 2D planimetry. The mean transvalvular gradient is measured by Doppler flow. See **Table 1.5** for echocardiographic figures of mitral stenosis relating to their severity
  - Cusp and subvalvular mobility and calcification, especially important when considering balloon valvotomy. The Wilkins' score is a system that grades mitral valve mobility, calcification, leaflet thickening and subvalvular thickening to determine the suitability for percutaneous balloon valvuloplasty
  - Any associated mitral regurgitation (if moderate or severe, this is a contraindication to balloon valvuloplasty)
  - Left atrial dimensions
  - The presence of left atrial or appendage thrombus is excluded on transoesophageal echocardiography, which also provides more detailed views of the mitral valve itself.
  - Estimated pulmonary arterial and right atrial pressures
  - Right ventricular size and systolic function.
- Cardiac catheterisation is only required when discrepancy exists after clinical assessment and echocardiography, or to rule out concomitant coronary artery disease in older patients undergoing surgical management of their MS

Always offer a management plan

Medical management of mitral stenosis includes:

- Antibiotic prophylaxis (see *Infective endocarditis*, p. 40).
- Anticoagulation: All patients with AF (paroxysmal or permanent) should receive anticoagulation. Patients in sinus rhythm should receive anticoagulation in the setting of a previous history of embolism, with a dilated left atrium (diameter >5 cm), or in the presence of left atrial or appendage thrombus or spontaneous echo contrast (signifying sluggish left atrial flow) on transoesophageal echocardiography
- Diuretics and nitrates to reduce left atrial filling pressures
- Beta-blockers to reduce heart rate and thus lengthen the duration of diastolic left ventricular filling across the stenosed mitral valve

Indications for intervention in mitral stenosis include:

- Symptomatic, severe mitral stenosis
- Asymptomatic patients but with high risk of embolism (e.g. previous embolism, recent or paroxysmal AF) or haemodynamic decompensation (specifically raised pulmonary artery pressure, defined as estimated peak systolic pressure of >50 mmHg on echocardiogram)
- Asymptomatic patients with severe MS who require optimisation prior to undergoing events with a high risk of haemodynamic disturbance, such as those considering pregnancy or prior to non-cardiac surgery

The decision regarding the percutaneous versus surgical (most commonly valve replacement) approaches to treating severe MS rests upon factors including the patient's functional status and comorbid burden, anatomical suitability for balloon valvuloplasty, and local expertise in both approaches.

Further reading

Vahanian A, Baumgartner H, Bax J, et al. Guidelines on the management of valvular heart disease: the task force on the management of valvular heart disease of the European Society of Cardiology. Eur Heart J 2007; 28:230–268.

Case 8: Aortic regurgitation

Instruction to the candidate

This 40-year-old man presents with exertional dyspnoea. Please examine his cardiovascular system.

Begin with a summary of positive findings

Peripheral signs in aortic regurgitation include:

- Collapsing ('water-hammer') pulse at the brachial artery with the patient's arm raised vertically
- Wide pulse pressure
- Thrusting (volume-loaded), laterally displaced apex beat
- Aortic thrill
- Look for associated aetiological features (see **Table 1.6** below): for example, Marfanoid habitus.

The auscultatory features of aortic regurgitation include:

- Early diastolic murmur: a high-pitched, decrescendo murmur heard loudest at the lower left sternal edge with the patient sitting forward in expiration
- Associated murmurs:
  - Systolic flow murmur
  - Ejection systolic murmur (mixed aortic valve disease)
  - Austin Flint murmur: a low-pitched, rumbling mid-diastolic murmur due to turbulent mixing of the retrograde AR and antegrade mitral valve forward flow in the left ventricular cavity
- An ejection click suggests a bicuspid aortic valve

The constellation of clinical signs in aortic regurgitation includes numerous eponymous signs. The important ones to know and seek to identify in the exam, include:

- Corrigan's sign – a visible carotid pulsation
- Quincke's sign – capillary pulsation in the fingernails
- Duroziez's sign – compressing the femoral artery with the stethoscope elicits murmurs of systolic forward flow and diastolic flow reversal
- Traube's sign – 'pistol-shot' sound heard on auscultation over the femoral arteries

- De Musset's sign – head nodding in time with systole

Of the clinical signs mentioned above, those that suggest severe aortic regurgitation include:

- A wide pulse pressure (noteably low diastolic blood pressure)
- A collapsing pulse
- Long duration of the early diastolic murmur
- The presence of signs of cardiac failure
- The presence of an Austin Flint murmur

Follow with a summary of relevant negative findings

The absence of stigmata of infective endocarditis and signs of cardiac failure are important to mention to the examiner. State that you would also want to check bilateral blood pressures to exclude dissection.

State the most likely diagnosis on the basis of these findings

'This young patient has signs consistent with severe aortic regurgitation, likely secondary to a bicuspid aortic valve given his age. He is clinically euvolaemic, and does not have any features of infective endocarditis. I would like to take a full history to establish his symptomatic status and my investigation of choice would be an echocardiogram to confirm the diagnosis and to rule out any associated aortic pathology.'

Offer relevant differential diagnoses

The differential of the causes of aortic regurgitation can be divided according to whether the lesion is congenital or acquired. The commonest cause of congenital aortic regurgitation is a bicuspid aortic valve. Acquired causes of aortic regurgitation are considered in **Table 1.6.**

It is also worth considering the differential diagnosis of a collapsing pulse, which can be a manifestation of other high-output states:

- Aortic regurgitation
- Patent ductus arteriosus
- Anaemia

Table 1.6 Aetiology of aortic regurgitation and associated clinical findings		
	Acute	**Chronic**
Valve leaflet	Endocarditis (review dentition, intravenous access, peripheral stigmata)	Rheumatic fever (check for concomitant mitral stenosis) Connective tissue diseases (e.g. rheumatoid arthritis – check joints)
Aortic root	Dissection (type A) Trauma	Dilatation – Idiopathic Marfan syndrome (check arm span, palate and eyes), Ehlers–Danlos syndrome, pseudoxanthoma elasticum Hypertension (check blood pressure) Aortitis Syphilis (check pupils for Argyll Robertson abnormality) Ankylosing spondylitis (check posture)

- Hyperthyroidism
- Fever
- Paget's disease
- Pregnancy

Demonstrate the importance of clinical context – suggest relevant questions that would be taken in a patient history

Relevant history questions include those aimed at identifying underlying cause and those regarding symptoms of cardiac failure.

Demonstrate an understanding of the value of further investigation

The key investigations include a 12-lead electrocardiogram, a plain chest radiograph, and a transthoracic echocardiogram. Additional investigations include CT, cMRI and cardiac catheterisation. The findings of such relevant investigations include:

- ECG:
  - Left ventricular hypertrophy
  - Left axis deviation
- CXR:
  - Cardiomegaly due to left ventricular dilatation
  - Pulmonary oedema if in heart failure
  - Aortic dilatation
- Echocardiography: the gold-standard diagnostic investigation. This demonstrates:
  - Severity by regurgitant orifice area, pressure half-time, regurgitant volume and fraction, jet width on colour Doppler and the presence of flow reversal in the descending aorta

  - Valve morphology: bicuspid versus tricuspid
  - Left ventricular cavity size and systolic function
  - Left ventricular wall thickness
  - Aortic root and ascending aorta dimensions, and associated aortic pathology, such as in the case of dissection or aneurysm
- CT: To visualise the thoracic aorta for associated abnormalities
- Cardiac MRI can be used to assess left ventricular volumes and aortic valve regurgitant fractions when echocardiography is unclear. This can also be used to visualise the thoracic aorta for associated abnormalities
- Cardiac catheterisation: for investigation of concomitant coronary artery disease in pre-operative patients. Aortic dimensions and visualisation of AR on aortogram can also be assessed

Always offer a management plan

Patient advice is important in aortic regurgitation. For patients with bicuspid aortic valve or Marfan syndrome, advice on family screening is relevant. Patients with mild and moderate aortic regurgitation should receive outpatient follow-up to monitor the natural history of the condition. For matters relating to antibiotic prophylaxis (see *Infective endocarditis*, p. 40).

Indications for specific medical therapies include:

- Acute severe AR: vasodilators (e.g. nitrates) are used to optimise prior to surgery
- Chronic severe AR with evidence of left ventricular dysfunction: ACE inhibitors

- Hypertension: vasodilators should be prescribed, including ACE inhibitors or dihydropyridine calcium channel antagonists
- Marfan syndrome: Beta-blockers and angiotensin receptor blockers (e.g. losartan) are used to slow the rate of aortic dilatation. (do not use beta-blockers in severe AR, as reducing heart rate lengthens diastole, consequently increasing regurgitant volumes)

Indications for surgery in cases of aortic regurgitation include:

- Symptomatic severe AR: requires aortic valve replacement
- Asymptomatic severe AR: aortic valve replacement is indicated in the following circumstances:
  - Resting left ventricular ejection fraction ≤50%
  - Significant left ventricular dilatation

(end-diastolic diameter >7 cm, end-systolic diameter >5 cm)
  - Patients undergoing other concomitant cardiovascular surgery (e.g. CABG, other valve surgery, aortic surgery)
- Aortic root disease: Surgical intervention is indicated in the following groups of patients (irrespective of AR severity) with an aortic root diameter of:
  - Marfan syndrome: ≥45 mm
  - Bicuspid valves: ≥50 mm
  - All other patients: ≥55 mm

Further reading

Vahanian A, Baumgartner H, Bax J, et al. Guidelines on the management of valvular heart disease: the task force on the management of valvular heart disease of the European Society of Cardiology. Eur Heart J 2007; 28:230–268.

Case 9: Pulmonary regurgitation

Instruction to the candidate

This 42-year-old man presents with dyspnoea. Please examine his cardiovascular system.

Begin with a summary of positive findings

Relevant positive findings in pulmonary regurgitation include auscultatory features and signs of severity.

The auscultatory features of pulmonary regurgitation include:

- A brief, early diastolic decrescendo murmur heard loudest at the upper left sternal edge typically on inspiration. The Graham Steell murmur describes the murmur of PR due to a dilated annulus secondary to a dilated pulmonary artery in severe pulmonary hypertension. It has a high-pitched quality, and can be present for the duration of diastole given the pressure gradient between the pulmonary artery and the right ventricle

- P2 is absent following pulmonary valvotomy or in cases of congenitally absent pulmonic valve
- P2 is loud and can be palpable at the upper left sternal edge in pulmonary hypertension

Signs of severity in pulmonary regurgitation include:

- When not caused by pulmonary hypertension, a shorter duration of the early diastolic murmur is related to increased severity of PR
- Examination findings of right heart failure

Follow with a summary of relevant negative findings

Important features which, if absent, are important to note, include:

- Signs of right heart failure: raised JVP, peripheral oedema and ascites
- Infective endocarditis: comment on the absence of peripheral stigmata, dental hygiene and the presence or absence of

indwelling intravenous access. It should be noted, however, that right-sided lesions usually cause pulmonary septic emboli rather than peripheral embolic phenomena. Peripheral stigmata of intravenous drug abuse should be carefully inspected given the propensity for right-heart valve endocarditis in these patients

- Scars indicating previous cardiothoracic surgery

Also note the presence or absence of concomitant tricuspid regurgitation. It can be due to a number of factors:

- Secondary to right ventricular dilatation, and thus consequent tricuspid annular dilatation, in the setting of chronic PR
- Clinically significant TR is found in approximately one-third of patients with repaired tetralogy of Fallot (either due to tricuspid annular dilatation or iatrogenic pulmonic valve injury following VSD repair)
- The tricuspid valve is the most commonly affected valve in carcinoid heart disease, and therefore patients with variable combinations of pulmonary regurgitation and stenosis are likely to have concomitant TR
- Patients with pulmonary hypertension causing PR may also have clinically significant TR due to right ventricular pressure-overload with or without volume-overload

State the most likely diagnosis on the basis of these findings

'This patient has signs consistent with severe pulmonary regurgitation secondary to pulmonary valvotomy, likely following repaired tetralogy of Fallot. He has clinical features of right heart failure, but does not have any features of infective endocarditis. I would like to take a full history to establish his symptomatic status, and my investigation of choice would be an echocardiogram to confirm the diagnosis.'

Offer relevant differential diagnoses

The differential diagnosis can be considered in the context of whether the lesion is congenital or acquired, anatomically and by acute versus chronic pathologies. Congenital causes include an absent pulmonary valve. For acquired causes see **Table 1.7**.

Demonstrate the importance of clinical context – suggest relevant questions that would be taken in a patient history

Patients are usually asymptomatic until right ventricular dilatation and dysfunction manifests. Once this occurs, symptoms will include:

- Exertional dyspnoea is usually the first symptom that is reported
- Peripheral oedema
- Palpitations: atrial and ventricular arrhythmias can occur, and are a risk factor for sudden cardiac death

Features suggesting aetiology of pulmonary regurgitation include:

- History of congenital heart disease and associated surgical or interventional treatment
- Infective endocarditis: intravenous drug abuse or long-term indwelling venous access, fevers or rigors, and recent dental procedures
- Carcinoid syndrome: flushing, diarrhoea, weight loss and wheeze
- History of childhood rheumatic fever

Demonstrate an understanding of the value of further investigation

The following investigations are key in the diagnosis and evaluation of pulmonary regurgitation:

- A 12-lead electrocardiogram demonstrates:
  - Any current arrhythmia
  - Widening of the QRS complex with RSR morphology in the right ventricular leads is reflective of dilatation of this chamber, and has prognostic implications with respect to the propensity for ventricular arrhythmia and sudden cardiac death
  - Right ventricular hypertrophy
  - Right bundle branch block, which is common in patients with a history of previous tetralogy of Fallot repair via a right ventriculotomy approach
- A plain chest radiograph may demonstrate evidence of right ventricular dilatation and/ or enlargement of the central pulmonary arteries
- Echocardiography with demonstrate the presence of pulmonary regurgitation, severity

Table 1.7 Aetiology of pulmonary regurgitation and associated clinical findings

	Acute	Chronic
Valve leaflet	Endocarditis (review for signs of intravenous drug abuse, intravenous access (especially in patients receiving renal replacement therapy, peripheral stigmata)	Rheumatic fever (check for other likely concomitant valvular abnormalities) Carcinoid syndrome (check for concomitant tricuspid valve and, less commonly, left-sided valve lesions, and flushed appearance) Congenital disease: bicuspid or quadricuspid valves
Functional (annular dilatation)		Pulmonary hypertension (the commonest cause in adults) Following intervention for tetralogy of Fallot (such as pulmonary valvotomy) or pulmonary stenosis (such as balloon valvuloplasty) Dilatation of the pulmonary trunk due to Marfan syndrome (check arm span, palate and eyes)

of the lesion, and any subsequent structural abnormalities:

- The valve morphology and underlying cause of pulmonary regurgitation is elucidated by looking at all structures that make up the pulmonary valve apparatus, including the valve leaflets, annulus, RVOT and pulmonary artery. However, previous surgical intervention can confer extra difficulty on echocardiographic assessment of the valve
- The severity of pulmonary regurgitation is assessed semi-quantitatively by colour Doppler and by the duration of pulmonary regurgitant flow in diastole
- The impact upon right ventricular cavity size and systolic function
- Cardiac MRI is currently the gold standard tool for quantification of pulmonary regurgitation, right ventricular size and systolic function. This technique also permits detailed imaging of complex treated or untreated congenital lesions
- Cardiac catheterisation is only required in patients undergoing transcatheter

intervention or for patients where haemodynamic quantification by non-invasive techniques remains suboptimal
- Functional data provided by serial CPEX testing can help determine the timing of surgery.

Always offer a management plan

Management of pulmonary regurgitation can be considered in terms of general advice, medical management, and intervention (whether surgical or percutaneous). Advice regarding antibiotic prophylaxis is considered in *Infective endocarditis*, p. 40). Medical management is limited to diuretics for relief of symptoms and treatment of the underlying cause. Surgery is indicated for moderate to severe PR with progressive right ventricular dilatation irrespective of symptomatology, and following the development of ventricular arrhythmias or syncope. Percutaneous pulmonary valve implantation is also a treatment option in this scenario.

Case 10: Mixed aortic valve disease

Instruction to the candidate

This 40-year-old man has been complaining of breathlessness on exertion. Please examine his cardiovascular system.

Begin with a summary of positive findings

The peripheral signs to identify in mixed aortic valve disease include:

- A bisferious (biphasic) pulse ('pulsus bisferiens') describes a palpable double peak in the pulse waveform during a single cardiac cycle. This is typically described in patients with mixed aortic stenosis and regurgitation when the regurgitant lesion predominates and is haemodynamically significant. However, it may also be found in isolated severe AR
- It is important to consider dominance, which can be determined before auscultation. If aortic stenosis is dominant, there will be a slow-rising pulse with a narrow pulse pressure. If the regurgitation is dominant, there will be a collapsing pulse with a wide pulse pressure. Likewise, thrills and the nature of the apex pulsation (heaving in stenosis versus thrusting in regurgitation) can assist to determine dominance.

Auscultatory features of mixed aortic valve disease include:

- A combination of ejection systolic and early diastolic murmurs in the aortic region and at the lower left sternal edge respectively
- An underlying bicuspid aortic valve can be identified by an aortic click

Follow with a summary of relevant negative findings

Important relevant negative findings include:

- Infective endocarditis: comment on the absence of peripheral stigmata, dental hygiene and the presence or absence of indwelling intravenous access
- Signs of cardiac failure, including pulmonary oedema, peripheral oedema, raised JVP and S3 gallop

In cases of rheumatic aortic valve disease, comment on the presence or absence of concomitant rheumatic mitral valve lesions.

State the most likely diagnosis on the basis of these findings

'This young patient has signs consistent with mixed aortic valve disease with predominant aortic regurgitation due to a bicuspid aortic valve. He is clinically euvolaemic, and does not have any features of infective endocarditis. I would like to take a full history to establish his symptomatic status, and my investigation of choice would be an echocardiogram to confirm the diagnosis and to rule out any associated aortic pathology.'

Offer relevant differential diagnoses

Key underlying diagnoses in mixed aortic valve disease include:

- Bicuspid aortic valve
- Rheumatic valve disease: note that concomitant mitral stenosis can cause a reduced stroke volume, thus leading to underestimated gradients across a stenosed aortic valve. Therefore, aortic valve area should be measured to provide a less load-dependent parameter of aortic stenosis

Demonstrate the importance of clinical context – suggest relevant questions that would be taken in a patient history

See *Aortic stenosis* (p. 2) and *Aortic regurgitation* (p. 19) for relevant history questions.

Demonstrate an understanding of the value of further investigation

Aortic stenosis (p. 2) and *Aortic regurgitation* (p. 19), outline the relevant investigations. As with all cardiology cases, the key investigations will include:

- A 12-lead electrocardiogram
- A plain chest radiograph
- Echocardiography

Always offer a management plan

The management of mixed aortic valve disease follows that of the predominant valvular lesion as for lone aortic stenosis or regurgitation. In situations in which balanced aortic stenosis and regurgitation manifest but neither individual lesion is severe, intervention is indicated when symptoms result or the mixed disease causes impairment of left ventricular function.

Further reading

Vahanian A, Baumgartner H, Bax J, et al. Guidelines on the management of valvular heart disease: the task force on the management of valvular heart disease of the European Society of Cardiology. Eur Heart J 2007; 28:230–268.

Case 11: Mixed mitral valve disease

Instruction to the candidate

This 45-year-old woman has been complaining of breathlessness on exertion. Please examine her cardiovascular system.

Begin with a summary of positive findings

Peripheral signs of mixed mitral valve disease include:

- Look for a scar overlying the femoral vein indicating previous vascular access for a percutaneous balloon mitral valvuloplasty. Increased mitral regurgitation is a frequent finding immediately post-procedure, with restenosis being a later complication
- Consider dominance, which is determined clinically before auscultation:
  - Dominant MS: a tapping, undisplaced apex beat with a loud first heart sound
  - Dominant MR: a thrusting, displaced apex beat with a soft first heart sound

Auscultatory features of mixed mitral valve disease include:

- Mixed pansystolic and mid-diastolic murmurs, best heard at the apex (with the bell of the stethoscope for the murmur of MS) on expiration in the left lateral position
- S3 is not heard with MS, and is a finding in LV dysfunction due to MR

Follow with a summary of relevant negative findings

Important relevant negative findings to comment on include:

- Arrhythmia (atrial fibrillation): comment on the rate, embolic complications and peripheral stigmata of anticoagulation
- Infective endocarditis: comment on the absence of peripheral stigmata, dental hygiene and the presence or absence of indwelling intravenous access
- Pulmonary oedema occurs in both mitral stenosis and regurgitation, albeit with differing underlying pathophysiology
- Signs of pulmonary hypertension, including:
  - Raised JVP
  - Left parasternal heave (pressure-loaded right ventricle)
  - Loud P2
  - Graham Steell murmur (rare)

In cases where there is a specific underlying cause, further relevant negative findings are pertinent. In cases of rheumatic mitral valve disease, comment on the presence or absence of concomitant rheumatic aortic valve lesions. In cases of Marfan syndrome and mitral regurgitation, rule out coexisting aortic regurgitation.

State the most likely diagnosis on the basis of these findings

'This woman has mixed mitral valve disease with predominant mitral regurgitation following valvuloplasty for rheumatic mitral stenosis. She is in rate-controlled atrial fibrillation with signs of pulmonary and peripheral fluid retention, but no stigmata of infective endocarditis. My investigation of choice to confirm the diagnosis and look for further complications is an echocardiogram.'

Offer relevant differential diagnoses

In the setting of mixed mitral valve disease, prior rheumatic fever is the likely cause.

Demonstrate the importance of clinical context – suggest relevant questions that would be taken in a patient history

See *Mitral regurgitation* (p. 5) and *Mitral stenosis* (p. 16) for relevant history questions.

Demonstrate an understanding of the value of further investigation

The key investigations will include a 12-lead electrocardiogram, a plain chest radiograph and a transthoracic echocardiogram. Further details can be found in *Mitral regurgitation* (p. 5) and *Mitral stenosis* (p. 16).

Always offer a management plan

The management of mixed mitral valve disease follows that of the predominant valvular lesion as for lone mitral stenosis or regurgitation. However, percutaneous balloon mitral valvuloplasty is contraindicated in mitral stenosis when moderate or worse regurgitation coexists.

In situations in which balanced mitral stenosis and regurgitation manifest but neither individual lesion is severe, intervention is indicated when symptoms result or predominant regurgitation causes impairment of left ventricular function.

Further reading

Vahanian A, Baumgartner H, Bax J, et al. Guidelines on the management of valvular heart disease: the task force on the management of valvular heart disease of the European Society of Cardiology. Eur Heart J 2007; 28:230–268.

Case 12: Prosthetic valves and cardiac surgery

Instruction to the candidate

This 60-year-old man has recently undergone cardiac surgery. Please examine his cardiovascular system.

Begin with a summary of positive findings

Positive peripheral clinical findings to look for include:

- Scars. When a scar is identified, run your finger over it to demonstrate to the examiner that you have noted it. Different scars include:
  - Midline sternotomy (CABG, valve replacement or repair, cardiac transplantation)
  - Lateral thoracotomy:
    - Cardiac causes: mitral valvotomy, coarctation repair, PDA ligation, Blalock-Thomas-Taussig shunt

○ Respiratory causes: lobectomy, pneumonectomy, lung transplantation, bullectomy, previous thoracoplasty for TB

- Inspect and palpate for either an infraclavicular or an abdominal (surgically implanted epicardial device) subcutaneous pacemaker in the cardiothoracic surgical patient. In one series of over 340 patients undergoing isolated aortic valve replacement, post-operative permanent pacing was required in 8.5% of patients
- Arterial (radial) or venous (saphenous and femoral) graft harvest scars. Remember that left internal mammary artery (LIMA) grafts are reflected from the internal thoracic wall. Therefore, a CABG is still a possibility in a patient with a midline sternotomy scar without saphenous vein or radial artery graft harvest scars
- Radial or femoral puncture scars from previous angiography. These tend to be on the right-hand side which is the conventional approach for performing these procedures

Before auscultating the chest, listen away from the chest without the stethoscope for the audible click of a metallic heart valve replacement. If this finding is present, state to the examiner that a mechanical valve prosthesis is in situ based upon the examination findings so far prior to confirming the type of prosthesis with the stethoscope. Auscultatory findings include:

- For tilting-disc or bileaflet valves, a soft opening click may be audible. A high-frequency metallic click at S1 indicates closure of a mechanical mitral valve replacement (MVR), or at S2 the closure of a mechanical aortic valve replacement (AVR)
- For caged-ball valves, a loud rumbling sound is heard on auscultation due to the ball rattling in the cage with forward flow of blood across the prosthesis. Opening and closing sounds in these valves are of low-frequency and equal in intensity
- Tissue valves have similar closing sounds to native valves
- Listen for soft flow murmurs across the valve. Such flow murmurs will be systolic for AVRs and diastolic for MVRs
- Auscultatory evidence of valvular incompetence is abnormal

> ### Prosthetic valve incompetence
>
> It is vital to identify auscultatory evidence of prosthetic valve incompetence.
> - In prosthetic aortic valves, a diastolic murmur indicates incompetence
> - In prosthetic mitral valves, a systolic murmur indicates incompetence

Follow with a summary of relevant negative findings

The following relevant negatives relate to those of prosthetic valves:

- Embolic complications: approximately 75% of complications experienced with prosthetic valves are due to thromboembolic phenomena and bleeding secondary to anticoagulation. Embolic complications can be due to:
  − Atrial fibrillation
  − From the valve prosthesis itself
  − As an immediate post-operative complication
- Bleeding from anticoagulation
- Dysfunction of the valve prosthesis can be due to thrombosis, degeneration, dehiscence, paravalvular leak or pannus formation. Valve thrombosis should be suspected when the patient presents with acute dyspnoea or syncope, possibly with a recent history of inadequate anticoagulation. Patients may report loss of the normal valve clicking, with muffled or absent prosthetic valve closing sounds on auscultation. Valve thrombosis can be treated medically (with heparin or thrombolysis) or surgically, depending on the degree of obstruction and the size of the thrombus, and the clinical condition of the patient. Such a decision requires a multidisciplinary approach. Valve failure can present acutely with cardiogenic shock, or subacutely with cardiac failure and/or valve haemolysis
- Prosthetic valve infective endocarditis: fever is the predominant clinical feature, and unexplained fever in a patient with a valve prosthesis should be treated as infective endocarditis until proven otherwise. Other presentations of prosthetic valve endocarditis include a new murmur, prosthetic valve failure, cardiac failure and embolic

phenomena. Typical peripheral stigmata of native valve endocarditis are often absent in prosthetic valve infection. Ask the examiner for the temperature and a urine dip (looking for microscopic haematuria), and comment on dental hygiene and the presence or absence of indwelling intravenous access as sources of infection

- Arrhythmia (atrial fibrillation): this is common post-cardiac surgery. Comment on the rate, embolic complications and peripheral stigmata of anticoagulation
- Anaemia (look for skin, conjunctival and mucosal pallor). This may be secondary to:
  - Anticoagulation
  - Prosthetic valve haemolysis due to paravalvular leak: this requires transoesophageal echocardiography for further evaluation, and potentially reoperation if the resultant anaemia is severely symptomatic or requires repeated transfusions

---

Prosthetic valve types

Mechanical valves can be divided into single-tilting disc, bileaflet (double-tilting disc) or caged-ball (Starr-Edwards) valves. The latter prosthesis is not used in the modern era (discontinued in 2007), and was notable for a high incidence of valve - related thrombosis and haemolysis. Prostheses vary in their relative thrombogenicity, and and hence the target INR for a patient with a mechanical prosthesis is dependent upon the prosthesis type itself, and patient-related risk factors (e.g. aortic position versus mitral position, AF, poor LV systolic function)

State the most likely diagnosis on the basis of these findings

The following three cases illustrate the range of possible presentations with scars and valve prostheses in MRCP PACES. They demonstrate the synthesis of the range of positive findings and relevant negatives that have been outlined above.

Case 1: Midline sternotomy with a metallic second heart sound

'This man has undergone a mechanical aortic valve replacement with coronary artery bypass grafting using saphenous vein grafts either with or without a left internal mammary artery graft. The most likely indication for this would be degenerative calcific aortic stenosis and coronary artery disease. Clinically, the valve appears to be well functioning with no evidence of infective endocarditis or cardiac failure. I would like to take a full history to establish the details of his intervention, and my investigation of choice would be an echocardiogram to review the valve function, orifice area and gradients.'

Case 2: Midline sternotomy with a metallic first heart sound.

'This woman has undergone a mechanical mitral valve replacement and is in rate-controlled atrial fibrillation. A possible indication for this procedure in a woman of this age is previous rheumatic mitral valve disease. Clinically, the valve appears to be well functioning with evidence of anticoagulation treatment. There is no evidence of infective endocarditis or cardiac failure. I would like to take a full history to establish the details of her intervention, and my investigation of choice would be an echocardiogram to review the valve function, orifice area and gradients.'

Case 3: Midline sternotomy with a metallic second heart sound and diastolic murmur

'This man has undergone a mechanical aortic valve replacement which is regurgitant as evidenced by an early diastolic murmur at the lower left sternal edge. He appears to be clinically well compensated, however, with no evidence of infective endocarditis or cardiac failure. He has also had coronary artery bypass grafting using saphenous vein grafts either with or without a left internal mammary artery graft. The most likely underlying indication for this operation would be degenerative calcific aortic stenosis and coronary artery disease. I would like to take a full history to establish the details of his intervention, and my investigation of choice would be an echocardiogram to determine if the regurgitation is valvular or paravalvular, the severity of the regurgitation and the impact upon left ventricular function.'

Offer relevant differential diagnoses

Once the appropriate form of cardiac surgery has been identified, give a differential diagnosis of the likely underlying disease condition(s) that would have warranted the intervention.

Demonstrate the importance of clinical context – suggest relevant questions that would be taken in a patient history

Questions would include symptomatic response to intervention, adequacy of anticoagulation in the case of mechanical prostheses, and any new symptoms that may warrant further investigation of valve replacements (e.g. fevers, rigors, dyspnoea, syncope).

Demonstrate an understanding of the value of further investigation

Relevant laboratory blood tests would include:

- A full blood count to identify anaemia
- LDH, haptoglobin and blood film to identify haemolysis
- Clotting studies for anticoagulation monitoring
- Serial blood cultures and inflammatory markers if there is suspicion of prosthetic valve endocarditis

Echocardiography is the central diagnostic modality for valve prostheses. Serial transthoracic studies can be used to follow-up prosthetic valve gradients and compared with a baseline post-operative study. Transoesophageal echocardiography is required in suspected infected prostheses, in prosthetic valve regurgitation or paravalvular leak, and when acoustic shadowing from the metallic prosthesis causing dropout of the ultrasound signal limits the data obtained by transthoracic study.

Always offer a management plan

Annual review by a cardiologist is required to review prosthetic valve function and rule out any complications, or review as soon as new symptoms of valvular dysfunction develop. Follow-up echocardiography parameters for the prosthetic valve should be compared to an initial baseline post-operative echocardiogram.

Lifelong anticoagulation is required for all patients with mechanical prostheses and in patients with tissue valve replacements who have a separate indication for anticoagulation (such as AF).

Antibiotic prophylaxis (see *Infective endocarditis*, p. 40).

The choice between a tissue valve replacement versus a mechanical prosthesis is an individualised decision taken with the patient and taking into consideration several patient-specific factors:

- Patient choice: having weighed up the advantages and disadvantages of each valve type
- Age and life expectancy: where life expectancy is expected to be less than the predicted time to valve degeneration, bioprostheses are acceptable. In contrast, mechanical valves are favoured in young individuals or patients with risks for accelerated tissue valve degeneration (e.g. renal impairment, hyperparathyroidism)
- Anticoagulation: patients with contraindications to anticoagulation or poor compliance are more preferable for a tissue valve replacement. Patients with other anticoagulation indications or already receiving anticoagulation (such as AF) would be more suitable for a mechanical prosthesis
- Women of childbearing age: this is a difficult decision with advantages and disadvantages for and against each type. This is an individualised decision that is reached following detailed discussion with the patient

Further reading

Vahanian A, Baumgartner H, Bax J, et al. Guidelines on the management of valvular heart disease: the task force on the management of valvular heart disease of the European Society of Cardiology. Eur Heart J 2007; 28:230–268.

Vongpatanasin W, Hillis LD, Lange RA. Prosthetic heart valves. N Engl J Med 1996; 335:407–416.

Dawkins S, Hobson AR, Kalra PR, et al. Permanent pacemaker implantation after isolated aortic valve replacement: incidence, indications, and predictors. Ann Thorac Surg 2008; 85:108–112.

Case 13: Cardiac failure

Instruction to the candidate

This 75-year-old woman presents with worsening dyspnoea and reduced mobility. Please examine her cardiovascular system.

Begin with a summary of positive findings

Peripheral signs to identify in cases of cardiac failure:

- Signs of poor perfusion such as cool and clammy peripheries, hypotension
- When palpating the pulse, feel for:
  - AF: present in up to 30–40% of patients with heart failure
  - Pulsus alternans: alternating strong and weak palpable arterial pulsations, a sign that confers a poorer prognosis
- Resting tachypnoea
- The apex beat may be displaced
- Raised JVP (state how high)
- An infraclavicular mass suggesting CRT, CRT-D, ICD alone, or bradycardia pacemaker (see *Infraclavicular mass*, p. 33)
- Bibasal reduced air entry (pleural effusions) and crepitations (state the level)
- Pitting peripheral and sacral oedema (state the level)
- Ascites
- Hepatomegaly

Auscultatory features which should be listened for include:

- An S3 with a gallop rhythm
- Murmurs indicative of valvular dysfunction. In the context of cardiac failure, mitral or tricuspid regurgitation may be causative or consequential lesions in heart failure. For example, MR may cause heart failure or be functional due to a dilated annulus. Similarly, TR can cause right heart failure or may occur due to congestive cardiac failure
- S4 in restrictive disorders

Follow with a summary of relevant negative findings

The presence or absence of signs of severity in cardiac failure should be commented upon, and include:

- Pulsus alternans
- Gallop rhythm
- Cardiac cachexia

State the most likely diagnosis on the basis of these findings

'This patient has signs consistent with congestive cardiac failure, likely secondary to coronary artery disease as evidenced by her midline sternotomy scar and saphenous vein graft harvest scars. She has increased right atrial pressure as evidenced by the raised JVP, and has peripheral fluid retention to the knees. I would like to take a full history to establish her symptomatic status, and my investigation of choice would be an echocardiogram to confirm the diagnosis.'

Offer relevant differential diagnoses. The differential diagnosis of the causes of cardiac failure is listed below, divided into those responsible for systolic heart failure, those that cause diastolic heart failure, and heart failure caused by a high-output state. They are accompanied where appropriate by clinical findings which may be elicited to suggest such diagnoses.

Systolic heart failure

- Ischaemic heart disease: signs would include a midline sternotomy, venous graft harvest scars, stigmata of CAD risk factors such as xanthelasma or evidence of diabetes
- Cardiomyopathy: including idiopathic dilated, alcohol-related (signs of chronic liver disease), peripartum cardiomyopathy (young female), chemotherapy-induced (especially having received anthracyclines or trastuzumab – note previous mastectomy and radiotherapy tattoos)
- Valvular heart disease
- Infection or inflammation: myocarditis, Chagas disease
- Arrhythmia ('tachycardiomyopathy')

Diastolic heart failure

- Restrictive cardiomyopathy: including infiltrative disorders (the examplar disease process being amyloidosis), sarcoid, haemochromatosis, connective tissue diseases
- Pericardial constriction (radiotherapy tattoos over the left hemithorax)

- Hypertrophic cardiomyopathy
- Hypertensive heart disease

High output cardiac failure

- Thyrotoxicosis
- Pregnancy
- Nutritional deficiencies: beriberi, thiamine deficiency
- Anaemia
- Paget's disease
- Systemic arteriovenous fistulae

Causes of a raised JVP

Aside from the aetiology of congestive heart failure, the differential diagnoses of key clinical signs need consideration, such as a raised JVP or peripheral oedema:

- Congestive cardiac failure versus isolated right-sided heart failure. Isolated acute right heart failure in the context of RV infarction or pulmonary embolism presents with a raised JVP but clear lung fields. In this setting, identification of isolated right heart failure is key, as treatment is aimed at fluid administration to support the right heart circulation rather than diuresis in the example of RV failure due to infarction
- Pulmonary hypertension
- Significant tricuspid regurgitation: giant 'v' waves
- Superior vena cava obstruction: non-pulsatile, distended JVP
- Cardiac tamponade and pericardial constriction: look for Kussmaul's sign, which is an increase in the level of the JVP on inspiration. The JVP usually falls on inspiration through increased venous return to the right heart, but in constriction and tamponade the right ventricle is unable to accommodate the increased inspiratory filling which is thus transmitted to the JVP

Be careful not to confuse Corrigan's sign (an arterial pulsation) in severe AR with a raised JVP. If congestive cardiac failure has resulted from severe AR, both signs may be present.

Peripheral oedema

The differential diagnosis of peripheral oedema includes:

- Cardiac failure
- Hypoalbuminaemia which can be due to impaired hepatic synthesis, malnutrition, gastrointestinal or renal losses
- Renal impairment
- Nephrotic syndrome
- Chronic venous insufficiency
- A pelvic mass with impaired lymphatic drainage

Demonstrate the importance of clinical context – suggest relevant questions that would be taken in a patient history

Important questions in a history regarding cardiac failure include:

- Dyspnoea: ask to quantify exercise tolerance and categorise according to NYHA class
- Orthopnoea and paroxysmal nocturnal dyspnoea
- Peripheral oedema: are shoes or trousers more difficult to fit?
- Palpitations or syncope suggestive of arrhythmia
- Angina
- Cardiovascular risk factors
- History of previous cardiovascular, renal or liver disease
- Medication history

Demonstrate an understanding of the value of further investigation

Important investigations in the assessment of cardiac failure include:

- Laboratory blood tests:
  - Full blood count for anaemia
  - Natriuretic peptides (BNP or NT-proBNP) as markers of myocardial stretch and thus volume overload
  - Urea, creatinine and electrolytes: deranged renal function has implications on prognosis and may be the result of cardiorenal syndrome or the deleterious impact of heart failure treatment. Renal impairment is an independent marker of poor prognosis in patients with heart failure, impacting upon both survival and the scope for certain medical therapies with known survival benefit. This is an important consideration in managing cardiac failure
- A 12-lead electrocardiogram may some or all of the following:
  - Evidence of previous ischaemia, arrhythmia, left ventricular hypertrophy
  - Poor R wave progression

- Left bundle branch block, the duration of the QRS complex being a criteria for cardiac resynchronisation therapy
- A normal ECG renders systolic heart failure unlikely (<10%) as the cause of the patient's symptoms
- A plain chest radiograph may show a variable combination of cardiomegaly, pleural effusions, alveolar pulmonary oedema , Kerley B lines, fluid in the fissure, and upper lobe blood diversion
- Echocardiography is the investigation of choice. It allows assessment of biventricular size, systolic and diastolic function, and can demonstrate evidence of a previous infarction. It also allows assessment of valvular aetiologies or consequences of cardiac failure and the impact of left heart failure on estimated pulmonary artery pressure
- Cardiac MRI allows additional assessment of myocardial (especially infiltrative) disease and viability when revascularisation is being considered
- Cardiac catheterisation is used to investigate coronary lesions responsible for impaired systolic function. It also allows assessment of haemodynamic parameters, such as left ventricular end-diastolic pressure, pulmonary capillary wedge and pulmonary arterial pressures. Endomyocardial biopsy is rarely required but can be considered in certain cases.

Always offer a management plan

General principles that should be applied include:

- Treat the underlying cause, such as targeted therapy for hypertensive heart disease or intervention on symptomatic valvular heart disease
- Fluid and salt restriction
- Immunisations (influenza, pneumococcal)

Symptomatic treatment includes diuresis with either oral or intravenous preparations. In cases of congested gut mucosa, bumetanide has superior oral bioavailability compared with furosemide. Metolazone can be combined with intravenous diuresis in severe cases of fluid retention, but warrants careful monitoring of renal function and electrolytes. Ultrafiltration can be used in cases of fluid overload refractory to diuretics. There is some evidence that this treatment modality may also 'reset' the sensitivity of the kidneys to diuretic therapy.

While diuretics only provide symptomatic benefit, several medications have evidence of mortality benefit. These include:

- ACE inhibitors, or angiotensin receptor blockers if intolerant of ACE inhibtors, in patients with systolic dysfunction (ejection fraction ≤40%)
- Beta-blockers in patients with systolic dysfunction (ejection fraction ≤40%)
- Mineralocorticoid receptor antagonists (potassium-sparing diuretics) in patients with systolic dysfunction (ejection fraction ≤35%) and NYHA class II–IV symptoms
- Adding ivabradine, an inhibitor of the I_f ion channel highly expressed in the sinoatrial node, is indicated in patients in sinus rhythm over 70 beats per minute who remain in NYHA classes II–IV with an EF ≤35% and on optimal therapy.
- The combination of hydralazine and isosorbide dinitrate (ISDN) may be considered to reduce the risk of heart failure or hospitalisation in patients intolerant of ACE inhibitors or angiotensin receptor blockers. One study (A-HeFT) showed a mortality benefit of this combination specifically in African-Americans.

These medications must be prescribed initially at an introductory dose and then up-titrated to the maximum tolerated dose, bearing in mind side effects (especially renal dysfunction and hypotension). Trial data for mortality benefit is derived from up-titration of medication to optimal doses rather than remaining on the introductory dose. This is where an MDT approach, with input from a community heart failure nurse specialist, is key.

Other ongoing treatment considerations which should be recognised include:

- Anticoagulation in the presence of AF or apical thrombus
- Devices: cardiac resynchronisation therapy (CRT, also known as biventricular pacing), implantable cardiac defibrillators (ICDs, with or without CRT) (see *Infraclavicular mass*, p. 33)
- Referral to a specialist centre for transplantation assessment and bridges to transplantation (ventricular assist devices)

Further reading

Dickstein K, Cohen-Solal A, Filippatos G, et al. ESC Guidelines for the diagnosis and treatment of acute and chronic heart failure 2008: the task force for the diagnosis and treatment of acute and chronic heart failure 2008 of the European Society of Cardiology. Developed in collaboration with the Heart Failure Association of the ESC (HFA) and endorsed by the European Society of Intensive Care Medicine (ESICM). Eur Heart J 2008; 29:2388–2442.

Case 14: The infraclavicular mass – pacemakers and implantable devices

Instruction to the candidate

This 60-year-old man previously complained of dyspnoea and reduced exercise tolerance. Please examine his cardiovascular system.

Begin with a summary of positive findings

The key positive finding in this case is an infraclavicular subcutaneous mass, the differential diagnosis of which includes:

- A conventional bradycardia pacemaker (single or dual chamber)
- CRT-P: cardiac resynchronisation therapy with biventricular pacing only
- CRT-D: biventricular pacemaker and an incorporated defibrillator device
- ICD: implantable cardiac defibrillator

> ### Which device?
>
> Examine and describe the pacemaker as you would any other mass found on examination. The interpretation of your findings will be putting the type of device into the context of the other examination findings (e.g. with signs of heart failure).

Additional findings may include:

- Signs of heart failure (such as poor perfusion with cool and clammy peripheries, displaced apex beat, raised JVP, bibasal reduced air entry and crepitations, pitting peripheral oedema – see preceding *Cardiac failure*, p. 30)
- An abdominal subcutaneous mass in patients with evidence of previous cardiothoracic surgery (such as a midline sternotomy scar), indicating a surgically-implanted epicardial pacemaker
- A left parasternal subcutaneous mass with an approximate size of a USB memory stick: this is an implantable recording device that continuously monitors cardiac rhythm

Follow with a summary of relevant negative findings

Important negative findings to note in their absence and comment on if positive include:

- Stigmata of infective endocarditis
- Complications of device implantation, such as erythema indicative of infection, haematoma formation or protruding wires
- It is important to always check the contralateral infraclavicular region for scars from previous device implantations

State the most likely diagnosis on the basis of these findings

'This patient has signs consistent with congestive cardiac failure and a subcutaneously implanted cardiac device in the infraclavicular region, the differential of which includes a bradycardia pacemaker, CRT device with or without defibrillator, or a standalone ICD. He has increased right atrial pressure as evidenced by the raised JVP, and has peripheral fluid retention to the knees. I would like to take a full history to establish his symptomatic status and the nature of the implanted device.'

Offer relevant differential diagnoses

As stated in the list of positive findings, an implanted device can be one of the following:

- A bradycardia pacemaker
- CRT-P
- CRT-D
- ICD
- Implantable loop recorder

While the size of the device cannot tell you definitively which device has been implanted, implantable loop recorders are the size of a USB stick. CRT and ICD devices tend to be larger than standard bradycardia pacemakers.

Demonstrate the importance of clinical context – suggest relevant questions that would be taken in a patient history

The exact questions which would be asked in a clinical history would depend upon the type of device in situ. Inform the examiner that you would ask for general symptoms of arrhythmia such as palpitations, dizziness, pre-syncope and syncope.

Further to this, if an ICD or CRT-D is in situ, patients should be asked about any delivery of device therapies noticed by the patient, i.e. shocks.

For patients with CRT devices, it is important to consider symptoms of cardiac failure and categorise according to NYHA class. Patients with CRT will, by definition, have had severe left ventricular dysfunction, so assessing their symptom burden and its change since device insertion is important.

Demonstrate an understanding of the value of further investigation

In a patient with an implanted device, the necessary investigations will depend upon the clinical presentation of the patient. For example, if a patient with an implanted device (of any type) presents with symptoms and/or signs of infection it would be important to take serial blood cultures and inflammatory markers with the suspicion of device-related infection or device-related infective endocarditis.

General investigations will include:

- A 12-lead electrocardiogram. The QRS duration is important because CRT is only implanted in patients with a broad QRS, indicating ventricular dysynchrony. Pacing spikes vary in location (atrial or ventricular) and amplitude (depending upon the lead implanted–more prominent in unipolar rather than bipolar leads)
- A plain chest radiograph will allow assessment of the number and type of leads from a device. An ICD lead and the left ventricular lead of a CRT device both have a different radiological appearance when compared to a conventional pacing lead. Chest radiography helps visualise lead placement and integrity, including lead fracture. AP and lateral views are required to check position
- Echocardiography guides the indications for CRT and ICD implantation through the assessment of severely impaired LV ejection fraction ($\leq 35\%$). LV dyssynchrony assessment has no role in the indications for CRT-P. Furthermore, current evidence for echocardiography in CRT optimisation is uncertain and hence is not recommended as standard practice
- Device interrogation is used to look for arrhythmia (ventricular or atrial), delivery of ICD therapies (including anti-tachycardia pacing and defibrillation episodes, and whether therapies were inappropriate or appropriate) and satisfactory device parameters (such as battery life, lead sensitivities and impedance)

Always offer a management plan

It is sensible to start off discussion of management of patients with implantable devices by discussing the indications for device implantation. CRT and ICDs both have a plethora of proven mortality benefit upon which the NICE guidelines are based, summarised below.

ICDs

ICDs have indications in both primary and secondary prevention settings (primary prevention with ICDs in heart failure are covered in the CRT section below).

Primary prevention

- Individuals who have a familial cardiac condition with a high risk of sudden death
  - Hypertrophic cardiomyopathy
  - Long QT syndrome
  - Brugada syndrome
  - Arrythmogenic right ventricular dysplasia (ARVD)
- Patients who have undergone surgical repair of congenital heart disease

Secondary prevention

Patients with proven previous serious ventricular arrhythmia in the absence of a treatable cause:

- Survivors of cardiac arrest caused by VT or VF
- Spontaneous sustained VT causing haemodynamic instability and/or syncope
- Sustained VT (regardless of syncope or cardiac arrest) in the presence of severe left ventricular dysfunction (defined as an ejection fraction $\leq 35\%$) and with heart failure symptoms no worse than NYHA class III.

CRT-P and CRT-D

As a treatment option for patients with heart failure and severe underlying left ventricular systolic dysfunction (defined as an ejection fraction $\leq 35\%$), ICDs, CRT-P and CRT-D are indicated depending upon NYHA class, QRS duration, and the presence/absence of LBBB (**Table 1.8**).

In addition to discussing the indications for device insertion, it is important to consider the advice that a patient should be given regarding their device. For example, the patient will be given a pacemaker identification card to keep after their device implantation. This will give details of the device manufacturer and of the model of device (information that is required

Table 1.8 Implantable device treatment options for patients with severe LV dysfunction (ejection fraction ≤ 35%) stratified by NYHA class, QRS duration, and the presence/absence of LBBB (reproduced from NICE guideline TA314)				
QRS interval	NYHA class			
	I	II	III	IV
<120 ms	ICD if there is a high risk of sudden cardiac death			ICD and CRT not clinically indicated
120–149 ms without LBBB	ICD	ICD	ICD	CRT-P
120–149 ms with LBBB	ICD	CRT-D	CRT-P or CRT-D	CRT-P
≥150 ms with or without LBBB	CRT-D	CRT-D	CRT-P or CRT-D	CRT-P

to select the correct equipment for device interrogation).

Implantable devices are followed-up in pacing clinics in order to check parameters such as battery life, satisfactory function and arrhythmia burden (e.g. AF burden for dual-chamber pacing or arrhythmic events recorded by ICDs). Device optimisation is also performed on an outpatient basis in the case of CRT devices.

Any implantable device has implications for vehicle licence holders, and all patients who have undergone any form of pacing or ICD device implantation must inform the DVLA (**Table 1.9**).

Patients can download information leaflets regarding bradycardia pacing, CRT and ICD devices from the British Heart Foundation (BHF) website. These contain a wide range of information covering the indications for the device, how the device works, the implantation procedure and post-procedural care, and advice regarding daily living with a device.

Further reading

National Institute for Health and Care Excellence (NICE). TA314: Implantable cardioverter defibrillators and cardiac resynchronisation therapy for arrhythmias and heart failure (review of TA95 and TA120). NICE, June 2014.

Table 1.9 Driving guidelines for patients with pacemakers and ICDs		
	Car or motorcycle driving licence holders (UK Group 1)	Heavy goods vehicle or passenger-carrying vehicle driving licence holders (UK Group 2)
Pacemakers	Patients can resume driving one week after the pacemaker has been implanted provided that they inform the DVLA, they do not have any recurrence of bradycardia symptoms (such as syncope or dizziness), they do not have any other medical condition that might preclude them from driving (e.g. recent myocardial infarction), and they continue to have their device checked regularly by the pacemaker clinic	Patients can usually resume driving after 6 weeks provided they have informed the DVLA and subsequently received clearance from them following a review of their case
ICDs	Primary prevention ICD: can resume driving 1 month after implantation. Secondary prevention ICD: can resume driving 6 months after implantation. Appropriate ICD device therapy: – can resume driving after 6 months provided that a new treatment strategy (either anti-arrhythmic medication or ablation) has been successfully implemented, or – can resume driving after 24 months if no new treatment strategy is implemented.	Unable to hold this licence following ICD implantation

Case 15: The irregular pulse: atrial fibrillation

Instruction to the candidate

This 65-year-old man complains of palpitations and exertional dyspnoea. Please examine his cardiovascular system.

Begin with a summary of positive findings

Comment on the pulse rate and irregular rhythm, measured both radially by palpation and apically by auscultation. The pulse difference between the apical and radial rates is an indicator of the degree of rate control: the higher the difference between the two (termed the pulse deficit), the poorer the rate control.

Clinical examination may also help identify the aetiology of atrial fibrillation. Such findings may include:

- A midline sternotomy scar and graft harvest scars which would indicate bypass grafting for underlying ischaemic heart disease, and previous cardiac surgery as a possible cause of AF
- Signs of thyrotoxicosis such thyroid eye disease, goitre, pretibial myxoedema
- Hypertension can be identified by asking for the patient's blood pressure
- Findings consistent with mitral valve pathology, such as mitral facies, murmurs
- Inspect for a permanent pacemaker: 'tachy-brady' syndrome, requiring 'pace and block' treatment
- Peripheral stigmata of alcoholic liver disease

Follow with a summary of relevant negative findings

The important relevant negatives to comment on in cases of atrial fibrillation pertain to the complications of atrial fibrillation itself and to complications of anticoagulation:

- Complications of atrial fibrillation include:
  - Embolic complications such as stroke. Approximately 20% of strokes result from atrial fibrillation, conferring significant importance on instigating appropriate anticoagulation strategies
  - Haemodynamic compromise, e.g. in atrial fibrillation with fast ventricular response. Request the patient's blood pressure to exclude this
  - Left ventricular dysfunction may be an associated finding, an aetiological factor, or indeed a consequence of long-standing uncontrolled ventricular rate (known as 'tachycardiomyopathy')
- An important complication of anticoagulation is bleeding, the stigmata of which include bruising. Additionally, while signs of previous stroke in a patient with atrial fibrillation are most likely to be due to embolic phenomena, over-anticoagulation may also cause haemorrhagic strokes

State the most likely diagnosis on the basis of these findings

'This patient has rate-controlled atrial fibrillation, with possible aetiologies including hypertension and previous cardiothoracic surgery for ischaemic heart disease. He has signs of recent venipuncture, likely in order to check adequacy of anticoagulation. He does not have any features of embolic complications'.

Offer relevant differential diagnoses

The differential of an irregularly irregular pulse includes:

- Atrial fibrillation
- Atrial flutter or atrial tachycardia with variable block
- Sinus rhythm with frequent atrial or ventricular extrasystoles. This can be ruled out on exercise which would abolish extrasystoles
- Sinus arrhythmia may also manifest as an irregularly irregular pulse.

Demonstrate the importance of clinical context – suggest relevant questions that would be taken in a patient history

Questions would relate both to any history of underlying causes and to current symptoms.

Demonstrate an understanding of the value of further investigation

The 12-lead ECG is the most important tool in diagnosing the cause of an irregular pulse. It is best to obtain a rhythm strip to accurately assess the cardiac rhythm.

Other investigations would include:

- Laboratory blood tests: thyroid function tests as a possible underlying aetiology, and clotting studies to assess the adequacy of anticoagulation. Cardiac biomarkers (e.g. troponin) may be elevated, but differentiation between arrhythmia or underlying ischaemia as the aetiology require further clinical evaluation.
- A 24-hour Holter monitor allows review of the AF burden in cases of paroxysmal AF and to assess for the adequacy of rate control in cases of permanent AF
- Echocardiography is used to rule out any structural cardiac lesion (e.g. mitral regurgitation) and to assess left atrial size and left ventricular function
- If ischaemic heart disease is a possibility, the relevant stress test should be considered

Always offer a management plan

There are two separate, principle considerations in managing AF. The first is anticoagulation, which is the only demonstrable intervention that reduces cardiovascular mortality in AF. Anticoagulation should be instituted according to risk profile for embolic stroke (CHADS-VASc score for non-valvular AF) and weighed up against bleeding risk (HAS-BLED score). Neither the nature of the AF (paroxysmal, persistent or permanent) nor the AF burden in paroxysmal AF should influence the indication for anticoagulation: they should all be managed in the same way with respect to anticoagulation. A target INR of 2–3 is indicated when treated with warfarin.

> Novel strategies for thromboprophylaxis in AF
> - The novel oral anticoagulants (e.g. Dabigatran) are effective alternatives to warfarin that can be considered, but their place in current practice is influenced by local policy. Whilst these agents do not require blood test monitoring, it should be remembered that they also do not have specific antidotes for reversal.
> - Left atrial appendage occlusion devices (e.g. Watchman) are also recommended by NICE in specific circumstances of non-valvular AF in which anticoagulation is not tolerated.

The second consideration is whether to pursue a rate or rhythm control strategy. For the former strategy, there is no evidence that strict rate control is beneficial against lenient rate control. Medical therapy for rate control includes beta-blockers, rate-limiting calcium channel blockers and digoxin (the latter preferably used as an adjunctive agent rather than as a standalone medication). In cases whereby medical therapy fails to provide adequate rate control, AV node ablation with permanent pacemaker implantation can be considered.

With regard to rhythm control, many trials have demonstrated that there is no evidence that mortality is improved by pursuing this strategy (the largest being the AFFIRM trial in 2002, consisting of 4,060 patients: this trial did not demonstrate any difference between rate- and rhythm-control groups for the primary end-point of all-cause mortality). In general, rhythm control should be considered particularly for young patients, individuals who are physically active, and patients who remain symptomatic despite adequate rate control. Rhythm control may be achieved by either medication or pulmonary vein isolation (so-called 'AF ablation'). Both have side-effects and potential for complications, hence the guidance for opting for rhythm control in individuals in whom the symptomatic burden of AF outweighs these disadvantages of treatment. In the absence of structural heart disease, Flecainide (a class 1c anti-arrhythmic) can be used usually in combination with a beta-blocker. The latter agent is to avoid rapidly conducted atrial flutter which is a common by-product of Flecainide when used to treat AF. In cases of structural heart disease (e.g. adult congenital heart disease, LV impairment), Amiodarone is generally recommended.

The examiner will want to feel that they can trust you to safely run and manage their acute unselected medical take. AF is the commonest arrhythmia encountered in this setting, either as the primary diagnosis or as an incidental finding or co-morbidity. Therefore, an appropriate scheme should be adhered to in order to prioritise the key management aspects of AF in the acute medical patient:

- Is the patient haemodynamically compromised? If so, arrange emergency DC cardioversion. Otherwise, decide how this can be managed medically.
- Decide upon the anticoagulation treatment regime in the acute setting

- Choose the most appropriate pharmacological strategy for either rate control, or rhythm control if the onset is within 48 hours
- Treat underlying cause, most commonly infection in the acute setting

Following the acute management of the patient, go on to investigate underlying causes and decide upon long-term anticoagulation and rate/rhythm control strategies.

Further reading

Fuster V, Rydén LE, Cannom DS, et al. 2011 ACCF/ AHA/HRS focused updates incorporated into the ACC/AHA/ESC 2006 guidelines for the management of patients with atrial fibrillation: a report of the American College of Cardiology Foundation/American Heart Association Task Force on Practice Guidelines developed in partnership with the European Society of Cardiology and in collaboration with the European Heart Rhythm Association and the Heart Rhythm Society. J Am Coll Cardiol 2011; 57:e101–198.

Camm AJ, Kirchhof P, Lip GY, et al. Guidelines for the management of atrial fibrillation: the task force for the management of atrial fibrillation of the European Society of Cardiology (ESC). Eur Heart J 2010; 31:2369–2429.

Case 16: Coarctation of the aorta

Instruction to the candidate

This 30-year-old woman was found to be hypertensive when attending her GP for abdominal pains. Please examine her cardiovascular system.

Begin with a summary of positive findings

Relevant peripheral signs to seek to identify include:

- Simultaneous palpation of radial and femoral pulses reveals the characteristic radio-femoral delay. Indeed, delayed and diminished pulses distal to the coarctation with differential limb blood pressures are the characteristic features of this condition. Auscultatory features are supportive
- Upper body systolic hypertension and lower body systolic hypotension with a difference of greater than 20 mmHg in favour of the upper limb is significant. Also check blood pressure in both arms as the left subclavian artery can be either part of the coarctation itself, or used in repair of the defect.
- Visible, palpable large collateral arteries develop over the left scapula, left chest wall and anterior abdominal wall

- A thrill over the suprasternal notch may be palpated
- A heaving (pressure-loaded), undisplaced apex beat indicates left ventricular hypertrophy
- An underdeveloped left arm may represent a coarctation at the level of the left subclavian artery. There may also be underdevelopment of the lower limbs.
- Auscultatory features of aortic coarctation include:
- A systolic murmur, typically heard posteriorly in the left infrascapular region but can also be auscultated in the left infraclavicular region
- The continuous murmurs of collateral vessels can be heard bilaterally across the thorax
- An ejection click (with or without concomitant ejection systolic and early diastolic murmurs) of an associated bicuspid aortic valve

Follow with a summary of relevant negative findings

It would be prudent to mention the absence of clinical features consistent with Turner's syndrome, as at least 35% of these patients also have aortic coarctation.

State the most likely diagnosis on the basis of these findings

'This patient has signs consistent with a coarctation of the aorta associated with a bicuspid aortic valve and evidence of aortic regurgitation. I would like to take a full history to establish her symptomatic status and my investigations of choice would be an echocardiogram and a CT or MRI of the aorta in the first instance to confirm the diagnosis and to look for associated pathology.'

Offer relevant differential diagnoses

In addition to offering the differential diagnosis of a systolic murmur (see *Aortic stenosis,* p. 2) it is important to consider associated valvar conditions:

- Bicuspid aortic valve: up to 85% of patients with aortic coarctation also have a bicuspid aortic valve with or without associated stenosis or regurgitation
- Other cardiac defects include VSD, patent ductus arteriosus, aortic stenosis and mitral stenosis due to parachute mitral valve, and other left ventricular outflow tract obstructive lesions (which can be part of the Shone complex of left-sided obstructive lesions)

Note from the relevant negatives that Turner syndrome is a genetic condition associated with aortic coarctation so this should be mentioned with regard possible aetiologies.

Demonstrate the importance of clinical context – suggest relevant questions that would be taken in a patient history

Many adult patients are asymptomatic, being diagnosed following the finding of hypertension. Those patients who are symptomatic patients may complain of:

- Headache
- Nosebleeds
- Dyspnoea
- Leg claudication
- Abdominal angina
- Cold feet

Other disease associations include: ascending aorta aneurysms (complicated by rupture or dissection), berry aneurysms of the circle of Willis (complicated by intracranial haemorrhage)

and premature coronary and cerebral artery disease.

Demonstrate an understanding of the value of further investigation

Relevant investigations in the diagnostic work-up of cases of aortic coarctation include:

- A 12-lead electrocardiogram demonstrating left ventricular hypertrophy with or without an accompanying strain pattern
- A plain chest radiograph may demonstrate:
  - Rib notching on the inferior borders of the posterior ribs, which represents the development of collaterals arising from intercostal arteries
  - The coarctation can appear as an indentation in the proximal descending thoracic aorta, giving rise to the so-called 'figure of 3' sign
- Echocardiography is important in confirming the diagnosis of coarctation with measurement of the pressure gradient across the lesion which can be made by 2D echo, colour Doppler and continuous-wave Doppler. Aortic dimensions and left ventricular function and wall thickness are also assessed and associated cardiac lesions are ruled out
- Cardiac catheterisation can also be used to measure the pressure gradient across the coarctation.
- CT and MRI are appropriate imaging modalities. The narrowing of the aorta occurs most commonly just distal to the left subclavian artery. These imaging modalities allow visualisation and measurement of the aorta in its entirety, as well as demonstration of collateral vessels

Always offer a management plan

Patients with aortic coarctation should be considered for referral to a specialist adult congenital heart disease (ACHD) centre for life-long follow-up.

Hypertension persists despite coarctation repair and may be due to baroreceptor dysfunction. There is also loss of aortic compliance. This requires lifelong monitoring. Regular ambulatory BP monitoring and stress testing for exercise hypertension (SBP >220 mmHg), should be performed. Intervention for lone coarctation may be performed by stenting (method of choice) or surgically.

Later complications such as aneurysm formation and recoarctation can occur.

Associated cardiac (such as bicuspid aortic valve, aortic aneurysm) or neurological (such as circle of Willis berry aneurysms) features would favour a surgical approach.

Further reading

Deanfield J, Thaulow E, Warnes C, Webb G, et al. Management of grown up congenital heart disease. Eur Heart J 2003; 24:1035–1084.

Case 17: Infective endocarditis

Instruction to the candidate

This 50-year-old man presented with fevers and dyspnoea. Please examine his cardiovascular system.

> **Likely cases for the PACES exam**
>
> Patients with active endocarditis are unlikely to present as a case in PACES, but knowledge of the clinical signs, management, risk factors and guidance on prophylaxis is relevant to many other stations where the patient may be at increased risk of developing this complication.

Begin with a summary of positive findings

The key clinical findings are fever and a murmur. While the patient in the exam will unlikely have an active fever (see text box above), such clinical information has been given in the instruction to the candidate. Therefore, in the clinical examination, the presence of a murmur will be the key clinical finding. This may either be the substrate for infection (e.g. native valve disease with superimposed endocarditis) or indeed the consequence of infection (e.g. valvular destruction due to infection with consequent incompetence).

Additional clinical signs to seek include:

- Vascular phenomena. These include splinter haemorrhages (nailfold infarcts), Janeway lesions (painless macular or nodular haemorrhagic lesions on the palms or soles)
- Immunological phenomena, such as Osler's nodes (tender raised subcutaneous

lesions in the fingers), Roth's spots (retinal haemorrhages), glomerulonephritis (microscopic haematuria on urine dipstick)
- Other signs of a more established (historically termed 'subacute') infection include clubbing, splenomegaly and anaemia

It is important to consider right-sided valvular lesions particularly in patients with indwelling venous catheters or stigmata of intravenous drug use.

Follow with a summary of relevant negative findings

If absent, comment on risk factors for the development of infective endocarditis such as stigmata of intravenous drug abuse, indwelling venous catheters, poor dental hygiene, and clinical evidence of high-risk cardiac conditions.

Additionally, it is important to show a consideration of the possible complications of infective endocarditis by commenting on the absence of signs of heart failure and of evidence of systemic septic emboli, such as cerebral events. Remember that right-sided lesions tend to cause pulmonary septic emboli.

State the most likely diagnosis on the basis of these findings

'This patient who has a history of a febrile illness has examination findings consistent with mitral regurgitation. This lesion is either a substrate for or consequence of infective endocarditis. He is clinically euvolaemic, and has evidence of poor dentition. I would like to take a full history to establish his symptomatic status, and my initial investigations would include serial blood cultures, inflammatory markers and transthoracic echocardiography.'

Offer relevant differential diagnoses

Report to the examiner that you would consider the differential diagnosis of the likely causative organisms of infective endocarditis, which includes *Staphylococcus aureus*, which is the most common aetiological organism, followed by *Streptococcus viridans* and coagulase-negative *Staphylococci*. *Staphylococcus aureus* is typically associated with nosocomial acquisition due to instrumentation (e.g. venous or urinary catheters) or community intravenous drug use. *Streptococcus viridans* is the most frequent causative agent in community-acquired infective endocarditis, being part of the normal oral flora.

HACEK organisms also constitute part of the oral flora, and are associated with endocarditis in patients with poor dentition or intravenous drug users due to the contamination of hypodermic needles with saliva.

Culture-negative endocarditis requires serology for *Bartonella*, *Chlamydia psittaci* and *Coxiella*.

Fungal endocarditis is associated with immunocompromised states, intravenous drug use and indwelling venous catheters (particularly in patients receiving total parenteral nutrition).

Demonstrate the importance of clinical context – suggest relevant questions that would be taken in a patient history

It is important to elicit whether the patient has a pre-existing cardiac abnormality or pre-existing endocarditis increasing the risk of subsequent episodes.

Demonstrate an understanding of the value of further investigation

The investigative strategy in cases of infective endocarditis is aimed at meeting the diagnostic criteria for the condition. The key principles are of gaining microbiological evidence and echocardiographic evidence of the disease.

Investigations will include:

- Blood cultures: three separate sets of aerobic and anaerobic cultures
- Serology: for *Bartonella*, *Chlamydia psittaci* and *Coxiella*
- Regular 12-lead electrocardiograms are essential to look for a prolonging PR interval indicating atrioventricular node involvement in cases of aortic root abscesses
- Transthoracic echocardiography is the first-line imaging modality, followed by transoesophageal echocardiography in either positive transthoracic studies (to look for abscesses and more accurately assess vegetation dimensions) or negative studies following which the clinical suspicion of endocarditis remains high

---

Diagnostic criteria for infective endocarditis

The modified Duke criteria (2000) establish a diagnosis of infective endocarditis if 2 major criteria, 1 major and 3 minor, or 5 minor criteria are present.

The major criteria are:

- Typical serial positive blood cultures (the number of cultures depending upon the organism identified)
- Typical echocardiography features (including independently mobile valvular, subvalvular or device related mass or masses, new valvular regurgitation, prosthesis dehiscence or abscess formation)

The minor criteria are:

- Fever > 38°C
- Predisposing factor (such as valve prosthesis, native valve lesion, intravenous drug user)
- Evidence of vascular phenomena (e.g. splinter haemorrhages)
- Evidence of immunological phenomena (such as glomerulonephritis)
- Positive blood culture result or serological evidence of a causative organism that does not meet major criterion

---

Always offer a management plan

The initial management of cases of infective endocarditis is appropriate antimicrobial therapy. The specific antimicrobial drugs used and the duration of treatment depends upon the identity and sensitivities of the organism isolated and the case itself. Factors to consider when starting empirical treatment include:

- Taking 3 sets of blood cultures 30 minutes apart prior to commencing therapy
- The appropriate antimicrobials will differ between cases of native and prosthetic valve endocarditis
- Local guidance regarding specific antimicrobials will be influenced by the prevalence of antibiotic-resistant organisms

The indications for surgical management of infective endocarditis are:

- Heart failure due to severe valvular regurgitation or fistula formation
- Persistent, uncontrolled infection refractory to antimicrobials
- To prevent systemic embolism in appropriate cases

Prophylaxis against endocarditis

Guidance for prophylaxis against endocarditis is now stratified according to the presence of pre-existing cardiac lesions that are deemed high-risk for the development of endocarditis, coupled with the medical procedure or intervention taking place. Firstly, the following conditions are common to NICE, ESC and AHA guidelines in being classified as high-risk for the development of infective endocarditis:

- Prosthetic cardiac valve or prosthetic material used for cardiac valve repair
- Previous infective endocarditis
- Congenital heart disease:
  - Unrepaired cyanotic congenital heart disease
  - Completely repaired congenital heart defect with prosthetic material or device prior to endothelialisation (judged as during the first 6 months after the procedure)
  - Repaired congenital heart disease with residual defects at the site or adjacent to the site of a prosthetic patch or device

In addition, NICE also classify the following two conditions as high-risk:

- Acquired valvular heart disease (stenosis or regurgitation)
- Hypertrophic cardiomyopathy

The AHA also specify cardiac transplantation recipients who develop cardiac valvulopathy as a separate high-risk group.

NICE no longer advises routine prophylaxis for high-risk patients undergoing respiratory, gastrointestinal or genitourinary procedures.

Instead, the guidance focuses upon appropriate antimicrobial cover for high risk patients undergoing gastrointestinal or genitourinary procedures where there is suspected concomitant infection. Furthermore, the importance of good dental hygiene should be conveyed to the patient.

For prophylaxis with respect to dental procedures that involve manipulation of the gingival mucosa or the periapical region of teeth or perforation of the oral mucosa, the guideline bodies differ in their advice. NICE guidance does not routinely recommend antibiotic prophylaxis in this scenario, with the benefits and risks of prophylaxis explained to high-risk patients. ESC and AHA guidelines state that antibiotic prophylaxis should, however, be considered in high-risk patients for such dental procedures. The pragmatic approach is to consult with local guidance and protocols. NICE do state that the guidelines do not overrule individualised treatment decisions appropriate to the patient by the clinician.

Further reading

Wilson W, Taubert KA, Gewitz M, et al. Prevention of infective endocarditis: guidelines from the American Heart Association: a guideline from the American Heart Association Rheumatic Fever, Endocarditis, and Kawasaki Disease Committee, Council on Cardiovascular Disease in the Young, and the Council on Clinical Cardiology, Council on Cardiovascular Surgery and Anesthesia, and the Quality of Care and Outcomes Research Interdisciplinary Working Group. Circulation 2007; 116:1736–1754.

Nishimura RA, Carabello BA, Faxon DP, et al. ACC/AHA 2008 Guideline update on valvular heart disease: focused update on infective endocarditis: a report of the American College of Cardiology/American Heart Association Task Force on Practice Guidelines endorsed by the Society of Cardiovascular Anesthesiologists, Society for Cardiovascular Angiography and Interventions, and Society of Thoracic Surgeons. J Am Coll Cardiol 2008; 52:676–685.

Habib G, Hoen B, Tornos P, et al. Guidelines on the prevention, diagnosis, and treatment of infective endocarditis (new version 2009): the task force on the prevention, diagnosis, and treatment of infective endocarditis of the European Society of Cardiology (ESC). Endorsed by the European Society of Clinical Microbiology and Infectious Diseases (ESCMID) and the International Society of Chemotherapy (ISC) for Infection. Eur Heart J 2009; 30:2369–2413.

Case 18: Pulmonary hypertension

Instruction to the candidate

This 50-year-old woman complains of a one year history of progressive exertional dyspnoea. Please examine her cardiovascular system.

Begin with a summary of positive findings

Peripheral signs to be identified in cases of pulmonary hypertension include a raised JVP (quantify how high), with giant V waves if significant tricuspid regurgitation is present. A parasternal right ventricular heave may also be identified.

Auscultatory features of pulmonary hypertension include:

- A loud P2
- Paradoxical splitting of the second heart sound
- An early diastolic murmur of pulmonary regurgitation (Graham Steell murmur)

Follow with a summary of relevant negative findings

If absent, signs of right heart failure, such as peripheral oedema and ascites should be noted. Additional relevant negative findings include stigmata of anticoagulation. Look for tunnelled lines and infusion pumps indicative of parenteral prostacyclin analogues.

State the most likely diagnosis on the basis of these findings

'This woman has signs consistent with pulmonary arterial hypertension, likely secondary to systemic sclerosis. She has signs of right heart failure, and is receiving formal anticoagulation. I would like to take a full history to establish her symptomatic status, and my screening investigation of choice would be an echocardiogram followed by right heart catheter to confirm the diagnosis.'

Offer relevant differential diagnoses

The causes of pulmonary hypertension can be divided clinically according to the WHO classification (Table 1.10).

WHO group	Description	Features to look for at examination
	Table 1.10 WHO classification of causes of pulmonary hypertension	
1	Pulmonary arterial hypertension (PAH): – Idiopathic – Familial – Associated with other diseases: – Connective tissue disease – Porto-pulmonary – Congenital heart disease with pulmonary-systemic shunts – HIV – Drugs (e.g. anorexigens)	Stigmata of systemic sclerosis or SLE Stigmata of portal hypertension Signs of congenital heart disease with a shunt Evidence of previous intravenous drug use
2	Associated with left heart disease	Signs of left ventricular systolic dysfunction Signs of diastolic dysfunction (e.g. hypertrophic cardiomyopathy) Signs of valvular heart disease (e.g. MS or MR)
3	Associated with lung disease	Signs of: COPD Interstitial lung disease Sleep apnoea
4	Chronic thromboembolic disease	Previous DVTs
5	Miscellaneous	

SLE, systemic lupus erythematosus; MS, mitral stenosis; MR, mitral regurgitation; DVT, deep vein thrombosis; COPD, chronic obstructive pulmonary disease.

Demonstrate the importance of clinical context – suggest relevant questions that would be taken in a patient history

Report to the examiner that history questions would seek to quantify breathlessness in terms of functional class, and identify known causes of pulmonary hypertension. A history of palpitations should be questioned, as atrial tachyarrhythmias are poorly tolerated. Syncope is an ominous sign that merits urgent work-up.

Demonstrate an understanding of the value of further investigation

Investigations in cases of pulmonary hypertension would include:

- A 6-minute walk test. This has prognostic value and also can be used to assess response to treatment
- Laboratory blood tests would include measurements of natriuretic peptides (BNP or NT-proBNP) as markers of myocardial stretch and thus volume overload. Additional blood testing can identify an underlying cause, e.g. markers of autoimmune disease, and urate and haematinics to assess for iron depletion
- A 12-lead electrocardiogram may demonstrate:
  - Atrial arrhythmia, which can be poorly tolerated in PAH
  - Right atrial enlargement
  - Right axis deviation
  - Right ventricular hypertrophy
- On a plain chest radiograph, look for dilated central pulmonary arteries with peripheral vascular pruning and right ventricular enlargement
- Echocardiography provides estimates (but not diagnostic measures) of pulmonary artery systolic pressure and right atrial pressure. Echocardiography also provides information on right ventricular systolic function, the response of which to raised pulmonary pressures is the essential determinant of survival (over and above the pulmonary arterial pressure value itself). Any causative left heart disease (systolic, diastolic or valvular dysfunction) or congenital lesions, and any

associated pathology (such as pericardial fluid) can also be evaluated
- Cardiac catheterisation: right heart studies are the gold standard for diagnosis (mean pulmonary artery pressure >25 mmHg, and pulmonary capillary wedge pressure <15 mmHg) and monitoring of response to treatment. Right heart catheterisation is also used to assess vasoresponder status. This has prognostic significance and alters management (can be treated with calcium channel blockers)
- Bubble echocardiography, transoesophageal echocardiography and cardiac MRI: these imaging modalities can be used to look for causative structural lesions, particularly intracardiac shunts

Investigations directed at an underlying cause include an autoantibody screen and HIV test. Liver ultrasound should be requested if porto-pulmonary hypertension is suspected. Investigate pulmonary function using pulmonary function tests, high-resolution CT chest, CTPA or V/Q scans.

Always offer a management plan

This needs to be directed at the underlying cause (hence the WHO classification).

In pulmonary arterial hypertension (WHO Group 1), therapies include:

- Those aimed at pulmonary arterial pressures (oral, inhaled and intravenous therapies):
  - Endothelin receptor antagonists: e.g. bosentan
  - Phosphodiesterase type 5 inhibitors: e.g. sildenafil
  - Prostacyclin analogues (administered parenterally using a syringe pump via tunneled lines): e.g. treprostinil
  - Also calcium channel blockers for those responsive to vasodilator studies
- Warfarin is considered in selected patients to prevent pulmonary thromboembolic disease
- Treating symptoms of right heart failure with diuretics and long term oxygen therapy where appropriate.

For WHO Group 4, pulmonary thromboendarterectomy is highly successful in appropriate patients (depending upon the suitability of the disease and the patient for surgery).

Lung transplantation should be considered in selected patients.

Further reading

Galiè N, Hoeper MM, Humbert M, et al. Guidelines for the diagnosis and treatment of pulmonary hypertension: the task force for the diagnosis and treatment of pulmonary hypertension of the European Society of Cardiology (ESC) and the European Respiratory Society (ERS), endorsed by the International Society of Heart and Lung Transplantation (ISHLT). Eur Heart J 2009; 30:2493–2537.

Case 19: Atrial septal defect

Instruction to the candidate

This 55-year-old woman presents with increasing exertional dyspnoea. Please examine her cardiovascular system.

Begin with a summary of positive findings

Seek to identify peripheral findings, auscultatory features and signs of severity:

- Peripheral signs include cyanosis if Eisenmenger's syndrome. The pulse may be sinus rhythm, AF or atrial flutter.
- Auscultatory features include a fixed split second heart sound (meaning that it does not vary with respiration). A systolic pulmonary flow murmur may also be present.
- Signs of severity include:
  - Right heart failure and arrhythmias
  - Severe pulmonary hypertension
  - Eisenmenger's syndrome

Follow with a summary of relevant negative findings

If negative, comment on the absence of:

- Arrhythmia (check for stigmata of anticoagulation)
- Signs of pulmonary hypertension
- Evidence of signs of stroke which would indicate cerebral (paradoxical) embolism from a right-to-left shunt
- Concomitant valvular heart disease. Associated lesions include all complex congenital heart disease, or isolated lesions such as pulmonary stenosis, mitral valve prolapse and aortic regurgitation in primum ASDs

- Associated hand findings: patients with Holt–Oram syndrome have upper limb abnormalities associated with secundum ASDs

State the most likely diagnosis on the basis of these findings

'This patient has signs consistent with an atrial septal defect, most commonly due to a secundum ASD. She is in rate-controlled atrial fibrillation and has no evidence of pulmonary hypertension. I would like to take a full history to establish her symptomatic status, and my investigation of choice would be an echocardiogram in the first instance to confirm the diagnosis and to quantitate the degree of shunting and estimate pulmonary arterial pressures.'

Offer relevant differential diagnoses

This anatomical nature of atrial septal defects can be divided as follows:

- Secundum: 80% of ASDs
- Primum: 15% of ASDs
- Sinus venosus: 5% of ASDs
- Unroofed coronary sinus: <1% of ASDs

Demonstrate the importance of clinical context – suggest relevant questions that would be taken in a patient history

It is worth noting that many patients are asymptomatic until after their fourth decade, beyond which symptoms may include exertional dyspnoea and palpitations. Peripheral oedema is present if right heart failure develops, although this tends to be a later presentation.

Demonstrate an understanding of the value of further investigation

Investigations in cases of atrial septal defect include:

- A 12-lead electrocardiogram which would demonstrate incomplete right bundle branch block or RSR, pattern in lead V1 alone. The axis is different depending on the anatomical nature of the lesion. There is right axis deviation in secundum lesions, while there is left axis deviation in primum defects
- A plain chest radiograph demonstrates increased pulmonary vascular markings , dilated pulmonary arteries and cardiomegaly if there is heart failure
- Echocardiography (transthoracic and transoesophageal) will provide:
  - Diagnosis, anatomical localisation and shunt quantification
  - Estimation of pulmonary arterial systolic pressure
  - Estimate of right ventricular size and function
  - Transoesophageal echocardiography allows visualisation of sinus venosus defects and anomalous pulmonary venous drainage, and improved characterisation of the ASD in terms of anatomical suitability for percutaneous device closure
- Cardiac catheterisation is indicated to determine pulmonary arterial pressures and PVR, and to determine shunt quantification from sequential blood oxygen saturations
- Cardiac MRI can provide further structural information, especially in more complex congenital lesions

Always offer a management plan

Patients should be referred to a specialist ACHD centre for follow-up (pre- and post-closure).

Closure of the ASD may be performed percutaneously (method of choice for secundum ASD) or surgically. ASD closure is recommended if the shunt ratio is greater than 1.5:1. Patient suitability for closure depends upon assessment of biventricular function and pulmonary arterial pressures. Closure is contraindicated in patients who have developed Eisenmenger's syndrome. Suitability for device closure depends upon anatomical considerations (e.g. suitable defect rims) on transoesophageal echocardiogram.

Antibiotic prophylaxis following device closure or in cyanotic patients: see *Infective endocarditis* (p. 40).

Atrial arrhythmias (fibrillation, flutter or tachycardia) can be ablated either prior to percutaneous closure or at the time of surgical closure.

Patients with AF should receive formal anticoagulation.

Further reading

Deanfield J, Thaulow E, Warnes C, et al. Management of grown up congenital heart disease. Eur Heart J 2003; 24:1035–1084.

Basson CT, Cowley GS, Solomon SD, et al. The clinical and genetic spectrum of the Holt-Oram syndrome (heart-hand syndrome). N Engl J Med 1994; 330:885–891.

Case 20: Patent ductus arteriosus

Instruction to the candidate

This 40-year-old man had an incidental murmur detected on an insurance medical. Please examine his cardiovascular system.

Clinical context for the PACES exam

In the adult patient, PDA is usually an isolated finding as associated congenital lesions predominate in the paediatric population.

Begin with a summary of positive findings

Seek to identify peripheral findings and auscultatory features to make a diagnosis, with additional clinical features to comment on severity:

Peripheral signs include:

- Differential cyanosis if the patient has Eisenmenger's syndrome. In such cases, the lower limbs are cyanosed whereas the upper

limbs are not. There will be toe clubbing, but not finger
- Differential peripheral oxygen saturations in the hands and feet if Eisenmenger's syndrome is present. Comment to the examiner that you would request pulse oximetry measurements to be taken from the fingers and toes
- Evidence of left ventricular failure

The key auscultatory feature is a continuous machinery murmur heard in the infraclavicular or infrascapular region.

The clinical presentation is related to the size of the PDA:

- Small PDA: no left ventricular volume overload, normal pulmonary artery pressures
- Moderate PDA with either predominant:
  - Left ventricular volume overload: left ventricular dilatation with or without impaired systolic function
  - Right ventricular pressure overload: pulmonary hypertension with ensuing right heart failure
- Large PDA: Eisenmenger's syndrome. The murmur disappears with Eisenmenger's syndrome, and hence differential cyanosis is the key clinical finding in this situation

Follow with a summary of relevant negative findings

It is important to comment on the absence of signs of pulmonary hypertension and left ventricular dysfunction.

State the most likely diagnosis on the basis of these findings

'This patient has signs consistent with a small patent ductus arteriosus. There are no features of left or right ventricular dysfunction, or pulmonary hypertension. I would like to take a full history to establish his symptomatic status, and my investigation of choice would be an echocardiogram in the first instance to confirm the diagnosis and to confirm the absence of left or right heart involvement and estimate pulmonary arterial pressures.'

Demonstrate the importance of clinical context – suggest relevant questions that would be taken in a patient history

History questions would be aimed at identifying symptoms of either pulmonary hypertension or left ventricular dysfunction.

Demonstrate an understanding of the value of further investigation

Investigations in cases of PDAs include:

- The results of a 12-lead electrocardiogram and plain chest radiograph relate to the complications of the PDA. A normal ECG and CXR would be expected with a small PDA with no cardiac sequelae. Right ventricular hypertrophy and prominent pulmonary vessels could be evident with shunts causing pulmonary hypertension. Cardiomegaly and pulmonary congestion may be evident with PDAs that have given rise to left heart failure
- Echocardiography (transthoracic or transoesophageal) provides useful information including:
  - Diagnosis, anatomical localisation and shunt quantification
  - Estimation of pulmonary arterial systolic pressure
  - Measurement of biventricular size and systolic function
- Cardiac catheterisation allows quantification of shunt and determination of pulmonary artery pressure and pulmonary vascular resistance
- Cardiac MRI provides further structural information, identification of complex congenital heart disease and ventricular function quantification

Always offer a management plan

Patients should be referred to a specialist ACHD centre for follow-up (pre- and post-closure).

Embolisation of the PDA may be performed percutaneously (method of choice for PDA with a device or coil) or surgically (for anatomically unsuitable or large PDAs not amenable to device closure). Closure is contraindicated at the extremes of the symptomatology spectrum, namely patients who have developed Eisenmenger's syndrome, or asymptomatic patients with small, haemodynamically insignificant lesions with no clinical evidence of shunt on examination.

Asymptomatic patients with clinical evidence of a PDA, signs of left ventricular volume overload or pulmonary hypertension should all be considered for closure. According to NICE guidelines, antibiotic prophylaxis is not routinely recommended unless cyanosis is present.

Further reading

Deanfield J, Thaulow E, Warnes C, et al. Management of grown up congenital heart disease. Eur Heart J. 2003; 24:1035–1084.

Case 21: Ebstein's anomaly: the cyanosed patient with a murmur

Instruction to the candidate

This 25-year-old man complains of exertional dyspnoea, ankle swelling and palpitations. Please examine his cardiovascular system.

Begin with a summary of positive findings

Patients can have a variety of symptoms and signs depending upon the severity of Ebstein's abnormality. Physical findings therefore can range dramatically from the well-saturated adult with a murmur of mild tricuspid regurgitation to the adolescent with severe right heart failure, arrhythmia and cyanosis.

Peripheral signs include features of right heart failure and those related to associated arrhythmia:

- Comment on cyanosis or clubbing, and request peripheral oxygen saturations. Cyanosis is indicative of a right-to-left shunt at the atrial or, less commonly, ventricular level and should trigger the candidate to look for signs of an atrial or ventricular septal defect
- Signs of right heart failure: the JVP will be raised with giant 'v' waves of TR; ascites and peripheral oedema will be present
- Arrhythmia: The patient could be tachycardic with either a regular or irregular rhythm if there is coexisting supraventricular tachycardia or AF respectively. Pre-excitation is associated with Ebstein's anomaly. Look for stigmata of anticoagulation therapy

Auscultatory features of Ebstein's' anomaly include

- The first heart sound will be split owing to late closure of the tricuspid valve. A pansystolic murmur of tricuspid regurgitation is heard maximally at the lower left sternal edge on inspiration
- A third heart sound is heard in the presence of right heart failure

Follow with a summary of relevant negative findings

The absence of a right ventricular heave in the presence of right heart failure is an important sign alluding to the diagnosis. Patients may have had corrective surgery so look for a midline sternotomy scar.

Comment on the absence of a neurological deficit. Paradoxical embolic phenomena are present if there is right-to-left shunting at the atrial level

Pathophysiology

This is a congenital malformation of the tricuspid valve with failure in the undermining process of the valve leaflets and chordae so they fail to reach the atrioventricular junction. This results in apical displacement of the tricuspid valve and atrialisation of the right ventricle. The anterior tricuspid leaflet often billows out like a sail, causing regurgitation of the valve

The most frequently associated anomalies include secundum ASD or patent foramen ovale with interatrial shunting, and accessory pathways such as Wolff–Parkinson–White syndrome. Other associated congenital abnormalities include VSD, PS, pulmonary atresia, tetralogy of Fallot, coarctation of the aorta, and disorders of the mitral valve

State the most likely diagnosis on the basis of these findings

'This young adult has features of right heart failure that include cyanosis, a raised JVP, a murmur of tricuspid regurgitation and ankle swelling. There is absence of a right ventricular heave. These findings are consistent with Ebstein's Anomaly with a right-to-left shunt. He has signs of venepuncture indicating that he is anticoagulated, probably for a supraventricular tachycardia such as atrial flutter.'

Offer relevant differential diagnoses

The two key differential diagnoses for Ebstein's anomaly are tricuspid atresia and tricuspid regurgitation.

Demonstrate the importance of clinical context – suggest relevant questions that would be taken in a patient history

Relevant questions would be those aimed at identifying symptoms of cyanosis and of right heart failure.

Demonstrate an understanding of the value of further investigation

The relevant investigations and the appropriate findings include:

On a 12-lead electrocardiogram one-third of patients have supraventricular tachycardia or atrial flutter, and many have accessory pathways leading to ventricular arrhythmia being a cause of death. Ebstein's anomaly is commonly associated with Wolff–Parkinson–White syndrome. Check for pre-excitation (e.g. delta waves) and right bundle branch block. P pulmonale, demonstrated by tall, peaked P waves may be observed indicating an enlarged right atrium. Notching within the RBBB is commonly associated with Ebstein's.

On a plain chest radiograph there is often gross cardiomegaly due to right atrial dilatation.

An echocardiogram will demonstrate the degree of valve malformation, degree of regurgitation, severity of right ventricular dysfunction and cavity loss. Additional congenital defects and the direction of shunting at atrial level (if a defect is present) can also be demonstrated.

Assessment of functional capacity, by CPEX for example, is important for symptom quantitation, degree of desaturation on exercise, arrhythmia provocation, and may guide interventional decision making.

Cardiac MRI is recommended to assess the valve leaflets and right heart volumes and function in more detail. The degree of shunting can also be determined.

Cardiac catheterisation is used infrequently, but a pressure study may be useful preoperatively.

Always offer a management plan

Treatment depends on the severity of the disease and associated structural or electrical defects. Specialist and multi-disciplinary team management is essential. It is important to realise that these patients can have very complex congenital heart disease and need to be assessed lifelong in a specialist ACHD centre. A multidisciplinary approach is essential as often the patient is a young adult with cyanosis and may require advice on pregnancy, contraception and genetic counselling. Other specialties such as electrophysiology are vital to the management of complex arrhythmia and structural defects.

Medical management includes diuretics and ACE inhibitors. Rate controlling agents such as beta-blockers, calcium channel blockers and digoxin are used to control tachycardia. Anticoagulation is indicated for atrial flutter.

Interventional techniques include electrophysiology studies and ablation of accessory pathways or arrhythmogenic substrate.

Surgical options in Ebstein's anomaly include:

- Repair of the tricuspid valve is more favourable than replacement. The Cone repair is the more contemporary method to reduce the degree of tricuspid regurgitation.
- Atrial reduction surgery
- Palliative creation of atrial shunt
- MAZE procedure for tachyarrhythmias
- Cardiac transplantation

Further reading

Deanfield J, Thaulow E, Warnes C, et al. Management of grown up congenital heart disease. Eur Heart J 2003; 24:1035–1084.

Case 22: Tetralogy of Fallot

Instruction to the candidate

Examine this 30-year-old man's cardiovascular system. He had repair of a congenital defect and now complains of palpitations and syncope.

Begin with a summary of positive findings

The four features of tetralogy of Fallot are:

- Right ventricular outflow tract obstruction
- Ventricular septal defect
- Aortic dextroposition
- Right ventricular hypertrophy

Morphologically, there is anterocephalad deviation of the interventricular septum that determines the degree of right ventricular outflow tract obstruction and the degree of cyanosis. Mild cases are described as 'pink Fallots'. Severe cases are cyanosed and classically 'squat' to increase their preload and subsequently cardiac output. Almost all Fallot lesions are repaired with transannular patch and pulmonary valvotomy in infancy. In the case of severe cyanosis, a neonate may undergo modified Blalock–Thomas–Taussig shunt to augment pulmonary blood flow via a thoracotomy. In adulthood it is therefore likely that the radial pulse will be weak. The major adverse sequela in adulthood is pulmonary regurgitation. This results in right ventricular dilatation and dysfunction. Additionally arrhythmias are the most common presentation in adulthood. Ventricular and atrial tachycardia are often poorly tolerated.

In keeping with the above features, the key clinical findings are:

- Atrial fibrillation or other tachyarrhythmia
- Raised JVP
- Right ventricular heave
- Infraclavicular mass, likely to be an ICD
- Auscultatory features include:
  - Decrescendo diastolic murmur at the upper left sternal edge, louder on squatting or inspiration and softer by Valsalva or expiration
  - A third heart sound may be heard in the presence of right ventricular hypertrophy or failure, and is louder on inspiration

The signs present on examination depend on what management, if any, the patient has undergone. If unrepaired (rare) the patient will demonstrate clubbing and cyanosis. The patient may have a midline sternotomy from a previous repair. If the patient has had a Blalock–Thomas–Taussig shunt performed, they will have an absent radial pulse.

Follow with a summary of relevant negative findings

Important signs to comment on in their absence, or include as positive findings if present, include:

- Stigmata of anticoagulation
- Stigmata of infective endocarditis. Look for peripheral stigmata, ask the examiner for the temperature and a urine dipstick (looking for microscopic haematuria), and comment on dental hygiene and the presence or absence of indwelling intravenous access
- Signs of right heart failure: The JVP will be raised, ascites and peripheral oedema will be palpated
- Ensure you have requested the patient's blood pressure, as associated aortopathy can lead to root dilation and regurgitation
- Features of Di George syndrome, with which tetratology of Fallot is associated

State the most likely diagnosis on the basis of these findings

'This man with a previous sternotomy and absent right radial pulse has had cardiac surgery for congenital heart disease. He has a right ventricular heave and a soft diastolic murmur consistent with pulmonary regurgitation. He is likely to have had repair of tetralogy of Fallot and now has right ventricular dysfunction. Given his symptom of palpitations, he needs to be assessed further for pulmonary valve replacement.'

Offer relevant differential diagnoses

The key differential diagnoses are pulmonary regurgitation, right heart failure and infective endocarditis.

Demonstrate the importance of clinical context – suggest relevant questions that would be taken in a patient history

Appropriate questions in a clinical history would include the age at diagnosis and intervention (including what type of procedure the patient had). Additionally, ask about current symptoms of cyanosis and breathlessness.

Demonstrate an understanding of the value of further investigation

Important investigations and the relevant results in cases of tetralogy of Fallot include:

- A 12-lead electrocardiogram to assess rhythm and for evidence of right ventricular hypertrophy. It is important to measure the QRS duration, as a duration greater than 180 ms is strongly related to a poorer prognosis and is an indication for ICD implantation
- Regular ambulatory Holter monitoring to assess arrhythmia burden
- Cardiopulmonary exercise testing. Serial measurements of VO_2max are useful for functional capacity and also may reveal ventricular arrhythmias and exertional desaturation
- Echocardiography allows quantification of pulmonary regurgitation and right ventricular function. The aortic root size should be measured as aortopathy results in dilatation and possibly regurgitation
- Cardiac MRI. Imaging of the right ventricle and measurement of volume and function is paramount in determining the timing for pulmonary valve replacement. Cardiac MRI is currently the gold standard tool for determination of right ventricular size and systolic function. This modality is also very useful for identification of complex

congenital heart disease. The aorta can also be monitored

Always offer a management plan

The main issues in management of tetralogy of Fallot are:

- Timing of pulmonary valve replacement, the choices including surgical bioprosthesis or percutaneous valve implantation (usually Melody or Edwards valves)
- Arrhythmia management, including medical and interventional approaches with input from electrophysiologists
- Branch pulmonary artery stenosis can be managed by surgical reconstruction
- Aortopathy and aortic root dilatation with or without valve regurgitation requires surgical root replacement
- Coronary artery disease should be evaluated and treated surgically at the time of surgery

Other considerations include:

- Assessment and follow-up should be conducted in a specialist ACHD centre
- Pregnancy is usually well tolerated but specialist care needs to be sought. There is an increased risk of cardiac defects in offspring of approximately 3%
- Assessment of the patient's condition is required prior to undertaking competitive sports

Further reading

Deanfield J, Thaulow E, Warnes C, et al. Management of grown up congenital heart disease. Eur Heart J 2003; 24:1035–1084.

Case 23: Eisenmenger's syndrome

Instruction to the candidate

This 33-year-old man complains of severely reduced exercise capacity, dizziness, breathlessness and palpitations. Please examine her cardiovascular system.

Begin with a summary of positive findings

Features of pulmonary hypertension predominate. These include:

- Central cyanosis
- Clubbing
- Plethora
- Scars: especially sternotomies and thoracotomies
- Pulse: may be absent if a subclavian artery was used to create a Blalock–Thomas–Taussig shunt.
- Raised JVP
- Right sided parasternal heave
- Loud S2 and P2 component
- Shunt murmurs and differential cyanosis. If shunt reversal occurs in the presence of a patent ductus arteriosus there will be differential cyanosis with marked clubbing and cyanosis in the feet and normal hands. The shunt usually occurs after the arm vessels branch off the aorta. This is easily demonstrated by checking the saturations in the hands and the feet, and emphasizes the importance of exposing feet fully. In the presence of unrepaired transposition of the great arteries with a patent ductus arteriosus, the differential cyanosis will be reversed. Shunt murmurs may become quieter and eventually inaudible as the pulmonary vascular resistance increases and the shunt reverses.

Other signs, categorised by system affected, include:

- Respiratory: breathlessness and tachypnoea
- Haematological: bruises, bleeding, conjunctival suffusion
- Abdominal: hepatosplenomegaly and jaundice
- Musculoskeletal: muscle wasting and gouty deposits
- Skin: plethoric facies. Venous changes especially in the lower limb
- Genetic abnormalities such as Down's syndrome

Aetiology

Uncorrected congenital shunts and palliative procedures with left-to-right shunt lead to Eisenmenger's syndrome. Initially there is an increase in pulmonary blood flow, but this subsequently leads to increased pulmonary vascular resistance and pulmonary hypertension. Ultimately this results in reversal of the shunt and cyanosis.
Common lesions include:
- Unrestricted VSDs
- Unrestricted ASDs
- Unrestricted PDAs
- Palliative surgical lesions such as Pott's, Waterston and Blalock–Thomas–Taussig shunts

Exercise capacity is reduced, as oxygen uptake cannot be increased through the pulmonary bed. There is also systemic vasodilation and this can lead to syncope, which is usually a poor prognostic symptom.

Long term prognosis can be variable. Eisenmenger's with simple lesions such as ASD can survive to the sixth decade. However, if pulmonary vascular resistance continues to increase rapidly and the right ventricle fails, the prognosis is poor. Multisystem comorbidities are common. Hypoxaemia, bleeding, sepsis (in particular cerebral abscesses) and arrhythmia contribute to the cause of death.

Follow with a summary of relevant negative findings

If no signs of intervention are present, this is important to note as a negative finding.

State the most likely diagnosis on the basis of these findings

'This patient with Down's syndrome has Eisenmenger's syndrome. The right radial pulse is absent and suggests the subclavian artery was used to create a Blalock–Thomas–Taussig shunt for pulmonary blood flow augmentation in lesions such as tetralogy of Fallot, for example. There are established features of pulmonary hypertension, cyanosis and haematological involvement with multiple bruises and plethora.'

Offer relevant differential diagnoses

The most relevant differential diagnoses are pulmonary hypertension and tetralogy of Fallot.

Demonstrate the importance of clinical context – suggest relevant questions that would be taken in a patient history

History questions would be aimed at identifying a history of intervention and current and past symptom burden, such as those of hyperviscosity.

Demonstrate an understanding of the value of further investigation

Important investigations and the likely results include:

- Laboratory blood tests:
  - Full blood count: for secondary erythrocytosis. Expect high haemoglobin. This does not need to be corrected with venesection unless the patient complains of hyperviscosity symptoms (usually occur with haematocrits >65%)
  - Iron studies: most patients are iron deficient and require replacement either orally or intravenously
  - Bleeding time is increased due to platelet dysfunction and thrombocytopaenia.
  - Liver function tests: check conjugated bilirubin
  - Natriuretic peptides (e.g. BNP or NT-pro BNP) for heart failure
  - Urate, as gout is common due to high cell turnover
- A 12-lead electrocardiogram may demonstrate right bundle branch block, right ventricular hypertrophy and/or right axis deviation
- A plain chest radiograph would be expected to show enlarged pulmonary vessels and an enlarged right heart
- Findings on echocardiogram would include:
  - Assessment of intracardiac congenital lesions and the degree and direction of shunting
  - Right ventricular function (a poor prognosis in context of failure)
  - Estimation of pulmonary artery pressure
- Cardiac catheterisation is useful to assess right heart pressures and to provide an assessment of the degree of shunting

Always offer a management plan

Inform the examiner that you would focus on patient education and a multidisciplinary approach.

Secondary erythrocytosis and both thrombotic and bleeding tendencies are the main points to discuss here. Patients are no longer venesected for erythrocytosis as this has shown to render them iron deficient, unless there are severe symptoms of hyperviscosity. Remaining well hydrated is paramount to their care and can avoid thrombus formation. Therefore intravenous fluids should be administered with a line filter to eliminate air in the presence of dehydration.

Options in medical therapy include:

- Oxygen: supplementary nocturnal oxygen may help symptoms but has no effect on outcome.

Supplemental oxygen may be required when travelling by commercial airlines
- Epoprostanil (prostacyclin analogue): A continuous intravenous infusion via central access. This has shown to improve symptoms and oxygenation from 65–85%. It can also reduce pulmonary vascular resistance and improve cardiac index
- Bosentan (endothelin receptor agonist): Improves NYHA class and 6 minute walk test. The BREATH-5 study showed safety in Eisenmenger population and improvement in WHO class and reduction in pulmonary artery pressure
- Sildenafil (phosphodiesterase inhibitor): Improves functional class and symptoms with a reduction in pulmonary pressures

Other considerations include:

- Anticoagulation. Although thrombus formation is common, anticoagulation needs to be carefully considered in the context of platelet dysfunction and bleeding tendency
- Contraception. The risk of fetal death is 25% and maternal mortality from pregnancy is 50%. Saturations less than 85% fare a worse outcome. Progesterone only contraception should be used either orally or with an intrauterine device (IUD).
- Specialist review and follow-up. The examiner will want to know that you appreciate that these are complicated patients and require ACHD and specialist pulmonary hypertension input. Their follow up should be 3–6 monthly in a specialist centre. Patients also need education to ensure their wellbeing. Patients should avoid:
  - Sudden fluid shifts, such as dehydration
  - Hot conditions that may promote vasodilation and syncope
  - Competitive sport and isometric exercise
  - Pregnancy
  - Poor oral hygiene as endocarditis is common and prophylactic antibiotics should be administered
  - Non-cardiac surgery without close cardiac input

Further reading

Deanfield J, Thaulow E, Warnes C, et al. Management of grown up congenital heart disease. Eur Heart J 2003; 24:1035–1084.

Case 24: Dextrocardia

Instruction to the candidate

This 50-year-old woman was referred by her GP after an incidental finding on cardiovascular examination. Please examine her and report your findings to the examiner.

> ### Understanding terminology in dextrocardia
>
> Demonstrate to the examiner that you understand the difference between:
> - Dextrocardia: the heart is in the right hemithorax with the base-apex axis pointing rightward and caudad
> - Dextroposition: the heart is displaced to the right hemithorax (e.g. with a diaphragmatic hernia) but the apex still points to the left
> - Levocardia: the heart is in the left hemithorax with the apex pointing leftward
> - Mesocardia: the heart is in the middle of the chest with the apex pointing leftward
> - Situs inversus: dextrocardia, trilobar left lung, bilobar right lung, right-sided stomach, left-sided liver, right-sided descending colon

Begin with a summary of positive findings

The key clinical finding is a right sided apex beat in the fifth intercostal space. The heart sounds are better heard on the right side than the left side of the chest, and are commonly normal.

Follow with a summary of relevant negative findings

It is important to comment on clear lung fields without crepitation. If present this may be suggestive of ciliary dysmotility which is present in Kartagener's syndrome. Ensure there are no stigmata of Turner's syndrome.

State the most likely diagnosis on the basis of these findings

'This patient has dextrocardia and is clinically well. I would like to examine the abdomen for situs inversus and my investigation of choice would be a chest radiograph to confirm my diagnosis.'

Offer relevant differential diagnoses

Dextrocardia is associated with:

- Kartagener's syndrome, comprising bronchiectasis, sinusitis and infertility (50% have situs inversus)
- Turner's syndrome
- Asplenia

Demonstrate the importance of clinical context – suggest relevant questions that would be taken in a patient history

In the absence of disease associations, the patient with dextrocardia is likely to be asymptomatic.

Demonstrate an understanding of the value of further investigation

Relevant investigations would comprise:

- A 12-lead electrocardiogram demonstrating mirror-imaged electrical activity, with P, QRS, and T waves in leads I, aVR, aVL that are reversed
- A plain chest radiograph will demonstrate the heart in the right hemithorax with the apex pointing to the right. Check the horizontal fissure of the right lobe and check sidedness of the gastric bubble. The descending aorta position will be reversed

Always offer a management plan

Dextrocardia in itself requires no specific management.

Chapter 2

Nervous system (station 3)

Case 25: Monocular blindness

Instruction to the candidate

This 64-year-old woman has been referred by her optometrist for urgent review. Please examine her visual fields and report your findings to the examiner.

Begin with a summary of positive findings

There is complete unilateral loss of vision affecting the right eye. The visual fields of the left eye are intact with no apparent deficit.

Additional examination findings, narrowing the level of the deficit:

- Relative afferent pupillary defect (RAPD) – the most useful additional finding in this situation. RAPD supports unilateral blindness secondary to pathology affecting the lens, retina, or optic nerve anterior to the optic chiasm
- Red reflex – where absent would suggest opacity of the visual axis
- Fundoscopy assessing for pale or swollen optic disc indicative of ischaemia

Follow with a summary of relevant negative findings

Pupillary responses, red reflex, and optic discs would be mentioned as important negative findings if they are examined and found to be normal.

State the most likely diagnosis on the basis of these findings

'This patient has monocular blindness. In the absence of lens pathology and the presence of a relative afferent pupillary defect monocular blindness is indicative of a CNS lesion anterior to the optic chiasm.'

Offer relevant differential diagnoses

A monocular field defect will always be due to disease anterior to the optic chiasm, before the nerve fibres cross. In order to confidently attribute monocular blindness to a CNS lesion, pathology of the lens, vitreous or retina must be excluded. Thus, the differential becomes:

If visual axis opacity (absent or poor red reflex) is present:

- Corneal opacity – traumatic (scarring, infection), corneal dystrophy
- Lens opacity – dense cataract

Vitreous opacity:

- Haemorrhage
- Inflammation
- Infection

If RAPD present:

- Inflammatory demyelination
- Central retinal artery occlusion
- Ischaemic optic neuropathy (anterior/posterior)
- Retinal detachment
- Advanced glaucoma
- Traumatic optic neuropathy
- Compressive optic neuropathy (e.g. optic nerve sheath meningioma). Interestingly this may give rise to Foster-Kennedy syndrome where optic atrophy is identified in the ipsilateral eye due to the compressive effect upon the optic nerve while in the contralateral eye papilloedema occurs due to the mass effect and raised intracranial pressure

Demonstrate the importance of clinical context – suggest relevant questions that would be taken in a patient history

When faced with a visual field deficit, attempt to establish the history of the visual loss in terms of onset, duration and progression. Enquire as to associated symptoms or visual phenomena including floaters (suggestive of retinal pathology) flashing lights halos around lights, suggesting lens pathology), or distorted colour vision.

Screen for systemic disease with potential for visual involvement, particularly diabetes, hypertension and those that increase the likelihood of ischaemia such as sickle cell disease. Where cataracts are suspected, consider congenital disease and family history (Myotonic Dystrophy and Lowe syndrome are good examples).

Consider extra-occular symptoms that may direct towards a specific diagnosis, particularly:

- Giant cell arteritis (GCA) – visual loss associated with headache, tender scalp over temporal artery, proximal weakness/stiffness of the upper girdle, and general malaise
- Migraines – visual loss may present with headaches as an ocular migraine

What effect has the visual deficit had on the patient's life? Consider independence and effect upon activities of daily living, work, driving, and resultant potential for depression.

Demonstrate an understanding of the value of further investigation

If recent onset, and ischaemic optic neuropathy suspected in a patient over 50 years of age, inflammatory markers should be requested to rule out giant cell arteritis as this can progress to bilateral blindness if treatment is not given.

If there is no obvious cause of blindness apparent in the eye, imaging of the orbit (contrast-enhanced CT or MRI with gadolinium) is indicated.

Visual-evoked potentials are useful in objectively evaluating optic nerve function.

Always offer a management plan

There may be no obvious underlying cause apparent, in which case the candidate may choose to discuss the management of a particular cause from the differential diagnosis. Focusing upon common causes, such as cataracts, or important causes where timely intervention reduces progression such as GCA, serves as a sensible approach.

Case 26: Homonymous hemianopia

Instruction to the candidate

This 60-year-old man complains of blurred vision. Please examine his visual fields and report your findings to the examiner.

Begin with a summary of positive findings

There is a visual field defect affecting the same side of the visual field of both eyes, namely the temporal field of the left eye and the nasal field of the right. The field defects respect the vertical midline.

When examining the visual fields, particular attention should be paid to the extent of the visual defect affecting each eye. Despite the description of a homonymous defect implying an identical field defect in each eye, in reality the extent of the visual field involved may vary between each side, in which case it is said to be incongruous. The degree of incongruity can be used to determine the likely site of the lesion. A lesion causing a congruous defect will be posterior (affecting the optic radiations, occipital cortex), while a lesion causing an incongruous defect will be more anterior, in the optic tract and lateral geniculate nucleus.

Follow with a summary of relevant negative findings

Pupillary responses, particularly the absence of a relative afferent pupillary defect.

State the most likely diagnosis on the basis of these findings

'The patient has visual field defects involving both eyes consistent with a left homonymous hemianopia indicating of a lesion affecting the right optic tract. The defect is more pronounced in the right eye than the left, and as such is considered incongruous suggesting the lesion is more anterior within the optic tract.'

Offer relevant differential diagnoses

Homonymous hemianopia is attributable to a lesion of the visual pathway posterior to the optic chiasm. The most common causes are considered secondary to infarction or as the result of a space-occupying lesion. Rarely homonymous hemianopia can be congenital, as the result of a porencephalic cyst for instance.

Demonstrate the importance of clinical context – suggest relevant questions that would be taken in a patient history

Focus upon extra-ocular symptoms consistent with either:

- Stroke – sudden onset with additional neurological deficit, commonly dysphagia or hemiparesis
- Space-occupying lesion – insidious onset with gradual deterioration in vision, but with the potential for acute deterioration (haemorrhage or oedema), associated with postural headache

Demonstrate an understanding of the value of further investigation

The most important investigation in this scenario is neuro-imaging with CT and/or MRI.

In the acute setting where clinical suspicion is of a cerebrovascular accident, priority will revolve around treatment options and

intervention based on the findings of neuro-imaging. It is vital however to highlight the importance of preventing disease progression and/or recurrence by optimising risk factors and identifying embolic sources, thus further investigation will include:

- Blood tests such as HbA1c and lipid profile
- Carotid Doppler ultrasound
- Transthoracic echocardiogram
- 24-hour ECG monitoring

Always offer a management plan

Treatment is directed towards the underlying cause. The management of, and scope for functional improvement or recovery from, homonymous hemianopia will depend upon the underlying cause.

Be prepared to demonstrate an understanding of the principles of cerebrovascular accident in the acute setting with need for urgent imaging and anti-platelet or thrombolysis therapy as appropriate, compared with the principles of rehabilitation and multi-disciplinary care in the longer term.

Any discussion relating to a space-occupying lesion should centre upon establishing the histopathology based on biopsy versus imaging guided diagnosis. The broad principles of treatment, dependent upon the nature of the mass, will be within a multidisciplinary setting and directed towards either aggressive resection or removal versus monitoring or palliation.

Case 27: Bitemporal hemianopia

Instruction to the candidate

This 43-year-old man has consulted with his general practitioner repeatedly over the preceding 12 months complaining of headaches. He has now experienced an acute deterioration in vision and has been referred for urgent assessment. Please examine his visual fields and report your findings to the examiner.

Begin with a summary of positive findings

There is a defect affecting the temporal visual field of both eyes.

Such a pattern of deficit is consistent with a lesion affecting the optic chiasm. Compression of the chiasm from below, classically due to a pituitary tumour, affects the lower nasal fibres in the first instance and may result in a denser upper field defect. Compression from above, classically due to a craniopharyngioma, affects the upper nasal fibres resulting in a denser lower field defect early in presentation. Both may progress to affect lower and upper fields equally and as such presentation will be variable and clinical discrimination subtle.

Follow with a summary of relevant negative findings

It would be prudent to perform fundoscopy assessing for pallor of the optic discs and assess pupillary responses for RAPD.

Where pituitary pathology is suspected relevant negatives would include acromegalic or Cushingoid features on gross inspection.

State the most likely diagnosis on the basis of these findings

'The patient has visual field defects of both temporal fields consistent with a bitemporal hemianopia, due to a lesion at the optic chiasm.'

Offer relevant differential diagnoses

Consider:

- Pituitary tumour
- Craniopharyngioma
- Meningioma
- Aneurysm of the internal carotid artery
- Metastasis from distal primary
- Granuloma (tuberculosis and sarcoidosis)

Demonstrate the importance of clinical context – suggest relevant questions that would be taken in a patient history

Clarify onset, duration and progression of visual symptoms. Thereafter, enquire as to associated symptoms, particularly those related to possible underlying pituitary adenoma. Commonly:

- Lactotrophic – (prolactinoma) with resultant glactorrhoea, gynaecomastia
- Somatotrophic – resulting in acromegaly with associated headaches, profuse sweating, and changes in physical appearance
- Corticotrophic – resulting in Cushing's disease with associated Cushingoid facies, centripedal and intrascapular adiposity, and thin skin

Where there is no evidence of pituitary involvement apparent, screen for granulomatous or neoplastic disease including risk factors and family history.

Demonstrate an understanding of the value of further investigation

Dedicated neuroimaging of the optic chiasm with MRI and appropriate endocrine investigations where pituitary adenoma suspected.

Always offer a management plan

Management would be directed to the underlying chiasmal lesion, but most discussions surrounding management of bitemporal hemianopia will centre on the management of pituitary adenomas.

Case 28: Homonymous quadrantanopia

Instruction to the candidate

Please examine the visual fields of this 60-year-old man.

Begin with a summary of positive findings

Examination demonstrates a visual field deficit of the right upper quadrants affecting both eyes. Lesions of the optic radiations:

- Temporal lobe lesions (superior quadrantanopias): 'pie in the sky defect'
- Parietal lobe lesions (inferior quadrantanopias): 'pie on the floor defect'
- Glaucoma can cause nasal defects which present as a quadrantanopia, sometimes binasal, and sometimes with a RAPD if unilateral
- A chiasmal lesion could give a bitemporal quadrantanopia

Follow with a summary of relevant negative findings

Pupillary responses and RAPD.

State the most likely diagnosis on the basis of these findings

'The pattern of deficit affecting the right upper quadrants is consistent with a homonymous quadrantanopia due to a lesion affecting the left temporal cortex.'

Offer relevant differential diagnoses

- Infarction
- Tumour
- Trauma

Demonstrate the importance of clinical context – suggest relevant questions that would be taken in a patient history

Clarify onset, duration and progression of visual symptoms.

Focus upon extra-ocular symptoms consistent with either:

- Stroke – sudden onset with additional neurological deficit, commonly dysphagia or hemiparesis
- Space-occupying lesion – insidious onset with gradual deterioration in vision, but with the potential for acute deterioration (haemorrhage or oedema), associated with postural headache

Demonstrate an understanding of the value of further investigation

- Neuro-imaging is useful to rule out an intracranial lesion
- Automated perimetry can more accurately map the visual field defect

Always offer a management plan

Management is directed to the underlying cause.

Case 29: Sixth nerve palsy

Instruction to the candidate

Please examine this 38-year-old woman complaining of blurred vision. Her husband reports that she has been squinting recently and has been experiencing difficulties driving.

Begin with a summary of positive findings

The eye is adducted in the primary position with horizontal diplopia. There is impaired abduction on the affected side.

Diplopia may be subtle when examined and apparent only when viewing distant objects. To limit diplopia patients will often assume

a compensatory posture, turning their head towards the side of the palsy.

Follow with a summary of relevant negative findings

There is no ptosis or proptosis, the uniocular visual acuity is normal, and there is no optic disc swelling. There is no evidence of fatiguability on repeated or sustained testing.

State the most likely diagnosis on the basis of these findings

'The patient has impaired eye abduction indicative of lateral rectus weakness. This is consistent with an isolated sixth nerve palsy.'

Offer relevant differential diagnoses

Differential diagnosis of a sixth nerve palsy

Consider the differential in relation to the course of the sixth nerve.

Where onset is spontaneous and sudden in the absence of other symptoms including headache and sensory disturbance the differential diagnosis is likely to include a microvascular occlusion commonly associated with poorly controlled diabetes or hypertension. Isolated palsies often indicate ischaemic pathology of the nucleus in the pons. That said the nucleus of the facial nerve is in close proximity and a combination of signs is often seen.

The nerve travels form its nucleus, through the subarachnoid space before passing over the petrous apex of the temporal bone and entering the cavernous sinus. Peripheral deficits at these points can be caused by anything that either directly compresses or stretches the nerve.

Papilloedema may suggest a space occupying lesion and raised intracranial pressure, resulting in stretching of the sixth nerve in the subarachnoid space (false localising sign, particularly if bilateral).

Sixth nerve palsy associated with hearing loss and facial pain due to involvement of fifth, seventh or eight nerves is caused by pathology at the petrous apex of the temporal bone. Consider trauma resulting in trauma. Also infectious, inflammatory or neoplastic processes.

Involvement of the sixth with any combination of third, fourth, or the ophthalmic branch of the fifth cranial nerve might suggest a cavernous sinus pathology. Look for a sixth nerve palsy together with Horner's syndrome and possibly a third or fourth palsy. Common causes include thrombosis, neoplastic disease or infiltration, or aneurysms of the carotid within the cavernous sinus.

Differential diagnosis of diplopia

The following conditions can cause diplopia which can mimic cranial nerve palsies affecting the extraocular muscles:

- Dysthyroid eye disease
- Myasthenia gravis
- Demyelination
- Ophthalmoplegic migraine
- Decompensated squint
- Monocular diplopia (can be due to cataract, corneal surface disease, iris abnormality, macular disease)

Diplopia: monocular or binocular?

Binocular diplopia is due to misalignment of the eyes. It disappears when one eye is covered. Monocular diplopia is due to a structural problem within one eye causing two focused images to be formed on the retina simultaneously. Occluding the fellow eye has no effect.

Demonstrate the importance of clinical context – suggest relevant questions that would be taken in a patient history

Clarify onset, duration, and ensure no associated deficit of visual acuity. In this case where the patient is relatively young, it would be important to be seen to explore symptoms consistent with raised intracranial pressure. Thereafter, focus on common co-morbidities associated with a sudden onset sixth nerve palsy - explore a history of diabetes and hypertension.

Demonstrate an understanding of the value of further investigation

Indications for neuro-imaging include:

- Suspicion of intracranial aneurysm – sudden onset sixth nerve palsy associated with headache, particularly in the young, demands evaluation for aneurysm
- Worsening signs on successive examinations
- Multiple cranial nerves involved including bilateral sixth nerve involvement
- Swollen optic discs
- Young patient (<50 years)

If any clinical suspicion of myasthenia gravis, antiacetylcholine autoantibodies can be checked, and either an ice pack test or an edrophonium test carried out to look for reversibility of signs.

Check the blood pressure and capillary blood glucose. Consider inflammatory markers and thyroid function tests.

Always offer a management plan

The underlying cause, if identified, should be treated. The commonest cause of third, fourth, and sixth nerve palsies is microvascular occlusion and the natural history is of spontaneous resolution. Spontaneous resolution would also be expected for an idiopathic palsy over weeks to months. Thus, failure to improve should prompt re-evaluation for persisting intracranial pathology.

Symptomatic management of diplopia can be achieved through occlusion of one eye, or by fitting an appropriate prism to the patient's glasses. An orthoptist can measure the angle of deviation and fit the correct prism. The angle of deviation should be monitored regularly and any worsening prompt reevaluation of underlying pathology.

Further reading

Murchison AP, Gilbert ME, Savino PJ. Neuroimaging and acute ocular motor mononeuropathies: a prospective study. Arch Ophthalmol 2011; 129:301–305.

Case 30: Fourth nerve palsy

Instruction to the candidate

Please examine this 70-year-old woman who has returned to clinic after successful cataract surgery complaining of new onset blurring of vision.

Begin with a summary of positive findings

The affected eye may be hypertropic (higher than the fellow eye) in the primary position with vertical diplopia. Diplopia may be subtle and only be apparent on looking down or on observing near objects. On examination of the eye movements, there is impaired downward gaze in adduction ('down and in') with diplopia. If long standing, there may be an over action of inferior oblique, with the ipsilateral eye shooting upwards in adduction.

Congenital or chronic deficit may be compensated by a head tilt away from the affected side to correct the deficit. Interestingly, in some cases a paradoxical tilt towards the side of the deficit is employed to widen the blurred images, allowing the patient to better suppress or ignore one image as a coping strategy.

Follow with a summary of relevant negative findings

There is no ptosis or proptosis, the uniocular visual acuity is normal, and there is no optic disc swelling. There is no evidence of fatiguability on repeated or sustained testing.

State the most likely diagnosis on the basis of these findings

'The patient has impaired vertical gaze, predominantly in adduction, indicative of superior oblique weakness. This is consistent with isolated fourth nerve palsy.'

Offer relevant differential diagnoses

Most fourth nerve palsies are either idiopathic or traumatic. Idiopathic palsy is generally expected to resolve, however while some traumatic palsies improve with time, the majority will not. Head injury resulting in a fourth nerve palsy is often not associated with loss of consciousness and need not be significant in force.

Infarction or microvascular occlusion secondary to diabetes should be excluded as resolution with treatment is common.

Raised intracranial pressure may cause a fourth nerve palsy but may be a false localising sign, especially if bilateral. That said consideration should be given to the possibility of direct compression of the fourth nerve by a space-occupying lesion. Associated cerebellar signs may raise suspicion of a space-occupying lesion affecting the fourth nerve nucleus.

Demonstrate the importance of clinical context – suggest relevant questions that would be taken in a patient history

Collateral history or old photographs are often useful in ascertaining a change in appearance with development of a characteristic head tilt.

Fourth nerve palsy, of any cause can develop insidiously and unnoticed as elderly patients gradually lose binocular function resulting from cataracts. Following surgical intervention and restoration of good vision, these patients become aware of diplopia and present with an apparently new deficit. Thus, timing in relation to cataract treatment can be a useful line of enquiry.

Demonstrate an understanding of the value of further investigation

Exclude medical conditions and consider neuro-imaging as appropriate.

Always offer a management plan

Oculomotor exercises or prism glasses may help restore concordant vision. In more severe cases, often congenital, surgical intervention is considered.

Case 31: Internuclear ophthalmoplegia – multiple sclerosis

Instruction to the candidate

A 30-year-old woman complaining of blurred vision has been referred by her GP who is concerned by the pattern of her recent consultations in which she has complained of a variety of symptoms. Please examine her eye movements and discuss your findings with the examiner.

Begin with a summary of positive findings

There is impaired adduction of the affected eye on looking to the opposite side (horizontal gaze). The contralateral eye abducts fully, but with nystagmus. The patient complains of horizontal diplopia.

Additional finding of bilateral optic atrophy on fundoscopy.

The neuroanatomy of conjugate gaze

The principle of conjugate gaze centres upon the coordinated movement of both eyes in the same direction, at the same time. Gaze palsies result in a lack of synchrony and result in diplopia.

Synchrony depends upon abduction of the ipsilateral globe through the action of lateral rectus mediated by the sixth cranial nerve together with adduction of the contralateral globe through the action of medial rectus mediated by the third cranial nerve. The medial longitudinal fasciculus (MLF) facilitates conjugate gaze by relaying signals between the cranial nerves and incorporating direction from the horizontal gaze centre of the brain, the paramedian pontine reticular formation. Additionally the MLF connects the vestibular nuclei with the third cranial nerve nucleus.

Lesions affecting the MLF are responsible for disrupting communication between the apparatus required to deliver conjugate gaze giving rise to an internuclear ophthalmoplegia.

Follow with a summary of relevant negative findings

The other eye movements are normal and importantly there is normal convergence to accommodation. Adduction in the affected eye is preserved in accommodation but not lateral gaze as the former does not require the MLF.

State the most likely diagnosis on the basis of these findings

'The patient has dissociated conjugate eye movements consistent with an internuclear ophthalmoplegia, suggesting a lesion in the medial longitudinal fasciculus on the side of the impaired adduction. A diagnosis of multiple sclerosis should be considered.'

Offer relevant differential diagnoses

- Demyelination – bilateral INO, together with optic atrophy is virtually diagnostic of multiple sclerosis in the young patient.
- Cerebrovascular accident – commonly in the elderly and often unilateral.
- Rarely space occupying lesion such as neoplasm (brainstem glioma) or vascular malformation (Arnold–Chiari)

Other conditions that may mimic an internuclear ophthalmoplegia include:

- Dysthyroid eye disease (but adduction with accommodative convergence equally impaired)
- Orbital myositis (again accommodative convergence equally impaired, and painful)
- Exotropia

Demonstrate the importance of clinical context – suggest relevant questions that would be taken in a patient history

Attempt to establish the pattern of disease on the basis of a history of symptoms commonly encountered in multiple sclerosis:

Relapsing-remitting	Characterised by relapses with subsequent full recovery in the early stages. Such remissions may last for months to years.
Primary progressive	Steady decline without remission. Generally later onset and poorer prognosis.
Secondary progressive	Initial relapsing remitting course followed by development of a progressive decline.
Progressive relapsing	Disease progression is a steady decline however clear, acute, relapses are superimposed.

> ### Common clinical symptoms in multiple sclerosis
>
> There are no clinical findings unique to multiple sclerosis but some are highly characteristic, classically disseminated in space and time.
> - Sensory or motor deficit of the limbs
> - Visual disturbance – including painful visual loss secondary to optic neuritis, and diplopia due to ocular palsy or INO
> - Impairment of facial sensation
> - Gait disturbance which may be related to poor coordination due to cerebellar deficit or vertigo
> - Bladder disturbance, usually in the first instance urgency
> - Generalised fatigue/exhaustion
>
> Ask specifically about:
> - Worsening of symptoms after a hot bath – Uhtoff phenomenon
> - Electric shock sensation radiating with neck flexion – L'hermitte sign

Demonstrate an understanding of the value of further investigation

The diagnosis of multiple sclerosis is predominantly a clinical one. However, imaging and investigations can be used to support the diagnosis, in line with the McDonald criteria.

A diagnosis can be made on the basis of 2 or more relapses and 2 or more objective clinical lesions.

- MRI – evidence of cerebral, classically periventricular, or cord plaques. There is no consensus on the role for serial imaging with MRI to monitor the response to treatment or progression of disease
- Evoked potentials relate to electrical signals generated in the central nervous system in response to sensory stimulation of peripheral nerves. Visual evoked potentials are slowed.
- Lumbar puncture with CSF analysis – oligoclonal IgG bands

Always offer a management plan

Relapsing-remitting disease

Acute exacerbations are treated with corticosteroids. Disease modifying therapy aims to reduce the rate and severity of relapses.
- Interferon beta

- Glatiramer
- Natalizumab – used in disease resistant to interferon and glatiramer

Progressive disease

Relapsing disease is associated with a better prognosis than progressive disease.

Progressive disease may be treated with an immunosuppressant such as mitoxantrone.

Symptom control

- Spasticity: baclofen or dantrolene, botulinum toxin and physiotherapy
- Tremor: clonazepam, gabapentin

- Fatigue: amantadine, selegiline
- Bladder disturbance: anti-cholinergics, e.g. oxybutinin or tolterodine, intermittent self-catheterisation or it may be that the switch from self-catheterisation to long-term or supraprubic catheterisation is necessary
- Impotence: sildenafil
- Depression: tricyclic or SSRI, consider counselling referral
- Pain and paroxysmal features: carbamazepine, gabapentin
- Visual problems: ophthalmology referral (exclude acute flare)
- Neuropsychological referral

Case 32: Ptosis, large pupil and ophthalmoplegia: third nerve palsy

Instruction to the candidate

Please examine this 40-year-old woman who complains of sudden onset double vision and a droopy eyelid.

Begin with a summary of positive findings

Ptosis of the right eye is evident, which is complete. To examine the remainder of the eye requires gentle manipulation of the eyelid, held open while assessing pupillary responses and eye movements.

The right pupil appears dilated and unreactive to light and accommodation. The anisocoria is accentuated by bright conditions and less noticeable in the dark.

In the resting position the right eye is found in abduction, slight depression and intorsion – 'down and out'. On examination of eye movements deficits of adduction, elevation and depression are noted:

- Adduction is limited and may not proceed past the midline

- Upward gaze is impaired
- On attempting downward gaze, the action of superior oblique causes subtle adduction and rotation

Follow with a summary of relevant negative findings

- The actions of superior oblique (IV) and lateral rectus (VI) are intact
- The uniocular visual acuity is normal
- There is no proptosis or displacement of the globe
- There is no optic disc swelling

State the most likely diagnosis on the basis of these findings

'The findings suggest weakness of the medial rectus, superior rectus, inferior rectus, and inferior oblique consistent with a third nerve palsy. Involvement of the pupil suggests a compressive aetiology and raises the suspicion of a cerebral aneurysm in the first instance.'

Offer relevant differential diagnoses

> ### The role of the pupil in determining the cause
>
> The parasympathetic fibres supplying the sphincter pupillae muscle originate from the Edinger–Westphal nucleus and are carried on the outside of the third nerve. The vasa nervorum supply blood to the nerve from the outside in. As such they are susceptible to external compression and relatively spared by ischaemic lesions. It follows that a third nerve with a dilated pupil is more likely to have a compressive ('surgical') cause, such as aneurysm of the posterior communicating artery, while preservation of the pupil is seen more often in ischaemic ('medical') causes, commonly microvascular occlusion secondary to diabetes.

The differential should consider pupil sparing and non-sparing pathology and whether the third nerve palsy is an isolated finding or found in the context of additional neurological deficit:

- Intracranial aneurysm of posterior communicating artery of circle of Willis. Also internal carotid and basilar artery aneurysms
- Cavernous sinus thrombosis associated with other cranial nerve deficit – commonly IV and VI
- Direct compression of third nerve by space occupying lesion (intracranial/intraorbital)
- Raised intracranial pressure (false localising sign, especially if bilateral)
- Peripheral ischaemic lesion due to microvascular occlusion. Commonly as the result of diabetes or hypertension
- Central/midbrain lesion – the most characteristic finding of a nuclear lesion is complete unilateral third nerve palsy. However, weakness affects both the ipsilateral and contralateral superior rectus and ptosis is bilateral due to the anatomy of the third nerve nuclei. The third nerve begins as a nucleus in the midbrain that consists of several subnuclei that innervate the individual extraocular muscles, the eyelids,

and the pupils. Each subnucleus, with the exception of the superior rectus subnucleus, supplies the ipsilateral muscle. Where due to infarction the palsy is often associated with contralateral hemiparesis and cerebellar ataxia. Other causes include space-occupying lesion and demyelination

- Giant cell arteritis
- Myasthenia gravis and thyroid eye disease may mimic pupil sparing third nerve palsy and should be considered in all patients

Demonstrate the importance of clinical context – suggest relevant questions that would be taken in a patient history

Pain is a common feature and is associated with most differentials including ischaemia. In the acute setting a third nerve palsy will usually result in diplopia, whereas a chronic palsy may be asymptomatic. Screen for conditions predisposing to ischaemia, particularly diabetes.

Demonstrate an understanding of the value of further investigation

Investigation centres upon imaging with contrast CT or MRI and consideration of angiography. Lumbar puncture may be required where imaging is inconclusive to rule out subarachnoid haemorrhage.

Always offer a management plan

Most cases of third nerve palsy recover. Those present at six months are likely to be persistent deficits.

Where appropriate, optimise vascular risk factors and consider anti-platelet therapy.

Diplopia in the short term may be treated with a patch/cover of the affected eye. Chronic, mild deficits may be corrected with a prism. Surgical intervention is rarely advocated due to the complexity caused by the involvement of four extra-ocular muscles and the resultant uncertainty of the outcome.

Instruction to the candidate

Please examine this patient's pupils and proceed as you feel appropriate.

Begin with a summary of positive findings

- Ptosis – Müller's muscle affecting both upper and lower lids (levator palpebrae unaffected)
- Miosis (constricted pupil) with dilation lag, a slow and delayed dilation of the pupil in darkness due to the loss of active radial pull of the dilator muscle.
- Anhidrosis (only in central/pre-ganglionic lesions. Post-ganglionic unaffected) a difficult clinical sign to detect on examination.

Additional findings

There may be apparent enophthalmos – an appearance of a sunken eye.

Anisocoria associated with heterochromia (different coloured irides either eye) suggests a congenital lesion (pigmentation in the first months of life is under sympathetic control).

Where Horner's syndrome suspected, the strong candidate will look to localise the lesion based on additional neurological deficit:

- Brainstem – diplopia, ataxia, weakness
- Spinal cord – weakness, long tract signs, sensory level, sphincter involvement
- Brachial plexus – hand weakness, wasting of small muscles, arm pain
- Cavernous sinus – VI nerve palsy with diplopia in the absence of brainstem signs
- Isolated Horner's syndrome may suggest head or neck pathology – soft tissue masses, lymphadenopathy

Follow with a summary of relevant negative findings

The visual acuity and the eye movements are normal.

State the most likely diagnosis on the basis of these findings

'Horner's syndrome – a lesion affecting the sympathetic nervous supply to the eye and orbit. The absence of diplopia and suspicion of anhidrosis suggests a preganglionic lesion' (see below).

Offer relevant differential diagnoses

Common potential causes of Horner's syndrome.

Central – lesions affecting brainstem and cervical/thoracic cord

- Stroke (lateral medullary syndrome)
- Tumour
- Demyelination

Pre-ganglionic – spinal cord, thoracic outlet, lung apex

- Pancoast tumour of the lung apex
- Brachial plexus lesion

Post-ganglionic

- Carotid artery dissection
- Cavernous sinus mass
- Middle cranial fossa tumour
- Migraine

Anhidrosis is present in central or pre-ganglionic lesions. The sympathetic fibres responsible for facial sweating and vasodilation separate from the remainder of the oculo-sympathetic pathway at the superior cervical ganglion. Thus, anhidrosis is not a feature of post-ganglionic Horner's syndrome.

Demonstrate the importance of clinical context – suggest relevant questions that would be taken in a patient history

Seek to correlate the history with the presentation to help differentiate the underlying cause.

Central

A history of possible dysarthria, dysphasia and vertigo in the context of diplopia, ataxia and weakness on examination.

Pre-ganglionic

Trauma or pain associated with the brachial plexus.

Cough, haemoptysis, weight loss on a background of significant smoking history suggestive of neoplasia, increasing suspicion of an apical lung lesion.

Post-ganglionic

- VI nerve palsy with diplopia
- Acute presentation with neck pain

As Horner's syndrome has the potential to be congenital or acquired, establishing onset of symptoms is important. Comparing old photographs, particularly from childhood may be of use.

Demonstrate an understanding of the value of further investigation

Confirming the diagnosis

Cocaine testing

Unaffected pupils dilate in response to cocaine drops. Cocaine inhibits noradrenaline re-uptake at the sympathetic nerve synapse and causes pupillary dilation in eyes with intact sympathetic innervation. Cocaine has no effect in eyes with impaired sympathetic innervation, regardless of the lesion location.

Apraclonidine testing

Affected pupils dilate in response to apraclonidine, as the result of denervation hypersensitivity, while unaffected pupils constrict. Thus in a positive test there is a reversal of the anisocoria. Apraclonidine is more widely available than cocaine and as such has

been proposed as an alternative test for Horner's syndrome where the diagnosis is in doubt.

Differentiating between central/pre-ganglionic and post-ganglionic lesions

Hydroxyamphetamine testing

The Horner's pupil caused by a central or pre-ganglionic lesion will dilate to hydroxyamphetamine but the Horner's pupil caused by a post-ganglionic lesion will not. Hydroxyamphetamine releases stored norepinephrine from the postganglionic adrenergic nerve endings, and therefore only relies on an intact post-ganglionic neurone for effect. 24 hours must be left after the cocaine test before performing this test.

Identifying underlying cause

Clinical examination, history and testing can direct investigations which may include:
- Chest X-ray
- MRI brain/brainstem/cord as appropriate
- CT/MRA/angiography to exclude carotid dissection

Always offer a management plan

Treatment is directed to the underlying cause. Emphasis may be placed on discussing acute presentations suggestive of carotid artery dissection or aneurysm requiring expedient vascular intervention.

Case 34: Bilateral ptosis with fatiguability: myaesthenia gravis

Candidate information

This 30-year-old woman has presented complaining of limb weakness and abnormal speech. Please inspect and proceed to an appropriate examination.

Begin with a summary of positive findings

On inspection, the patient has classic myasthenic facies:
- Bilateral ptosis

- Expressionless face with flat affect – bilateral lower motor neuron facial weakness with myasthenic snarl when asked to smile

Examination of eye movements reveals weakness and diplopia in a pattern that does not conform to individual nerves or muscles suggesting a 'complex' opthalmoparesis/plegia.

Be sure to demonstrate an appreciation of fatiguability (incremental weakness with repetitive testing of muscle strength) and in doing so consider generalised involvement:

- Levator palpebrae superioris – fatiguability with sustained upward gaze
- Fatiguable, 'nasal' speech due to weakness of pharyngeal and tongue muscles
- Fatiguable proximal limb weakness (upper limb more pronounced that lower limb)

Follow with a summary of relevant negative findings

The pattern of disease – occular versus generalised is an important consideration. Thus, the presence of occular signs without evidence of proximal weakness or vice versa would be important.

The absence of a 'second-wind' phenomenon which, if present, would shift the likely diagnosis towards Lambert–Eaton syndrome.

State the most likely diagnosis on the basis of these findings

'This patient displays bilateral ptosis, fatiguability and proximal weakness consistent with neuromuscular junction pathology. The likely diagnosis is one of generalised myasthenia gravis (MG).'

Occular versus generalised myasthenia

There are two clinical forms of myasthenia gravis: ocular and generalised.
- In ocular myasthenia, the weakness is limited to the eyelids and extraocular muscles
- In generalised disease, the weakness commonly affects ocular muscles, but it also involves a variable combination of bulbar, limb, and respiratory muscles

---

Offer relevant differential diagnoses

The differential diagnosis of fatiguable weakness includes myasthenia gravis and Lambert–Eaton syndrome. Fatiguable proximal muscle weakness is also seen in myopathies.

Where there is predominantly ocular manifestation, consider alternative causes of complex ophthalmoplegia such as thyroid eye disease.

Demonstrate the importance of clinical context – suggest relevant questions that would be taken in a patient history

How do her symptoms affect her function and activities of daily living?

- Involvement of speech and/or swallowing – enquire as to episodes of dysphagia possibly complicated by aspiration pneumonia
- Difficulty with mastication
- Limb weakness, classically proximal – difficulty walking up stairs, rising out of a chair unaided, or lifting arms above head
- Progressive worsening of symptoms towards the end of the day or after exercise?

Does she have any other autoimmune diseases – rheumatoid arthritis/SLE?

Ask specifically about previous myasthenic crises and admissions to HDU/ITU with or without ventilatory support. Shortness of breath, indicating diaphragmatic involvement is an important consideration in neuromuscular disease.

Demonstrate an understanding of the value of further investigation

Blood tests

- Antibodies to the post-synaptic cholinergic receptors at the neuromuscular junction (AChR antibodies) are the pathological mechanism for weakness. Serological tests for these antibodies are the key diagnostic investigation and are positive in the majority (>90%) of cases
- Antibodies to muscle specific kinase (MusK) are found in up to 50% of generalised Myasthenia patients who are AChR antibody negative
- Seronegative cases, where AChR and MusK antibodies are absent are rare but more commonly associated with occular myasthenia
- ESR/CRP to help exclude an inflammatory myopathy
- Thyroid function profile

Neurophysiological testing

- Bedside investigation with a Tensilon (edrophonium) test may be performed where a short-acting anticholinesterase inhibitor is administered to the patient. A positive result involves a transient improvement in power of affected muscle groups due to the prolonged presence of acetylcholine in the neuromuscular junction
- Repetitive nerve stimulation (RNS) shows decrement at high frequency stimulation with a 10% drop being significant
- Single fibre electromyography (EMG) shows 'jitter' which is a characteristic finding

Further consideration

Other investigations include a CT Thorax to identify any thymic enlargement and forced vital capacity (FVC) when diaphragmatic involvement suspected.

Always offer a management plan

Understanding of the pathophysiological mechanism of MG can act as an aide memoire as to the management of MG.

Due to auto-antibodies causing blockade at the neuromuscular junction (NMJ), symptomatic treatment involves cholinesterase drugs which inhibit the breakdown of acetylcholine at the NMJ. These drugs include neostigmine and pyridostigmine (Mestinon).

As MG is an auto-immune disorder, corticosteroid therapy has a large role to play. Steroid-sparing therapies (azathioprine and mycophenolate) are also used in cases where the side-effect burden of corticosteroids is large. Biological treatment with rituximab is possible.

If a thymoma or thymic hyperplasia is present, the patient undergoes thymectomy. Thymectomy is also occasionally considered as a therapeutic option for symptom control in severe generalised MG.

If disease is severe and/or in a myasthenic crises, plasmapheresis and intravenous immunoglobulin (IVIG) can be used. Plasmapheresis involves removing the causative auto-antibodies from the circulation. IVIG has a similar mechanism of action.

Avoidance of medications which worsen weakness and predispose to a mysthenic crisis including:

- Aminoglycoside and quinolone antibiotics
- Beta-blockers
- Procainamide
- Quinine
- Phenytoin

Case 35: Relative afferent pupillary defect (RAPD)

Instruction to the candidate

Please examine this patient's vision.

Begin with a summary of positive findings

On general inspection the pupils are equal with no evidence of anisocoria.

Examination of the individual pupillary responses to light appears normal. Light shone in each eye results in constriction with both a direct and consensual response.

Performing the swinging light test, moving the light source quickly between each eye with only a brief pause, reveals a deficit. The affected eye paradoxically dilates when light is moved from the fellow eye to the abnormal eye. This is caused by dysfunction of the afferent pathway of the affected eye (from the optic nerve to the optic chiasm), such that the consensual pupillary response from the fellow eye predominates.

To help narrow the differential diagnosis test also for:

- Impaired colour vision
- Reduced visual acuity
- Reduced eye movement or pain on eye movements

Look for:

- Optic disc swelling
- Optic atrophy

RAPD

The swinging light test compares the function of one optic nerve to that on the contralateral side. It relies on the principle that the pupillary constriction response to light has an equal relaxation response when the light source is removed. The term afferent refers to the optic nerve being the afferent limb of the pupillary light reflex arc; the efferent limb is the parasympathetic fibres of the third cranial nerve. The presence of a relative afferent pupillary defect suggests a disrupted reflex arc due to either dysfunction of the retina or the optic nerve anterior to the optic chiasm.

Pitfalls in assessing for RAPD:

- Room too bright – a subtle RAPD can only be seen in a dimly lit room
- Expecting RAPD in bilateral disease – RAPD only indicates asymmetry in optic nerve function. If each eye has significant but equal disease, no deficit is observed
- False positive – hippus is a physiological fluctuation in papillary constriction under steady illumination. It is usually bilateral

---

Follow with a summary of relevant negative findings

Remember to check for signs of temporal arteritis if it is a possibility (age >50 years, sudden loss of vision with RAPD). Signs of temporal arteritis can include:

- Tender temporal arteries
- Absent temporal artery pulses
- Scalp tenderness
- Ischaemic ulceration of scalp

State the most likely diagnosis on the basis of these findings

'This patient has a relative afferent pupillary defect.'

Offer relevant differential diagnoses

RAPD indicates an impaired optic pathway, compared to the collateral side, anterior to the chiasm. This is most commonly caused by ischaemia, particularly in the elderly (e.g. ischaemic optic neuropathy, central retinal artery occlusion), and inflammation, particularly in younger patients (e.g. optic neuritis or retrobulbar neuritis, which are often due to demyelinating disease).

Less commonly seen causes are:

- Compressive optic neuropathy (e.g. optic nerve sheath meningioma, other orbital tumour)
- Advanced glaucoma
- Severe retinal disease (macular degeneration, retinal detachment, retinitis) where a significant proportion of retinal nerve cells are damaged
- Traumatic optic neuropathy
- Radiation optic neuropathy
- Inherited optic neuropathy such as Leber's
- Very dense amblyopia (visual acuity worse than 6/60)

Demonstrate the importance of clinical context – suggest relevant questions that would be taken in a patient history

Screen for past medical history as outlined in the differential diagnosis.

Demonstrate an understanding of the value of further investigation

- Formal slit lamp examination to assess the retina
- Consideration of MRI where ischaemia or demyelination suspected

Always offer a management plan

Treatment is directed to the underlying cause.

Case 36: Unilateral large pupil in a young woman – Holmes–Adie pupil

Instruction to the candidate

Please examine this 32-year-old woman, sent by her new GP concerned about the appearance of her pupils on the background of a history of minor head injury.

Begin with a summary of positive findings

On general inspection there is anisocoria with the appearance of a grossly dilated right pupil. The main clinical question in the patient with anisocoria is deciding whether the larger pupil or the smaller pupil is the problem. The key differentiating signs are:

- The pupillary reaction to light
- The pupillary response to accommodation
- The reaction of relative pupillary size in the light and in the dark

In this case, the right pupil constricts poorly or not at all to light but reacts better to accommodation. Having initially appeared larger than the left pupil, following constriction with accommodation the right pupil remains tonically constricted and smaller than the left. Subsequent relaxation is slow and sustained.

Anisocoria: which pupil is abnormal?

In cases of anisocoria (unequal pupils), it can be difficult to ascertain which is the abnormal pupil.

- Measure both pupils in normal room lighting, and then in dim lighting
- If the abnormal pupil is the larger, it will remain large in normal room lighting while the other constricts
- If the abnormal pupil is the smaller, it will remain small in dim lighting while the other dilates

Additional findings:

- On close examination (with the slit lamp, or high magnification direct ophthalmoscope) there are vermiform movements of the iris – the iris is seen to 'wriggle'. This is attributable to segmental palsy
- Loss of corneal sensation – absent corneal reflex
- Loss of deep tendon reflexes in the legs

Follow with a summary of relevant negative findings

- Visual acuity is intact
- No restriction of eye movements, and no diplopia
- No ptosis

State the most likely diagnosis on the basis of these findings

'Findings of a unilateral tonic pupil, impaired corneal sensation and loss of lower limb reflexes are consistent with Holmes–Adie syndrome. Pupillary dilatation is due to parasympathetic denervation at the ciliary ganglion with tonicity as the result of iris sphincter hypersensitivity.'

Offer relevant differential diagnoses

- Argyll Robertson pupils. Normally Argyll Robertson pupils are bilateral and constricted. Holmes–Adie can rarely be bilateral, and the pupils can become constricted and unreactive over time.
- Third nerve palsy (if ptosis and diplopia along with dilated pupil)
- Pharmacological mydriasis (is the patient on any anticholinergics such as atropine, ipratropium, scolpamine)
- Local disorders within the orbit affecting the ciliary ganglion including tumor, inflammation, trauma, surgery, or infection

Demonstrate the importance of clinical context – suggest relevant questions that would be taken in a patient history

Speed of onset and collateral history or objective evidence with old photographs for change in appearance. Screen for symptoms of blurred vision or headaches.

Demonstrate an understanding of the value of further investigation

The pupil can be tested for its response to pharmacological agents:

- Denervation hypersensitivity will result in constriction to a weak pilocarpine drop. After the administration of dilute 0.1% pilocarpine, a more miotic response will be seen compared with the fellow, normal, eye
- The response to mydriatic drops such as tropicamide will be normal

Always offer a management plan

No treatment usually required. The Adie's tonic pupil is benign, and most patients only require reassurance once the diagnosis is confirmed. Although patients with Adie's syndrome may complain of difficulty reading due to accommodative paresis, this usually improves spontaneously. Where blurred vision requires correction, contact lenses with an artificial pupil can be considered in the appearance conscious patient.

Case 37: Bilateral small pupils: Argyll Robertson pupils

Instruction to the candidate

Please examine this 45-year-old man's pupils.

Begin with a summary of positive findings

The pupils are small and irregular. Varying degrees of anisocoria may be seen but both pupils are constricted. They react poorly to light but appropriately to accommodation.

Follow with a summary of relevant negative findings

There is no evidence of ptosis and the visual acuity is intact with normal eye movements.

State the most likely diagnosis on the basis of these findings

'The findings suggest a diagnosis of Argyll Robertson pupils consistent with a lesion affecting the periaqueductal gray matter of the midbrain.'

Offer relevant differential diagnoses

Classically Argyll Roberston pupils have been associated with late syphilitic infection (tabes dorsalis).

Non syphilitic causes

- Diabetes mellitus
- Multiple sclerosis
- Wernicke's encephalopathy
- Lyme disease
- Sarcoidosis
- Other midbrain pathology including tumours and ischaemia

Conditions capable of mimicking the presentation:

- Miotic eye drops used for the treatment of glaucoma may result in an iatrogenic presentation. Previous cataract surgery can result in irregular, albeit usually dilated, pupils. Note that miotic pupils – small, regular pupils, are normal in the elderly
- Uveitis (inflammation in the eye can result in posterior synechiae, sticking the pupil edge to the lens, giving small, irregular, unreactive pupils)

Demonstrate the importance of clinical context – suggest relevant questions that would be taken in a patient history

Screen for systemic disease and behaviours increasing risk of syphilis.

Demonstrate an understanding of the value of further investigation

General screen to reflect the range of conditions as outlined in the differential. Syphilis serology may help to confirm the diagnosis due to the strong association.

Always offer a management plan

Directed towards underlying cause. High dose intravenous or intramuscular penicillin is used to treat late stage syphilis infection. Treatment will prevent further progression, but will not reverse existing damage.

Case 38: Facial weakness

Candidate information

Please examine this 40-year-old man's cranial nerves.

Begin with a summary of positive findings

The patient has an asymmetrical face on inspection with sagging of the eyebrow, loss of naso-labial fold and drooping of the corner of the mouth towards the right side at rest. On testing, weakness is observed to involve the entirety of the right sided of the face including:

- Paucity of blinking with difficulty closing and/or resisting eye opening on the right (orbicularis oculi)
- Inability to prevent deflation of the cheek when puffed out and external pressure applied (buccinator). The patient is unable to grimace, show teeth or pucker their lips
- Importantly, loss of ability to raise eyebrow and wrinkle forehead on the right side (occipitofrontalis)

Follow with a summary of relevant negative findings

Nerve lesions that occur proximal to the geniculate ganglion cause impairment of lacrimation, taste and salivation thus relevant negatives include:

- Intact cornea with no evidence of ulceration or infection
- Moist mucus membranes and tongue

on inspection. On history, see below, no alteration of taste

There are no vesicles around the external auditory meatus and there is no associated ipsilateral hearing loss.

There is no mass associated with the ipsilateral parotid gland.

State the most likely diagnosis on the basis of these findings

'This patient has signs consistent with a lower motor neuron facial nerve deficit.'

Offer relevant differential diagnoses

As with any lower motor neuron weakness, the lesion can be anywhere from the anterior horn cell to the innervated muscle, however the causes include:

Common
- Idiopathic – Bell's palsy
- Infection – Ramsay Hunt (herpes zoster oticus)

Rare
- Infection – Lyme disease
- Inflammatory:
  - Guillain–Barré syndrome
  - Sarcoidosis
- Malignant parotid tumours are often associated with indolent, slowly progressive facial nerve palsy

- Cerebello-pontine angle tumours possible, with a similar presentation, commonly acoustic neuroma

> ### Upper neuron facial nerve weakness
>
> Facial nerve weakness where the forehead is spared implicates upper motor neuron pathology due to the bilateral nature of cortical innervation from the facial nucleus in the brain stem. Orbicularis occuli may also be relatively spared in central lesions for the same reason. The differential diagnosis should focus upon stroke, with consideration given to a cerebellopontine angle lesion or inner ear causes where vertigo, ataxia, and hearing loss feature.
>
> During their examination the strong candidate will take the time to assess for any associated limb weakness. As a common cause for upper motor neuron facial weakness is stroke, it is important to identify any associated upper motor neuron limb weakness. By identifying these, the strong candidate can present the examiner with a diagnosis and differential that more accurately reflects the patient's underlying condition including any associated risk factors such as AF, carotid bruits and evidence of anti-coagulation.

Demonstrate the importance of clinical context – suggest relevant questions that would be taken in a patient history

Important questions would include:

- The speed of onset of symptoms
- Any recent flu-like symptoms
- Any pain or discharge from the ipsilateral ear
- Does the patient have a past medical history of diabetes?

Screen for related symptoms:

- Hyperacusis
- Altered taste sensation on anterior two-thirds of tongue

Demonstrate an understanding of the value of further investigation

Patients with a typical presentation of Bell's palsy with no worrying features do not typically require further investigation unless no improvement or resolution is observed within 4 months, at which point the diagnosis should be reconsidered.

Neurophysiology is predominantly used to assess severity, identifying the degree of residual nerve function, and predict outcome.

Neuro-imaging with MRI should include brain, temporal bone and parotid gland. Inflammatory markers and autoimmune screen if a systemic and/or vasculitic cause suspected.

Serological testing for Lyme disease where suspected.

Always offer a management plan

Bell's palsy can be expected to recover with conservative management within 6–8 weeks.

There is good evidence for the use of corticosteroids and aciclovir within 24 hours of onset of Bell's palsy:

- Steroid – link to neuroanatomy with the course of the seventh nerve through the temporal bone, and narrowing at the internal acoustic meatus. Swelling thus results in potential ischaemia, and necrosis. Reduction in the extent of inflammation may thus be protective
- Aciclovir – link to serological evidence suggesting herpes-simplex virus activation as the cause of Bell's palsy in most cases

Eye care is advisable with use of taping or a patch, particularly at night, and drops to prevent drying.

Case 39: Conductive hearing loss

Candidate information

Please examine the hearing of this 45-year-old man who has been experiencing difficulty hearing in his right ear.

Begin with a summary of positive findings

Gross assessment of hearing by rubbing fingers by the patient's ears in turn confirms hearing loss in the right ear.

Weber's test localises to the right ear (the affected ear).

When Rinne's test is performed at the right ear, bone conduction is better than air conduction. That is to say, the patient hears the sound better when the tuning fork is placed on the mastoid process rather than when it is held close to the external auditory meatus.

Weber's and Rinne's tests

Begin by understanding the findings of each test where no pathology exists.

Weber's test

A tuning fork (256 or 512Hz) is vibrated and placed in the midline of the forehead. Where no pathology exists, sound is perceived equally in each ear.

Rinne's test

The tuning fork is initially placed on the mastoid process. Patients in whom there is no deficit affecting the inner ear will report hearing sound conducted through bone, bypassing the auditory canal and tympanic membrane. When the patient reports no further sound from the fork, which is still vibrating, it is moved from the mastoid process to the pinna. At this point, where no conductive problem is present sound is once again heard, indicating air conduction superior to bone conduction.

Pathology

Thereafter consider the affect of pathology on the tests:

Weber's test
- Unilateral conductive loss – the sound will localise to the affected ear
- Unilateral senorineural loss – the sound will localise to the unaffected ear

Rinne's test
- Conductive hearing loss is indicated where bone conduction is perceived to be better than air conduction as evidenced by no perception of sound once the tuning fork is moved from the mastoid process to close to the pinna
- Sensorineural loss is suggested when both bone conduction and air conduction are reduced, however normally air conduction will remain superior to bone if the deficit is not complete

Follow with a summary of relevant negative findings

No evidence of associated cranial nerve lesions.

State the most likely diagnosis on the basis of these findings

'This patient has signs of conductive deafness.'

Offer relevant differential diagnoses

Conductive hearing loss is attributable to pathology affecting the outer ear, predominantly the outer auditory canal, or the middle ear, impacting upon the tympanic membrane or ossicles, preventing the transmission of sound to the functioning inner ear.

Causes of conductive deafness attributable to outer ear pathology include

- Cerumen (wax) accumulation
- Infection – otitis externa, often due to trauma to the inner ear and subsequent introduction of bacteria or fungus with increased risk in the diabetic population
- Chronic psoriasis causing recurrent local irritation with resultant scar tissue impeding conduction
- Local tumours (squamous cell)

Causes attributable to middle ear pathology include

- Infection – otitis media (OM) – chronic/recurrent may result in permanent hearing loss particularly if complicated by cholesteatoma
- Eustachian tube dysfunction/blockage, often secondary to an upper respiratory tract infection, may result in perceived hearing impairment similar to that associated with change in air pressure (flying/diving)
- Trauma to tympanic membrane
- Otosclerosis where abnormal bone growth affecting the middle ear results in reduced mobility of the stapes impacting upon its ability to transmit sound to the inner ear

Overall the most common causes of conductive hearing loss are wax accumulation and infection.

Demonstrate the importance of clinical context – suggest relevant questions that would be taken in a patient history

Important questions include establishing the timing and onset of the hearing loss – acute versus gradual. Thereafter look to identify precipitating events, including:

- Infection
- Head trauma
- Barotrauma (recent SCUBA diving for instance)

Seek to elicit associated symptoms such as tinnitus or headaches and assess the impact on activities of daily living.

Demonstrate an understanding of the value of further investigation

Investigation in the first instance centres upon clinical evaluation and direct visualisation with otoscopy. The external ear is inspected for obstruction or infection. Thereafter, examination of the tympanic membrane for perforation, evidence of secretion or drainage suggestive of otitis media, or signs consistent with choleasteatoma.

Disorders of the tympanic membrane or middle ear apparatus such as chronic OM or otosclerosis may require formal audiological testing. Tympanometry is useful for assessing middle ear pathology.

Where head trauma, cholesteatoma or a benign/malignant growth is suspected it would be considered prudent to perform CT or MRI.

Always offer a management plan

Causes are treated:

- Otitis media - upon resolution of the acute infection a large proportion of patients with hearing deficit will continue to experience problems for up to 6 weeks. In a small number of patients, hearing deficit due to residual fluid in the middle ear preventing free movement of the tympanic membrane and diminishing movement of the ossicular chain, require myringotomy and grommet (tympanostomy tube) placement or aspiration.
- Cerumen impaction removal, often with suction.
- Consideration can be given to the benefit of surgical removal of masses, such as benign or malignant growths, blocking the eustachian tube or ear canal.

Where the hearing deficit is permanent and/or severe, or where reversible causes have been treated without resolution, refer to a hearing loss specialist for further investigations and management, including adaptations to deal with hearing loss.

Case 40: Sensorineural hearing loss

Instruction to the candidate

Examine the hearing of this 40-year-old man recently discharged from the ITU.

Begin with a summary of positive findings

Gross assessment demonstrates gross hearing loss in the right ear. Weber's test suggests that the sound from the tuning fork is heard best in the contralateral, left, ear. When Rinne's test is performed, air conduction is heard better than bone conduction in both ears albeit reduced in the right compared with the left.

Follow with a summary of relevant negative findings

Cranial nerve deficits, commonly:

- V – Loss of facial sensation and weak jaw clench
- VII – Weakness or asymmetry of the face and abnormal sense of taste

Cerebellar signs, which may suggest compressive lesions at the cerebellopontine angle e.g. schwannoma.

State the most likely diagnosis on the basis of these findings

'The patient displays signs of sensorineural hearing loss.'

Offer relevant differential diagnoses

Inner ear (sensory) or auditory nerve (neural) lesions resulting in hearing deficit include:

Inner ear

Congenital causes:

- Infection: maternal rubella, CMV, toxoplasmosis
- Maternal use of ototoxic drugs commonly in the treatment of TB, historically thalidomide

Acquired:

- Noise exposure/presbycusis
- Ototoxicity: aminoglycosides, vancomycin, loop diuretics

- Infection: childhood measles/mumps
- Autoimmune disorders: RA/SLE
- Ménière's
- Trauma with base of skull fracture

VIII nerve

Congenital causes:

- Infection: maternal rubella, CMV, toxoplasmosis
- Neurofibromatosis type 2

Acquired:

- Tumours affecting the cerebello-pontine angle
- Demyelinating disease

Demonstrate the importance of clinical context – suggest relevant questions that would be taken in a patient history

Screen for medical conditions with the potential for hearing loss, as above, and review medication for current of previous use of drugs with known ototoxicity.
Look to identify associate symptoms:

- Tinnitus
- Pain/headache
- Vestibular symptoms – dizziness, vertigo often worse in the dark

Demonstrate an understanding of the value of further investigation

Formal audiological testing:

- Pure tone and speech threshold testing will quantify the level of hearing loss
- Speech discrimination, while reduced in both, is often worse in neural than in sensory deficit
- An absent acoustic reflex may indicate a lesion of the auditory nerve

Red flags indicating the need for imaging include unilateral sensorineural hearing loss and abnormalities of cranial nerves other than VIII (commonly V and VII). MRI with contrast for soft tissue or vascular masses or CT where bony lesions are suspected.

Always offer a management plan

Identify and treat reversible causes. Sensory hearing loss, due to pathology of the inner ear, is often reversible and rarely life-threatening unlike lesions affecting the auditory nerve which a rarely reversible and may be due to intracranial masses such as cerebello-pontine tumours.

Steroids may be beneficial in patient with autoimmune disease.

Minimising the impact of ototoxic drugs, particularly antibiotics, where possible. Vigilant testing for peak and trough levels to guide dosing and monitoring renal function prudent.

Where the hearing deficit is permanent and/or severe, or where reversible causes have been treated without resolution, refer to a hearing loss specialist for further investigations and management, including adaptations to deal with hearing loss.

Case 41: V, VII, VIII cranial nerves – cerebellopontine angle

Instruction to the candidate

This 74-year-old man has been referred to the neurology outpatient clinic with difficulty in balance. Please assess him and present your findings to the examiner.

Begin with a summary of positive findings

Examination reveals cerebellar signs:

- Ataxic gait
- Nystagmus on the right
- Past-pointing on the right
- Right-sided dysdiadochokinesia

General inspection suggests right-sided facial weakness and formal examination reveals:

- Right-sided lower motor neuron facial weakness
- Hemi-facial loss of sensation on the right. Candidates should also offer to examine for a corneal reflex which is absent.

Facial weakness in this context should prompt assessment of hearing, demonstrating a sensorineural deafness as evidenced by:

- Assessment demonstrates gross hearing loss in the right ear
- With Weber's test the sound from the tuning fork is heard best in the contralateral, left, ear
- When Rinne's test is performed, air conduction is better than bone conduction. The patient hears the sound better when the tuning fork is held outside the external auditory meatus than when held against the mastoid process

Additional signs:

- Nerves IX, X, XI and XII may be affected
- Long tract signs would indicate involvement of the brain stem

Facial sensory loss

In the neurology station – as in this case – abnormalities of facial sensation are most likely to present in the context of other cranial nerve lesions rather than as an isolated clinical sign. When considering facial sensory loss, the following points on anatomy should be considered should be considered:

- Highly focal deficits attributable to an individual branch of the trigeminal nerve – either ophthalmic (VI), maxillary (V2) or mandibular (V3) are generally distal to the ganglion while hemisensory loss is indicative of pathology affecting the ganglion itself.
- Lesions of the lower pons, medulla, or upper cervical cord, will produce a dissociated sensory loss of pain and temperature, with preservation of normal light touch, vibration and proprioception in a classical 'balaclava' or 'onion skin' distribution. As the lesion extends up the brainstem, the sensory deficit spreads incrementally towards the nose.

When as part of a constellation of clinical signs, facial sensory loss can present in a number of ways:

- As in this case, lesions at the cerebellopontine angle are often associated with a disturbance in ipsilateral facial sensation and a reduced corneal reflex. An isolated ophthalmic division deficit is often an early sign of a cerebellopontine angle lesion prior to onset of facial weakness with VII and VIII involvement.
- Supranuclear lesions (e.g. cerebrovascular, demyelination, neoplastic) may result in facial sensory loss associated with ipsilateral pyramidal weakness, ipsilateral upper motor neuron facial weakness, or other cortical signs such as dysphagia, inattention, apraxia, and hemianopia.
- Involvement of III, IV, and VI would suggest a cavernous sinus lesion often associated with ophthalmic and maxillary branch involvement.
- Concomitant Horner's syndrome would suggest a lateral brainstem or upper cervical lesion. Think of lateral medullary syndrome.

Follow with a summary of relevant negative findings

Note the absence of bilateral signs.

State the most likely diagnosis on the basis of these findings

'The pattern of signs, with unilateral involvement of the V, VII and VIII cranial nerves along with cerebellar signs, is consistent with a diagnosis of a cerebello-pontine angle lesion. The likely cause is an acoustic neuroma.'

Offer relevant differential diagnoses

Any mass lesion is capable of producing a cerebello-pontine angle syndrome. The commonest CPA lesion is an acoustic neuroma (schwannoma). Note bilateral acoustic neuromas are common in neurofibromatosis type 2.
Other lesions at the CPA include:

- Menigiomas
- Arachnoid cysts
- Vascular malformations
- Cholesteatomas
- Lipomas
- Granulomas

Demonstrate the importance of clinical context – suggest relevant questions that would be taken in a patient history

Symptoms can be divided into those due directly to cranial nerve involvement and other symptoms caused indirectly.

Symptoms associated with individual cranial nerve lesions

- V nerve symptoms: numbness
- VIII nerve symptoms: slowly progressive unilateral hearing impairment with or without tinnitus
- Additionally, there may be a vestibular element with dizziness

  Cerebellar involvement: slurred speech, balance issues, incoordination.

Indirect symptoms

Blurred vision and headache can occur due to false-localising signs as a result of raised intracranial pressure.

Demonstrate an understanding of the value of further investigation

This patient would warrant urgent intracranial imaging, likely a CT head in acute presentations, followed by MRI with contrast in all.
Other investigations would include:

- Audiometry to confirm and grade the degree of sensorineural hearing loss
- CSF analysis where TB or sarcoidosis is suspected

Always offer a management plan

Management depends on the underlying cause but any mass lesion, which is amenable to surgical excision, should be removed where possible. It is important to look behind the patient's ear for evidence of previous surgical intervention.

Case 42: Dysphasia

Instruction to the candidate

Please examine this 60-year-old man's speech.

Begin with a summary of positive findings

The examination is remarkable for speech that is non-fluent with the slow production of short phrases. It is hesitant and stutters with apparent significant effort required to communicate. The ability to convey meaning is impaired with the use of inappropriate words. Naming objects and repetition are both impaired. There is a poverty of descriptive speech and the use of neologisms (made up words used to convey meaning) evident.

Comprehension is intact as evidenced by the ability to follow a three-stage command – asked to point to their head, pick up a pencil, and stand up for instance.

Variations in presentation of dysphasia

Expressive (non-fluent) dysphasia
The patient demonstrates incomprehensible speech. Expressive dysphasia due to a deficit in Broca's (frontal lobe) speech area of the brain.

Receptive (fluent) dysphasia
There is evidence of abnormal comprehension of language and inability to recognise auditory or visual stimuli. Receptive dysphasia due to a deficit in Wernicke's (posterosuperior temporal lobe) language area of the brain.

Mixed/global dysphasia
There is evidence of both abnormal comprehension of language and production of incomprehensible speech. Given that the damaged area of brain this presentation is relatively large, one would expect to find additional visual field or long-tract signs.

Conduction dysphasia
The patient displays normal comprehension of language and is capable of fluent speech but appears confused and is nonsensical. There is a failure of repetitive speech. Conductive dysphasia due to a defect in the arcuate fasciculus that links Broca's area to Wernicke's area.

Follow with a summary of relevant negative findings

Evidence of motor cortex involvement – Broca's area sits anterior to the motor cortex in the posteroinferior frontal lobe.

State the most likely diagnosis on the basis of these findings

'Expressive dysphagia in the context of right hemiparesis consistent with a lesion affecting Broca's area in the left frontal hemisphere.'

Offer relevant differential diagnoses

In any case of cerebrovascular accident be prepared to discuss the likely territory affected and the relevant vascular anatomy.

Causes of damage to areas of the brain required for speech can be considered generally as one of:
- Infarction
- Tumour
- Trauma
- Degeneration

Demonstrate the importance of clinical context – suggest relevant questions that would be taken in a patient history

Evaluate speed of onset and assess for impairment of written language, which may affect both reading and writing. Understanding, as with verbal speech, is intact.

Screen for cardiovascular risk and evidence of previous transient ischaemic attacks.

Demonstrate an understanding of the value of further investigation

Acute stroke demands urgent CT head with subsequent consideration of thrombolysis and transfer to a stroke centre. Aside from imaging, the investigations required will depend on the likely underlying cause.
Ischaemic stroke
- Blood tests to assess cardiovascular risk, including HbA1c and lipid profile
- A 12-lead electrocardiogram to ensure to rule out atrial fibrillation. Other, less common pieces of useful information would include the presence of sustained ST elevation post-MI which may be suggestive of left ventricular aneurysm formation which can predispose to left ventricular mural clot formation

- A trans-thoracic echocardiogram will identify any structural abnormalities of the heart and, in the setting of atrial fibrillation, give information about the size of the left atrium, which is important for consideration of cardioversion
- A 24-hour tape will potentially identify any underlying arrhythmias
- Carotid Doppler images will identify any carotid stenosis. It is worthwhile reviewing the indications for carotid endarterectomy in the setting of cerebro-vascular events

MRI with contrast should be considered where signs of raised intracranial pressure suggest a space-occupying lesion.

Always offer a management plan

In the first instance, evaluation of potential for thrombolysis in acute stroke. Thereafter, secondary stroke prevention – anti-hypertensive, anti-platelets, anti-coagulation, statin therapy, and attending to reversible causes of thromboembolism including anticoagulation and/or rhythm control of atrial fibrillation or endarterectomy for critical carotid disease

Functional impairment is often significant with rehabilitation and recovery dependent upon a multi-disciplinary team.

Consideration of treatment options for neoplastic disease, including palliative options.

Case 43: Dysarthria – bulbar palsy

Instruction to the candidate

Please assess this 60-year-old woman who has been experiencing difficulties with her speech for over 12 months.

Begin with a summary of positive findings

On inspection wasting of the tongue, with fasciculations, evident. Speech is quiet with a nasal quality sometimes described as flaccid dysarthria. Hoarseness suggests vocal cord involvement. Excessive salivation with drooling and as a consequence regular forced swallowing of saliva is noticeable with occasional choking.

Examination of the upper and lower limbs suggests weakness with mixed upper and lower motor neuron signs. Importantly, these mixed signs are also observed within the same limb.

Bulbar versus pseudo-bulbar palsy

Bulbar palsy is due to diseases affecting the nuclei of cranial nerves IX–XII in the medulla. The clinical manifestation is one of lower motor neuron signs. Pseudo-bulbar (cortico-bulbar) palsy is due to lesions affecting the cortico-bulbar tracts. The tongue is small and spastic. There are no fasciculations. Speech is weak, slow and deliberate,
and difficult to hear. Jaw jerk is pathological. More common than bulbar palsy, pseudo-bulbar palsy is commonly caused by:
- Multiple sclerosis
- Motor neuron disease
- Tumours affecting the brainstem

Follow with a summary of relevant negative findings

Examination reveals pure motor weakness with no sensory deficit or cerebellar signs.

There is no involvement of the extra-ocular muscles.

State the most likely diagnosis on the basis of these findings

'Bulbar palsy secondary to amyotrophic lateral sclerosis (ALS).'

Offer relevant differential diagnoses

Of bulbar palsy
- Motor neuron disease (MND)
- Guillan–Barré
- Syringobulbia
- Myasthenia gravis
- Poliomyelitis

Of motor neuron disease

Amyotrophic lateral sclerosis is the most common form of MND. Variants of ALS include:

- Progressive muscular atrophy – presentation with only lower motor neuron dysfunction, which may progress to involve upper motor neuron degeneration
- Primary lateral sclerosis – presentation with only upper motor neuron dysfunction, which may progress to involve lower motor neuron degeneration
- Progressive bulbar palsy – upper and lower motor neuron dysfunction of the cranial nerves which often spreads to the upper limbs. Where mixed findings involve the cranial nerves an alternative diagnosis to MND is unlikely

Various disorders may resemble MND in the early stages. These disorders should be considered, not least due to the potential for treatment and improvement as compared with the poor prognosis associated with MND. Conditions with the potential for pure motor involvement include:

- Cervical myelopathy – upper and lower signs within the upper limb but with a characteristic pattern and associated signs
- Nueromuscular junction disorders – MG
- Myopathies
- Polymyositis/dermatomyositis
- Spinal muscular atrophy – lower motor neuron signs with bulbar involvement
- Infections – Lyme disease, HIV, syphilis may produce MND-like symptoms

Demonstrate the importance of clinical context – suggest relevant questions that would be taken in a patient history

The history should be consistent with a progressive upper and lower motor neuron dysfunction affecting one area of the body, such as the bulbar region, and spreading to involve a combination of limbs, axial and respiratory weakness over a period of months to years.

In relation to the bulbar palsy, evaluate involvement of difficulties with mastication and dysphagia, reduced gag reflex increases the potential for aspiration pneumonia. The patient may complain of nasal regurgitation.

Screen for emotional lability which may indicate an ALS-plus picture with cognitive impairment.

Demonstrate an understanding of the value of further investigation

EMG and nerve conduction studies to rule out NMJ dysfunction or demyelination.

MRI of the brain and cord to exclude alternative diagnoses where ALS is suspected, including structural lesions – such as spondylosis, herniation, and syrinx.

Always offer a management plan

Riluzole can be beneficial. It is postulated to increase survival by several months, particularly in those patients with bulbar involvement and difficulty swallowing. Riluzole does not reverse existing damage or deficit but slows progression, particularly in relation to the eventual need for ventilatory support.

Multidisciplinary support. Speech therapists can provide invaluable support particularly in developing strategies to improve speech and prepare for potential loss with alternative communication skills. Practical measures such as suction devices. Consideration should be given to the eventual requirement for non-invasive ventilation and palliative care planning.

Symptomatic relief can be achieved with:

- Baclofen – spasticity
- Quinine – cramps
- Anti-cholinergic – salivation
- Amitriptyline – emotional lability

Case 44: Lateral medullary syndrome

Instruction to the candidate

A 58-year-old type II diabetic presented with a sudden onset of speech, swallowing difficulties, ataxia, hemifacial sensory and contralateral hemisensory temperature loss.

Begin with a summary of positive findings

Ipsilateral findings:

- Hemi-facial sensory loss to pain and temperature
- Hemi-facial pain
- Arm and leg ataxia
- Gait ataxia
- Nystagmus
- Vertigo
- Horner's syndrome

Contralateral findings:

- Hemi-sensory loss of pain and temperature sensation

Follow with a summary of relevant negative findings

Absence of cardiovascular signs, which may point to an embolic source:

- Atrial fibrillation
- Valvular heart disease

Absence of xanthelasma which may indicate hyperlipidaemia

State the most likely diagnosis on the basis of these findings

'This patient has signs consistent with lateral medullary syndrome.

'The diagnosis is evidenced by involvement of the facial and vestibular nuclei as well as nucleus ambiguous (dysphagia). There is additional evidence for damage to the spinothalamic tract, the descending sympathetic fibres (Horner's syndrome) and midline cerebellar structures (gait ataxia).'

Offer relevant differential diagnoses

Lateral medullary syndrome is the most common and important syndrome related to intracranial vertebral artery occlusion. The majority of occlusive lesions are atherlosclerotic. Other possible causes of lateral medullary syndrome include:

Cardiovascular embolus sources

- AF, valvular heart disease, LV aneurysm, atrial myxoma
- Rarer causes of vertebro-basilar emboli including vertebral artery dissection
- Thrombophilic/procoagulent states (OCP and pregnancy) can be contributory factors

Non cardiovascular causes

Demyelinating plaques can occasionally occur in exactly this anatomical distribution
If the lateral medullary syndrome evolves relatively slowly, consider:

- Neoplastic lesions such as primary gliomas and secondary metastases
- Rarely, infectious processes leading to local abscesses

Demonstrate the importance of clinical context – suggest relevant questions that would be taken in a patient history

Speed of onset of symptoms:

- Previous TIAs with vestibulocerebellar symptoms or elements of lateral medullary syndrome. The most common symptoms is dizziness
- Screen for cardiovascular risk

Demonstrate an understanding of the value of further investigation

Imaging

MRI of the brain. There is no role for CT of the brain in these circumstances as the resolution for this technique in the posterior fossa is poor. MR angiogram of extra-cranial vertebral arteries is useful in excluding dissection.

Cardiac investigations

- Echocardiogram
- ECG
- Holter monitoring

Always offer a management plan

In the first instance evaluation of potential for thrombolysis in acute stroke. Thereafter, secondary stroke prevention including anti-hypertensive, anti-platelets, anti-coagulation, statin therapy.

Consideration of treatment potions for neoplastic disease, including palliative options.

Case 45: Jugular foramen syndrome

Instruction to the candidate

Please examine this 64-year-old man who has complained of progressive difficulty swallowing and problems with his speech, worsening over a period of 3 months.

Begin with a summary of positive findings

Examination of the cranial nerves reveals:

- Decreased/absent palatal movement on the left
- Decreased power of left sternocleidomastoid and trapezius with some wasting
- Left sided tongue wasting and some fasiculations. Tongue deviates to the right on protrusion

Additional findings

Albeit difficult to test within a PACES environment, information may be included in the case vignette alluding to altered taste involving the posterior 1/3 of the tongue on the left.

Follow with a summary of relevant negative findings

- No contralateral signs – all signs are lateralised
- No lymphadenopathy or masses palpable within the soft tissue of the neck

State the most likely diagnosis on the basis of these findings

'This patient has involvement of the IX, X and XIth cranial nerves constituting a left sided 'jugular foramen' syndrome. The additional involvement of the XIIth nerve on the same side suggests a lesion at the base of the skull.'

Offer relevant differential diagnoses

Causes of a jugular foramen syndrome include:

- Glomus jugulare tumour
- Base of skull metastases commonly from a prostate cancer, or plasmacytoma
- Lymphoma, TB, sarcoidosis
- Carotid artery dissection (rare)
- Focal anterior horn cell disease (MND) can produce a similar presentation but the presence of sensory signs exclude this

Demonstrate the importance of clinical context – suggest relevant questions that would be taken in a patient history

- Speed of onset
- Systemic features of disease and relevant risk factors
- Consequences of dysphasia

Demonstrate an understanding of the value of further investigation

Investigation revolves around imaging:

- MRI/MR venogram to visualise the jugular bulb and venous structures
- CT skull base
- Blood tests: ESR, serum electrophoresis, Bence Jones proteins, serum ACE, TB ELISPOT, lactate dehydrogenase

- Lymph node excision/biopsy, if lymphadenopathy present

Always offer a management plan

- Removal of glomus jugulare tumour or treatment of metastases
- Anti-microbials for TB or other infections
- Corticosteroids for sarcoid
- Haematology–oncology management of lymphoproliferative disorders

Case 46: Myotonic dystrophy

Instruction to the candidate

This 20-year-old man has recently been diagnosed with diabetes. He has presented complaining of weakness. Please inspect the patient and examine as appropriate.

Begin with a summary of positive findings

Inspection reveals classical facial features of myotonic dystrophy including:

- Frontal balding
- Temporalis wasting
- Bilateral ptosis

Focusing examination on the bilateral ptosis may be tempting, but given the likely differential of myotonic dystrophy and myasthenia gravis the strong candidate will consider examination of the upper limbs in the first instance. Examination reveals:

- Muscle weakness with myotonia. Myotonia is a slowed relaxation following a normal muscle contraction and can be demonstrated by slow grip release after an introductory handshake with the patient. Alternatively, firm percussion of the thenar eminence (specifically abductor pollicis brevis) will result in abduction of the thumb followed by slow relaxation. Predominantly affects the facial, jaw, tongue and hand muscles. Importantly, myotonia tends to fade as muscle weakness worsens with progression of disease, thus avoid dismissing

the diagnosis where there is difficulty demonstrating it
- Wasting of the intrinsic muscles of the hand and distal muscles of the arm

Other positive findings may include additional evidence of myotonia such as:

- Cataracts
- The presence of a pacemaker device in the infraclavicular fossa indicative of AV node involvement
- Finger prick marks from blood glucose testing indicating diabetes mellitus
- Testicular atrophy

Follow with a summary of relevant negative findings

No evidence of fatiguability.

State the most likely diagnosis on the basis of these findings

'The patient has muscle weakness with evidence of transiently increased tone in response to voluntary contraction or percussion. This is consistent with a diagnosis of myotonic dystrophy.'

Offer relevant differential diagnoses

Myopathies, which may be inherited or acquired:

- Hereditary – facio-scapulo-humeral, limb girdle
- Acquired – neuromyotonia (anti-voltage gated potassium channel antibodies) paraneoplastic myopathies
- Myasthenia gravis (anti-acetylcholine receptor antibodies)
- Mitochondrial myopathies (these can also have diabetes and cataracts as part of the spectrum)

Demonstrate the importance of clinical context – suggest relevant questions that would be taken in a patient history

Muscle pain is common affecting the legs more than the arms. Myotonia is often referred to by patients merely as muscles stiffness and they may not fully appreciate the nature of the symptom. Symptoms may be aggravated by cold and stress.
Screen for systemic symptoms:

- Respiratory complications are common – screen for shortness of breath and pneumonias
- Gastrointestinal symptoms due to involvement of smooth muscle may present as colicky abdominal pain often with bloating and constipation as pseudo-obstruction
- Diabetes
- Palpitations associated with arrhythmias, commonly atrial fibrillation or flutter. Aortic valve disease is also prominent

Given the autosomal dominant nature of the disorder, be sure to explore a thorough family history (see below).

Demonstrate an understanding of the value of further investigation

The diagnosis of myotonic dystrophy can be readily established when there is muscle weakness and clinical myotonia in the context of a positive family history. Confirmation centres upon electromyography, and genetic testing.

Neurophysiology

EMG may be used to demonstrate myotonia where uncertainty exists as to clinical findings, and to distinguish from the fatiguability seen in myasthenia.

Genetic testing

Specific genetic testing to demonstrate the presence of an expanded CTG repeat in the myotonic dystrophy protein kinase (DMPK) gene on chromosome 19 is the gold standard for the diagnosis. The size of the expansion length is linked to severity of disease as well as contributing to anticipation with successive generations having more severe disease.

Maternal inheritance may suggest mitochondrial disease which can be tested for by genetic analysis of mitochondrial DNA.

Also consider specific testing to investigate the spectrum of associated conditions:

- Oral glucose tolerance testing
- 12-lead ECG, echocardiogram
- Formal slit lamp evaluation

Always offer a management plan

There is no disease-modifying therapy available for the treatment of myotonic dystrophy. Thus, treatment is directed towards symptom control.

- Pain management will often require neuropathic modulating agents such as gabapentin and amitriptyline
- Physiotherapy, specifically late in disease where distal weakness becomes more prominent. The use of orthoses for foot drop and wrist weakness is common
- Particular care should be taken in relation to anesthesia with the chance of respiratory failure precipitated by sedatives and neuromuscular blocking agents

Genetic counselling is paramount since prenatal diagnosis is possible.

Case 47: Cervical myelopathy

Instruction to the candidate

Please examine the upper limbs of this 80-year-old woman with severe rheumatoid arthritis.

Begin with a summary of positive findings

Examination of the upper limbs reveals:

- Wasting of the deltoids and biceps evident on general inspection with fasciculations visible from the end of the bed. Testing confirms weakness of shoulder abduction and elbow flexion as expected and additionally suggests weakness of supination consistent with brachioradialis involvement
- Triceps reflex is pathologically brisk whereas biceps and supinator reflexes are absent. Inversion of reflexes is noted
- Dermatomal sensory loss is noted in C5–7 distribution. There is profound loss of vibration sense and proprioception is absent – pseudoathetosis (writhing movements) of the fingers may be observed when the patent is asked to close their eyes

The strong candidate will examine the lower limbs to confirm spastic paraparesis and sensory deficit:

- Markedly increased tone with clasp-knife spasticity
- Pyramidal weakness of the lower limbs bilaterally. No evidence of muscle wasting. Pathologically brisk reflexes with clonus at the ankle and knee. Extensor plantar response
- Sensory deficit evident. Impairment of vibration sense and sensory level. Proprioception, pain and temperature sense are spared

Inversion of reflexes and the mid-cervical reflex pattern

Paradoxical contraction of triceps with elbow extension when testing biceps reflex, and flexion of the fingers when testing supinator jerk, occurs. Biceps and supinator reflexes in of themselves are absent due to a lesion affecting their roots at C5–6, while the reflex arcs for triceps and finger jerks lie below the level of the lesion and are pathologically brisk. Together this is termed the mid-cervical reflex pattern.

Additional signs on general inspection

Deformity of the cervical spine or evidence of rheumatological conditions, such as RA, OA or ankylosing spondylitis, which may result in degenerative change. The patient may be wearing a supportive c-spine collar.

Follow with a summary of relevant negative findings

- No wasting of the small muscles of the hand – no involvement of C8/T1
- Absence of cerebellar signs

State the most likely diagnosis on the basis of these findings

'Evidence of lower motor neuron weakness and sensory disturbance in a dermatomal distribution of C6–7 with inverted reflexes is consistent with a diagnosis of cervical myelopathy. This is further supported by the findings of spastic paraparesis and dorsal column deficit in the lower limbs.

'The patient is likely suffering from spondylitis of the cervical spine as a consequence of her rheumatoid arthritis.'

Offer relevant differential diagnoses

- Cervical spondylosis
- Tumours
- Trauma
- A common cause of cervical myelopathy in younger patients is demyelination

Demonstrate the importance of clinical context – suggest relevant questions that would be taken in a patient history

Confirm an insidious onset of weakness and sensory symptoms:

- Assess involvement of bladder/sphincter control, albeit rare
- Neck pain possible

Demonstrate an understanding of the value of further investigation

CT myelography and/or MRI to assess the stenosis of the spinal column and establish the underlying cause.

Always offer a management plan

Consultation with a neurosurgeon for consideration of surgical intervention to reduce impingement or stabilise the cervical spine. Conservative management with supportive collar, analgaesia and physiotherapy/occupational therapy input.

Case 48: Unilateral arm weakness – neuralgic amyotrophy

Instruction to the candidate

A 28-year-old female teacher presents with a painful right shoulder and weakness in the arm on that side evolving over a few days. Please examine them appropriately and present your findings to the examiner.

Begin with a summary of positive findings

Peri-scapular muscle wasting and occasional fasiculations visible affecting the deltoid of the right shoulder. Weakness of some but not all muscle groups supplied by C5 and C6 on right. Diminished right bicep and supinator jerks but preserved tricep jerks.

Follow with a summary of relevant negative findings

- There is an absence of objective sensory loss
- Examination is normal in other limbs
- The absence of Horner's syndrome
- There are no long tract signs or suggestion of sphincter dysfunction

State the most likely diagnosis on the basis of these findings

'This patient has a predominantly motor syndrome with patchy involvement of muscles supplied by C5–6 roots on the right. With pain also being a feature the most likely diagnosis is brachial neuritis (neuralgic amyotrophy).'

Offer relevant differential diagnoses

- Multiple radiculopathies
- Infiltrative radiculopathies/plexopathy in the context of a carcinomatous mass
- Mononeurits multiplex due to vasculitis
- Hereditary neuropathy with liability to pressure palsies (HNPP)

Demonstrate the importance of clinical context – suggest relevant questions that would be taken in a patient history

In addition to enquiring about the exact nature and timing of symptoms, screen for potential causes and triggers:

- Any history of malignancy such as lung, breast, or ovarian cancer, and lymphoma
- Any history of a preceding upper respiratory tract or gastrointestinal infection, which may suggest a viral cause

Demonstrate an understanding of the value of further investigation

Blood tests:

- ESR
- Serum electrophoresis
- Autoimmune screen
- Anti-ganglioside antibodies

EMG and nerve conduction studies will demonstrate post-dorsal root ganglionic nerve dysfunction. Rarely, a nerve biopsy may be considered in the context of a vasculitis

MRI of the cervical spine and/or the brachial plexus to rule out a compressive or infiltrative process.

CSF analysis is indicated if a more generalised immune process is suspected.

Always offer a management plan

Symptomatic relief with neuropathic modulating agents such as gabapentin, pregabalin, or amitriptyline. Steroids may be of limited benefit. Treatment is directed to the underlying cause.

Case 49: Resting tremor – Parkinsonism

Instruction to the candidate

This 70-year-old man has been suffering with a worsening tremor. Please examine his upper limbs.

Begin with a summary of positive findings

Examination of the upper limbs reveals tremor, rigidity, and bradykinesia.

Tremor

Unilateral resting tremor, classically pill rolling in nature.

Distraction with repetitive movements of the contralateral arm may accentuate/augment a mild tremor or uncovers a latent one. This phenomenon is often observed when assessing gait. Excitement, stress or anxiety may also worsen the tremor.

The tremor is predominantly resting however action and postural tremor possible, albeit less severe.

The latter is associated with a re-emergent tremor – a postural tremor that manifests after a latency of several seconds with identical features to the resting tremor. The re-emergent tremor of Parkinson's differs from that of an essential tremor in which no latency is observed.

Rigidity

Cogwheel rigidity is prominent – tremor superimposed upon rigidity and/or lead piping. Tonic resistance throughout passive movement.

Bradykinesia

Slowness of initiation of voluntary movement. Affecting manual dexterity of the fingers. Movements may become less coordinated, with frequent hesitations or arrests as disease progresses.

Additional findings:

- Paucity of facial expression:
  - Hypomimia
  - Reduced blink rate
- Stooped posture
- Characteristic shuffling gait

Follow with a summary of relevant negative findings

Tremor of the legs, lips, jaw, and tongue are also commonly seen with Parkinsonism whereas tremor of the head is rare. Tremor of the head would suggest essential tremor.

Signs of a Parkinson's-plus syndromes

Multisystem atrophy:
- Autonomic deficit
- Cerebellar ataxia
- Severe akinesia
Progressive supranuclear palsy:
- Vertical gaze palsy
- Pyramidal signs
- Dementia

State the most likely diagnosis on the basis of these findings

Idiopathic Parkinson's disease.

Offer relevant differential diagnoses

Secondary Parkinsonism

- Iatrogenic – anti-psychotics and anti-emetics
- Toxin mediated
- Metabolic
- Infection
- CVA – vascular Parkinsonism due to multiple infarcts. Postulated to be associated with the late onset of a Parkinson-like gait due to infarcts of the basal ganglia

Neurodegenerative disorders

Parkinson's disease may be mimicked by other neurodegenerative disorders, including:

- Dementia with Lewy bodies – early dementia with parkinsonism
- Corticobasal degeneration – most closely resembles Parkinson's disease with asymmetrical signs however often displays limb apraxia/dystonia/alien limb phenomenon
- Multi-system atrophy – autonomic symptoms generally more severe, symmetrical symptoms, lack of tremor, and poor response to levodopa. Cognitive deficit unusual
- Progressive supranuclear palsy – vertical supranuclear palsy with downward gaze abnormalities and postural instability with unexplained falls. Again, tremor is rare. Cognitive deficit is severe
- Wilson's disease
- Huntington's disease

Features suggestive of an alternative diagnosis to idiopathic Parkinson's disease

- Poor response to levodopa
- Symmetrical presentation of tremor, bradykinesia and rigidity
- Rapidly progressive course
- Absence of tremor
- Early falls with autonomic component
- Early or rapidly progressing dementia
- Supranuclear gaze
- Cerebellar signs

Demonstrate the importance of clinical context – suggest relevant questions that would be taken in a patient history

Assess the impact of symptoms on function. A history of falls is common and would suggest postural instability.

Screen for non-motor symptoms:

- Cognitive dysfunction and dementia
- Psychosis and hallucinations
- Mood disorders including depression, anxiety
- Sleep disturbances
- Fatigue

Demonstrate an understanding of the value of further investigation

Diagnosis relies upon clinical evaluation. It is generally accepted that bradykinesia, plus one of the other two cardinal manifestations, tremor and rigidity, must be present in order to make the diagnosis of idiopathic Parkinson's disease. Response to treatment with dopamine based treatment all but confirms the diagnosis.

Investigations may, however, give supporting evidence. Such investigations may include:

- MRI brain for vascular changes
- DaT scan for dopamine content in basal ganglia

Always offer a management plan

Management should take place in the context of a multi-disciplinary team with involvement of specialist nursing, physiotherapy and occupational therapy. The mainstay of medical management is dopamine replacement.

Drugs used in Parkinson's disease:

- LevoDopa is given with a peripheral dopa-decarboxylase antagonist to minimise both the systemic side effects of dopamine and its breakdown by hepatic metabolism. Systemic side effects include nausea, vomiting and postural hypotension. The main central side effect is that of dyskinesia. In the longer term, patient's

can develop a so-called 'on-off' syndrome, where they are rigid without L-dopa, but dyskinetic with it
- Ergot dopamine agonists such as bromocriptine are almost never used in modern clinical practice. Non-ergot-derived examples, including ropinerole and pramipexole, are less likely to cause retro-peritoneal or cardiac valve fibrosis
- Amantadine – preferential effect on rigidity
- Apomorphine – acts as a dopamine agonist. Used in Parkinson's where severe

rigidity 'freezing' is a problem. Usually administered by continuous infusion
- COMT inhibitors (entacapone) reduce the metabolism of levodopa
- MAO inhibitors (selegiline) act to inhibit MAO-A and MAO-B to reduce the breakdown of dopamine and thus increase levels

Neurosurgical interventions in Parkinson's disease include deep brain stimulation and stereotactic surgery, however these are very much second line therapies.

Case 50: Intention tremor and problems with co-ordination – cerebellar syndrome

Instruction to the candidate

Please examine this 30-year-old woman with a tremor.

Begin with a summary of positive findings

Intention tremor and past-pointing of the right hand best elicited by performing 'nose-to-finger' testing. The patient should be made to fully extend their arm to maximally elicit any tremor present, which worsens as it approaches the target at the extremes of reach. A postural tremor is also seen with the arms held against gravity and rebound phenomenon is observed on testing with the patients eyes closed reinforcing dysmetria.

Thereafter, examination of the cerebellar system reveals:

- Nystagmus of eye movements towards the right side (the fast phase travels towards the right)
- Speech disturbance highlighted by an inability to articulate 'British Constitution'. Speech is described as scanning which relates to hesitancy at the beginning of a word or syllable. Also interrupted, staccato, and slurred
- Dysdiadochokinesia on the right side with profound dysmetria
- Generalised hypotonia may be subtle

Gait disturbance is observed. The patient is ataxic, with a wide-based, unsteady gait. Multiple falls or loss of balance towards the right side. Ataxia is exacerbated, and often subtle signs revealed, by walking heel to toe.

Localisation of cerebellar symptoms

Unilateral cerebellar symptoms can be localised to the ipsilateral cerebellar hemisphere, which control finely co-ordinated movements, predominantly of the upper limbs.

Symptoms resulting from dysfunction of the midline cerebellar vermis include truncal ataxia – unsteadiness when sitting down.

The archicerebellum together with the vestibular nuclei maintains equilibrium and balance serving to coordinate eye, head, and neck movement.

Follow with a summary of relevant negative findings

- There is no resting tremor
- There are no contralateral signs

Romberg's test is negative – imbalance does not get worse when the patient closes their eyes. Signs of chronic liver disease (a full abdominal examination is not necessary, but a scan for easily visible signs such as clubbing, jaundice, leuconychia and spider naevi will elicit sufficient evidence if such signs are present).

State the most likely diagnosis on the basis of these findings

'This patient has signs consistent with cerebellar syndrome. The ipsilateral nature of the symptoms suggests a lesion affecting the right hemisphere.'

Offer relevant differential diagnoses

Lesion of the ipsilateral cerebellar hemispheres

- Demyelination
- Ischaemia
- Space-occupying lesion

Lesions affecting the vermis or global cerebellar dysfunction

- Chronic alcohol abuse
- Iatrogenic – phenytoin, amiodarone, lithium
- Vitamin deficiency – B12 and vitamin E
- Infections – varicella (cerebellitis), Lyme disease, TB
- Paraneoplastic – breast, ovarian and lung cancer, and lymphoma. Often bilateral and rapidly progressive.
- Hypothyroidism
- Degenerative – multiple system atrophy (MSA)
- Hereditary ataxias:
  - Freidreich's – the most common hereditary ataxia
  - Ataxia telangiectasia
  - Ataxia with vitamin E deficiency
  - Spinocerebellar ataxias

Demonstrate the importance of clinical context – suggest relevant questions that would be taken in a patient history

- Clarify onset and speed of progression
- Screen for associated past medical history guided by the differential diagnosis

Demonstrate an understanding of the value of further Investigation

Principles of investigation include both intracranial imaging and tests to provide evidence of the underlying cause.

- Blood testing: full blood count for MCV (alcohol). B12 and folate levels.
- Imaging: MRI is the gold standard imaging investigation for cerebellar dysfunction

Always offer a management plan

Given the significant functional impairment caused as a result of cerebellar dysfunction, management would take place in a multi-disciplinary setting with input from physiotherapy, occupation therapy, neurology specialists and alcohol liaison teams as appropriate.

The exact management depends on the underlying cause, but principles include removing any offending toxins. If the cause is thought to be a medication, this can be changed to an alternative. If this is impossible, the dose can be adjusted to give the maximal balance between treatment benefits and side effect.

Case 51: Central cord syndrome – syringomyelia

Instruction to the candidate

Please examine this 30-year-old woman referred by her GP with a 2-year history of worsening neck and shoulder pain and progressive weakness of the upper limbs.

Begin with a summary of positive findings

Examination of the upper limbs reveals:

- Weakness of the hands and arms bilaterally

- Muscle wasting of the small muscles of the hand and arm
- Reflexes are reduced or absent
- Loss of pain and temperature sensation in a cape-like distribution over the shoulders, neck and upper thorax but preservation of light touch, vibration sense and proprioception

Additional signs:

- Weakness of legs (spastic paraparesis) usually less pronounced than the upper limbs. Look for walking aids in the room to support involvement without the need for formal examination
- Multiple small cuts and burns to the pulps of the fingers/hands suggestive of sensory loss
- There may be scoliosis

Follow with a summary of relevant negative findings

Damage to the sympathetic chain may produce Horner's syndrome.

Extension of the lesion rostrally results in syringobulbia, signs of which include:

- Dysarthria
- Wasting of the tongue
- Facial sensory disturbance with sparing of central areas (nose and mouth)
- Nystagmus

State the most likely diagnosis on the basis of these findings

'The patient displays signs of limb weakness consistent with lower motor neuron pathology. There is a dissociated sensory loss consistent with a lesion affecting the central cord. These signs are consistent with a diagnosis of syringomyelia.'

Neuroanatomy underlying the clinical signs in central cord syndrome

A syrinx arises centrally, most commonly at the level of C5/6, and impinges the decussating spinothalamic tracts while the lateral dorsal columns and posterior tracts are spared (**Figure 2.1**).

Syrinx extension into the anterior horns of the spinal cord damages motor neurons, resulting in lower motor neuron signs, with diffuse muscle atrophy beginning in the hands and progressing proximally to include the forearms and shoulder girdles.

Offer relevant differential diagnoses

Common causes of central cord lesions include:

- Syringomyelia most commonly occurs in the setting of an Arnold–Chiari malformation – congenital herniation of cerebellar tissue into the spinal cord, thus associated with cerebellar signs.
- Tumours of the central cord
- Cervical spondylosis – central cord syndrome may be the initial presentation of a progressive cervical myelopathy.
- Trauma

Lumbar syringomyelia

Lumbar syringomyelia can occur and is characterised by atrophy of both proximal and distal leg muscles. A dissociated sensory loss occurs, affecting the lumbar and sacral dermatomes. Lower limb reflexes are reduced or absent and commonly sphincter function is impaired.

Demonstrate the importance of clinical context – suggest relevant questions that would be taken in a patient history

Seek to establish the speed of onset which is normally insidious/slowly progressive. Rapid development may be suggestive of syringobulbia. Painless burns or cuts may be the first symptom alerting the patient to an underlying problem. Deep aching of the neck and shoulders can also be an early sign.

In considering the underlying cause, rule out recent trauma, including hyper-extension injuries of the cervical spine.

Demonstrate an understanding of the value of further investigation

Localisation of a spinal cord lesion can usually be achieved through clinical evaluation and this is useful in directing the level of the cord to be imaged. MRI should be used to differentiate between the possible causes and fully appreciate the extent of cord involvement. Gadolinium-enhanced images are indicated if a tumor is suspected.

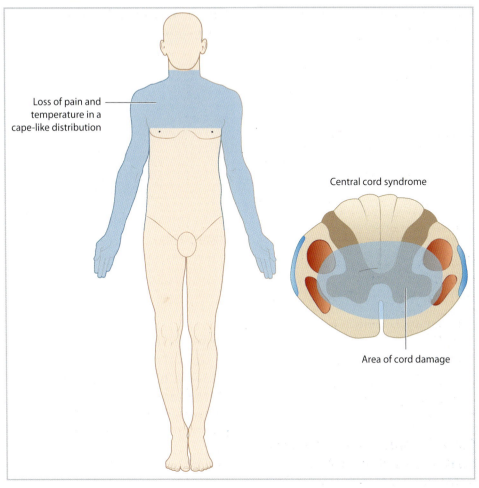

Loss of pain and temperature in a cape-like distribution

Central cord syndrome

Area of cord damage

Figure 2.1 Central cord syndrome. Cape-like distribution of deficit with lower motor neuron weakness of the hands, forearms and shoulder girdle with loss of pain and temperature (spinothalamic tracts) in the same distribution, but sparing light touch, vibration and proprioception (dorsal columns and posterior tracts). Commonly associated with pathology affecting the cervical spine.

Always offer a management plan

The clinical course is often stable and chronic however surgical decompression with fenestration and/or shunt placement may be indicated dependent upon severity/progression of symptoms.

Medical treatment for syringomyelia is limited however steroid use may be beneficial, particularly with cervical spondylosis. Muscle relaxants and analgaesia are a prudent consideration for symptom control.

Case 52: Brown–Séquard (hemi-cord) syndrome

Instruction to the candidate

Please examine the lower limbs of this 36-year-old woman who complains of weakness in her left leg and changes in sensation.

Begin with a summary of positive findings

Ipsilateral examination findings

Pyramidal loss of power in the left leg with brisk knee and ankle jerks and extensor plantar response. Sensory examination reveals loss of fine touch, proprioception and vibration.

Contralateral findings

No weakness on motor examination of the right leg but loss of pain and temperature is evident. Additional signs:

- Inspect surgical scars over the spine to suggest a history of trauma or surgery
- Loss of ipsilateral autonomic function can result in Horner's syndrome

Follow with a summary of relevant negative findings

- Examination of the upper limbs is unremarkable
- There are no brainstem signs

State the most likely diagnosis on the basis of these findings

'The patient has signs consistent with a right hemi-cord (Brown–Séquard) syndrome most probably secondary to demyelination.'

Neuroanatomy underlying the clinical signs in hemi-cord syndrome

- Interruption of the lateral corticospinal tract results in ipsilateral spastic paralysis below the level of the lesion
- Interruption of posterior column results in ipsilateral loss of tactile discrimination, as well as vibratory and position sensation, below the level of the lesion

---

Interruption of lateral spinothalamic tract results in contralateral loss of pain and temperature sensation which usually manifests clinically 2–3 segments below the level of the lesion (**Figure 2.2**).

Most cases are incomplete and as such the clinical presentation of Brown–Séquard syndrome may range from mild to severe neurologic deficit.

Offer relevant differential diagnoses

- Cord compression – trauma, disc herniation or tumour
- Demyelination
- Inflammatory – SLE or sarcoidosis
- Infection – Lyme disease, TB, HIV, HTLV-1

Demonstrate the importance of clinical context – suggest relevant questions that would be taken in a patient history

- Rule out a history of trauma
- Speeds of evolution – inflammatory lesions generally occur over a period of days as compared to neoplasm typically over a period of weeks to months
- Screen for a history of previous neurological events consistent with demyelination and multiple sclerosis

Demonstrate an understanding of the value of further investigation

Traumatic injury or history of acute pain demands urgent MRI spine to visualise abnormality/lesion at a level directed by the clinical findings.

Non-traumatic presentation will still require imaging but consideration of other tests may precede MRI:

- Blood tests (inflammatory/immunological screen)
- Serological testing (viral antibodies)
- CSF examination (culture, oligoclonal bands)

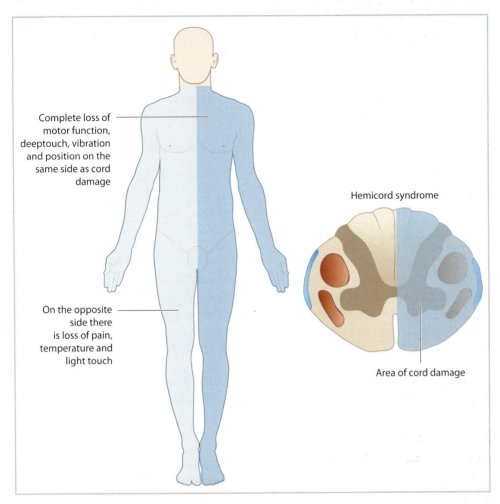

Complete loss of
motor function,
deeptouch, vibration
and position on the
same side as cord
damage

Hemicord syndrome

On the opposite
side there
is loss of pain,
temperature and
light touch

Area of cord damage

Figure 2.2 Hemi-cord syndrome. Ipsilateral motor weakness with loss of vibration sense and proprioception, and contralateral loss of pain and temperature loss.

Always offer a management plan

Cord compression will require urgent referral to neurosurgeons for consideration of decompression. Thereafter treatment is directed to the cause including corticosteroid for demyelinating lesion or anti-microbial therapy as appropriate (antibiotics, anti-virals, anti-retrovirals). Symptom control may revolve around pain management – neuropathic modulating agents and a multi-disciplinary approach to rehabilitation for persisting deficits.

Case 53: Anterior cord syndrome

Instruction to the candidate

Please examine the lower limbs of this 69-year-old man returning to clinic for follow up.

Begin with a summary of positive findings

Examination findings:

- Bilateral spastic paraparesis with brisk reflexes and extensor plantar response
- Bilateral loss of pain and temperature sense
- Bilateral retention of fine touch, proprioception and vibratory sense

Follow with a summary of relevant negative findings

Sparing of proprioception and vibratory sense is crucial.

State the most likely diagnosis on the basis of these findings

'Loss of motor function and a sensory deficit consistent with a lesion affecting the anterior columns of the spinal cord, while retaining those of the posterior column is consistent with an anterior cord syndrome' (**Figure 2.3**).

Offer relevant differential diagnoses

The most common cause of anterior cord syndrome is infarction caused by occlusion of the anterior spinal artery. However, any direct or indirect injury to the spinal cord can cause the syndrome, including:

- Trauma with crush injury
- Hyperflexion injury with bony instability, which may result in quadriplegia due to the vulnerability of the cervical spine
- Compression from a hematoma or disc herniation
- Ischemia secondary to compression of the anterior spinal artery

Demonstrate the importance of clinical context – suggest relevant questions that would be taken in a patient history

Screen for underlying causes. Focus upon risk profiling for stroke and a history of trauma.

Demonstrate an understanding of the value of further investigation

MRI is the optimal modality for imaging the spinal cord.

Always offer a management plan

Optimisation of risk factors for secondary prevention of stroke. Treatment may involve stabilisation or removal of any structure that exerts increased pressure on the anterior aspect of spinal cord demanding neurosurgical input.

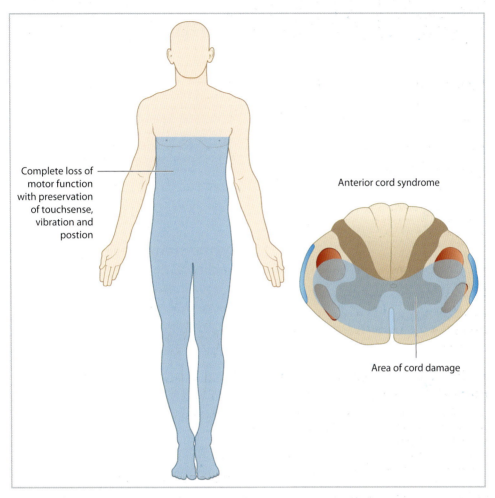

Complete loss of
motor function
with preservation
of touchsense,
vibration and
postion

Anterior cord syndrome

Area of cord damage

Figure 2.3 Anterior cord syndrome. Upper motor weakness as evidenced by bilateral spastic paraparesis with associated loss of pain and temperature sense (spinothalamic tracts), but sparing of fine touch, vibration and proprioception (dorsal columns and posterior tracts).

Case 54: Spastic paraparesis

Instruction to the candidate

Please examine the lower limbs of this 30-year-old woman.

Begin with a summary of positive findings

Examination is remarkable for:

- Increased tone and weakness bilaterally affecting distal and proximal muscles in a pyramidal pattern, with flexors weaker then extensors. No evidence of wasting
- Pathologically brisk reflexes, extensor plantars and clonus at the knee and ankle
- Sensory level at the xiphisternum – affecting dorsal columns (spinothalamic sparing)

Additional findings:
Assessment of gait confirms spasticity with circumduction and scissoring.

Follow with a summary of relevant negative findings

Where demyelination forms a working diagnosis:

- Cerebellar signs
- Cranial nerve involvement
- Evidence of bladder dysfunction

Evidence of B12 deficiency

State the most likely diagnosis on the basis of these findings

'There is evidence of transverse myelitis with a cord lesion at the level of T6. The most likely cause is demyelination with a diagnosis of multiple sclerosis.'

Offer relevant differential diagnoses

Cord lesions can be either intrinsic or extrinsic.

Intrinsic

- Demyelination – transverse myelitis is most commonly due to multiple sclerosis, also consider acute disseminated encephalomyelitis (ADEM) and Devic's disease

- Metabolic – B12 deficiency, important due to the potential for reversibility, copper deficiency
- Vascular – arterial occlusion
- Infectious – HIV, TB, HTLV-1-associated myelopathy, neurosyphilis
- Inflammatory – sarcoidosis, SLE, Behçet's

Extrinsic

- Neoplastic compression
- Traumatic cord injury/spondylosis

Demonstrate the importance of clinical context – suggest relevant questions that would be taken in a patient history

Establish onset of lower limb weakness. Onset and speed of development can be useful in establish both cause and prognosis.

Screen for features of underlying disease, particularly in relation to multiple sclerosis, previous weakness, sensory disturbance, and visual deficit. Ask specifically in relation to sphincter disturbance.

Demonstrate an understanding of the value of further investigation

Investigation of demyelination:

- MRI spine and brain to assess for demyelination both at the suspected spinal level and of the entire neuroaxis
- Evoked potentials (visual and sensory to confirm central conduction delay)
- CSF analysis for oligoclonal bands

Approach to spastic paraparesis where differential is wide:

- Blood tests – ESR/CRP, vitamin B12, serology – HIV/HTLV-1/VDRL, auto-antibodies, culture
- Lumbar puncture – CSF analysis, culture, acid-fast bacilli
- Imaging – MRI/CT-myelogram
- Electromyelography/nerve conduction studies

Always offer a management plan

Treatment is directed towards the underlying cause. High dose steroid in the acute setting may be of therapeutic benefit.

Case 55: Proximal myopathy

Instruction to the candidate

Please examine the lower limbs of this 50-year-old woman who has presented complaining of increasing difficulty climbing the stairs in recent months.

Begin with a summary of positive findings

On examination of the lower limbs there is generalised muscle weakness bilaterally, most marked in the hip flexors (there is weakness on straight-leg raising). The weakness is of a lower motor neuron pattern, with normal or absent knee and ankle reflexes. There is a flexor plantar response.

On walking, the patient displays a waddling gait, with excessive hip swing. When asked to rise from a seated position with arms crossed, the patient has insufficient strength to stand.

The pattern is suggestive of proximal myopathy. Strong candidates will move swiftly to an assessment of the upper limbs and of neck flexion to confirm a similar pattern of weakness.

Candidates should be alert to signs of underlying causes on general inspection:

- Centripedal obesity, purple striae, characteristic facial appearance – Cushingoid
- Heliotrope rash and Gottron's papules. Muscles may be painful – dermatomyositis
- Scleroderma/SLE
- Irregular pulse of atrial fibrillation, profuse sweating, in a thin patient – thyrotoxicosis
- Ptosis and fatiguability – myasthenia gravis

Follow with a summary of relevant negative findings

Signs consistent with upper motor neuron pathology – mixed upper and lower motor neuron signs would be highly suggestive of motor neuron disease.

There is no associated sensory loss, which would favour peripheral nerve pathology.

State the most likely diagnosis on the basis of these findings

'This patient displays clinical signs in the lower limbs of lower motor neuron dysfunction suggestive of a proximal myopathy.'

Offer relevant differential diagnoses

Common myopathies causing proximal weakness include:

- Polymyositis or dermatomyositis
- Thyrotoxicosis
- Cushing's syndrome
- Alcoholic myopathy

Demonstrate the importance of clinical context – suggest relevant questions that would be taken in a patient history

Screen for conditions producing fatigue that may be misunderstood or reported as weakness. Consider cardiac failure, chronic respiratory conditions, or malignancy, amongst others, which may cause cachexia but not true weakness. Patients with true weakness usually complain not of feeling weak but of an inability to perform specific tasks. Thus, explore activities in which weakness proves most problematic.

Clinical patterns of weakness are often reflected in patterns of disability:

- Proximal weakness impairs reaching upward, ascending stairs, or getting up from a sitting position.

  As opposed to:
- Distal weakness which impairs tasks such as stepping over a curb often due to foot drop. Manual dexterity is impacted and simple actions such as holding a cup, buttoning a shirt or writing may prove problematic.

If signs pointing to a likely underlying cause are elicited, then the candidate can offer questions relating to a focused history for that condition. Candidates should be alert to screening for underlying malignancy in a patient with proximal myopathy and heliotrope rash in whom the most likely diagnosis is dermatomyositis.

Demonstrate an understanding of the value of further investigation

Blood work utilised as a screen for common causes of weakness would include:

- Full blood count to exclude anaemia
- Electrolytes including bone profile and magnesium
- Thyroid function
- ESR
- Creatinine kinase and LDH will be raised as evidence of muscle breakdown and supported further by a urine dip
- Serology for antibodies is warranted – ANA, ANCA and ENAs

EMG and nerve conduction studies are useful to distinguish between neuropathy, neuromuscular junction, and myopathy.

Biopsy to differentiate between the myopathies where the cause is not clear.

Imaging with MRI has a limited role where the suspicion is one of lower motor neuron dysfunction but can be useful to direct biopsy to affected muscle as evidenced by atrophy and inflammation.

Testing of respiratory function should always be considered in cases of muscle weakness due to the potential for respiratory failure.

Always offer a management plan

In the acute setting, where true muscle weakness is suspected it is important to demonstrate an appreciation of the need to exclude diaphragmatic involvement that would require ventilatory support. Thereafter, treatment would be directed at the cause as determined by relevant investigations. In general terms it would be prudent to discuss management in the context of a multi-disciplinary team and stress the importance of occupational therapy and physiotherapist support in adapting to potential disability where full function may not be expected to be regained despite treatment.

Case 56: Glove and stocking distributions – sensory polyneuropathy

Instruction to the candidate

Please examine this 50-year-old patient's lower limbs and perform further neurological testing as appropriate.

Begin with a summary of positive findings

There is sensory deficit in the distal aspect of the lower limbs bilaterally to approximately 5 cm above the medial malleoli bilaterally. This applies to light touch, pin-prick, proprioception and vibration sense. There is areflexia (sensory limb of reflex arc interrupted) and a Romberg's test is positive.

The strong candidate, despite only being asked to examine the lower limbs, will briefly examine the upper limbs to assess whether there is an associated 'glove' sensory deficit to match the 'stocking' sensory deficit in the lower limbs.

Patients with long-standing sensory polyneuropathies may develop tropic changes such as hair loss, nail changes, and cool extremities.

Follow with a summary of relevant negative findings

- No deficit in tone or power
- Commonly sensory peripheral neuropathy will affect the lower extremities before the upper extremities. Thus, an absence of upper limb deficit may correlate with early or mild disease and warrant discussion as a relevant negative finding
- No sign of Charcot's joint – destruction or deformity of a joint would be indicative of both the chronicity and severity of any sensory deficit and should be commented upon as such
- Comment on the presence or absence of signs consistent with an underlying cause

State the most likely diagnosis on the basis of these findings

'The patient has signs consistent with a diagnosis of a sensory polyneuropathy.'

Offer relevant differential diagnoses

It is important to appreciate that this list is not exhaustive. When approaching the differential diagnosis of a sensory polyneuropathy the aim should be to impress upon the examiner an understanding of the diffuse nature of the peripheral nerve damage. A range of systemic diseases commonly causes symmetrical, distal neuropathy indiscriminately.

Important causes of a sensory polyneuropathy include:

Metabolic
- Diabetes
- Alcohol
- Amyloidosis
- Porphyria

Iatrogenic (drugs)
- Isoniazid
- Amiodarone
- Metronidazole
- Chemotherapy (vinca alkaloids)

Nutritional
Vitamin deficiency – B1, B3, B6, B12 and E

Connective tissue and inflammatory disorders
- Rheumatoid arthritis
- SLE
- Sarcoidosis

Hereditary
- Hereditary sensory neuropathy (HSN)
- Freidreich's ataxia

Infection
- HIV
- Leprosy
- Lyme disease (Borreliosis)

Demonstrate the importance of clinical context – suggest relevant questions that would be taken in a patient history

The past medical history is important in identifying the diseases and medications listed above that are known causes.

Screen for symptoms, which often precede or accompany peripheral neuropathy, including pain – often burning or shooting pain worse at night. Consider resultant loss of function due to poor co-ordination.

Speed of onset can be useful in narrowing the differential diagnosis, acute versus insidious.

Demonstrate an understanding of the value of further investigation

Confirm nerve damage with nerve conduction studies.

Screen for common and easily identifiable causes, such as diabetes and alcohol misuse, with specific testing directed by clinical suspicion.

Always offer a management plan

Treatment is directed at the underlying cause. The strong candidate will realise that, by advocating cessation of a neuropathy-inducing medication, an alternative treatment for the initial condition must be sought.

Case 57: Friedreich's ataxia

Instruction to the candidate

Please examine the lower limbs of this 30-year-old man.

Begin with a summary of positive findings

On inspection of the patient's lower limbs, there is bilateral pes cavus – high-arch deformity of the foot.

Examination reveals:

- Reduced power in all muscle groups – spastic paraparesis
- Reduced knee and ankle jerks bilaterally
- Bilateral extensor plantar reflexes

Examination of sensation reveals decreased vibration sense and loss of proprioception. Pain and temperature sensation are retained.

Additional findings include cerebellar signs with ataxia of all four limbs. Often patients become wheelchair bound but an ataxic gait would be expected.

Additional signs on inspection include marked kypho-scoliosis of the spine. Involvement of the autonomic nervous system may result in bladder dysfunction and presence of a long-term catheter. The upper limbs may be notable for wasting of the small muscles of the hands.

Follow with a summary of relevant negative findings

- Evidence of cardiac disease – cardiomyopathy
- Suspicion of intellectual impairment
- Signs of diabetes

State the most likely diagnosis on the basis of these findings

'This patient has signs consistent with a diagnosis of Friedreich's ataxia as evidenced by:

- Pes cavus
- Pyramidal weakness and extensor plantar reflexes
- Loss of deep tendon reflexes
- Posterior column deficit
- Cerebellar ataxia

Offer relevant differential diagnoses

The differential diagnosis of pes cavus includes:

- Friedreich's ataxia
- Sensorimotor neuropathy (Charcot–Marie–Tooth disease)
- Syringomyelia
- Hereditary spastic paraplegia
- Spinal cerebellar ataxia

Demonstrate the importance of clinical context – suggest relevant questions that would be taken in a patient history

Friedreich's ataxia has autosomal recessive inheritance requiring a detailed family history.

The predominant clinical manifestations of the disease are neurological deficit, cardiomyopathy and diabetes. Thus, screen for cardiac failure with questions pertaining to breathlessness, orthopnoea, and paroxysmal nocturnal dyspnoea.

Assess functional impairment.

Demonstrate an understanding of the value of further investigation

Investigations would centre on genetic testing to provide a diagnosis.

> ### Summary of key points
>
> - Inherited condition
> - Autosomal recessive
> - Due to a triplet repeat expansion affecting the frataxin gene, 9q13
> - Implication of mitochondrial iron accumulation
> - Onset of symptoms in adolescence and progressive

MRI typically reveals spinal cord and, in some cases, cerebellar atrophy.

Always offer a management plan

No disease modifying treatment exists. The principles of management in Friedreich's ataxia are those of supportive care in the context of a multi-disciplinary team with appropriate genetic counselling. The prognosis is poor albeit improved with late onset disease.

Case 58: Charcot–Marie–Tooth disease (hereditary sensorimotor neuropathy – type 1)

Instruction to the candidate

Please examine the lower limbs of this 40-year-old woman.

Begin with a summary of positive findings

On inspection significant symmetrical wasting in the distal lower limbs is evident, giving an appearance of inverted champagne bottles and the patient has gross pes cavus.

On examination:

- Reduced power in distal muscle groups
- Absent or markedly diminished deep tendon reflexes
- Sensory disturbance predominantly affecting proprioception and vibration sense
- Given the inherent difficulty in mobilising, requests to assess gait may be declined by the examiner. However on walking, the patient may demonstrate a bilateral high-stepping gait, due to foot drop, and is clumsy due to muscle weakness and sensory deficit

Additional findings:

- Wasting of the small muscles of the hands/upper limbs
- Kyphosis/scoliosis

Follow with a summary of relevant negative findings

Clinical signs associated with a minority of cases of HSMN type 1 should be looked for and commented upon where absent:

- Palpable peripheral nerves, which are present in approximately a quarter of cases of HSMN type 1

- Essential tremor
- Ataxia

  No upper motor neuron pathology.

State the most likely diagnosis on the basis of these findings

'This patient has signs consistent with a diagnosis of hereditary sensorimotor neuropathy, also known as Charcot–Marie–Tooth disease.'

Offer relevant differential diagnoses

Peripheral neuropathy, which if long standing may produce pes cavus, however weakness would be expected to be less pronounced and sensory deficit more significant with a stocking distribution.

Offer a differential diagnosis of neuromuscular disease resulting in pes cavus:

- HSMN
- Muscular dystrophy
- Friedreich's ataxia
- Syringomyelia
- Cerebral palsy
- Hereditary spastic paraplegia

Demonstrate the importance of clinical context – suggest relevant questions that would be taken in a patient history

Attempt to clarify the age of onset of symptoms, commonly in childhood with difficulties walking, frequent falls and recurrent ankle sprains due to weakness. Obtain a detailed family history due to inherited nature of disease. Assess the impact upon the patient's functional capacity.

Demonstrate an understanding of the value of further investigation

Electromyography, nerve conduction studies and nerve biopsy. Nerve conduction studies (NCS) show severe slowing of conduction velocity in both the motor and sensory nerves. Histology on biopsy confirms demyelinating disease of peripheral nerves with characteristic 'onion bulb' formation.

Consideration may be given to genetic testing – be aware of the association of different mutations within the same gene giving rise to various clinical phenotypes/spectrum of disease.

Always offer a management plan

Principles of management include supportive care in the context of a multi-disciplinary team, with appropriate genetic counselling.

Early implementation of physiotherapy, stretches and foot orthoses/splints can improve function and significantly delay ankle contracture. Surgical intervention for foot deformity may be required later in disease.

Case 59: Shuffling gait – Parkinson's disease

Instruction to the candidate

This 70-year-old man has been suffering with recurrent falls and difficulty mobilising. Please examine his gait and proceed as appropriate.

Begin with a summary of positive findings

The patient has difficulty standing-up from a chair. Thereafter, a slow shuffling gait is evident with a narrow base. There is difficulty starting, turning, and stopping.

Tremor

Tremor of the upper limb may be exacerbated on assessment of gait either as a product of distraction or due to anxiety/stress.

Rigidity

Decreased arm swing, and the typical stooped posture, result, at least in part, from rigidity.

Bradykinesia and postural instability

Effects of bradykinesia and postural instability on gait include:

- Shuffling, short steps
- Dragging of the legs
- Freezing, particularly when initiating a turn

- Festination may develop – quickening of steps, often into a run, to avoid falling

Postural instability is tested clinically with the pull test, firmly pulling the patient by the shoulders from behind. Where postural reflexes are intact, balance is normally maintained with minimal retropulsion. Patients with postural instability however, are likely to fall or take multiple steps backwards.

Further examination should focus on the upper limbs.

Follow with a summary of relevant negative findings

Postural instability is a late sign in Parkinson's disease. As such, where falls or instability are a prominent feature, and occur early in the context of parkinsonism, the patient is more likely to be suffering from a Parkinsonian syndrome. Look for evidence of progressive supranuclear palsy or multiple system atrophy.

State the most likely diagnosis on the basis of these findings

'Parkinson's disease or Parkinsonism.' For discussion in relation to differential diagnosis, history, investigation and management see *Resting tremor* (p. 90).

Case 60: Ataxic gait

Instruction to the candidate

Please examine this 57-year-old patient complaining of dizziness when walking. Perform a gait assessment and proceed to relevant further examination before discussing the case with the examiner.

Begin with a summary of positive findings

A broad based unsteady gait, which at times lurches to one side. Efforts to compensate by slowing the speed of movement and shortening the length of stride may be evident.

Additional findings on subsequent cerebellum examination may include:

- Nystagmus
- Slurring of speech
- Intention tremor
- Past-pointing (dysmetria)
- Dysdiadochokinesia
- Generalised hypotonia

Follow with a summary of relevant negative findings

Rule out evidence of spasticity and upper motor neuron weakness.

A paucity of cerebellar symptoms on further examination may be indicative of either sensory or vestibular ataxia as a culprit for the changes in gait.

State the most likely diagnosis on the basis of these findings

'This patient has an ataxic gait, with associated signs of cerebellar disease.'

Differential diagnosis, history, investigation and management

See *Intention tremor* (p. 92)

Case 61: Unilateral high-stepping gait

Instruction to the candidate

A 28-year-old man has been experiencing difficulty with his gait having recently been involved in an accident. He complains of limping and tripping. Assess his gait and examine the lower limbs.

Begin with a summary of positive findings

Examination of gait reveals:

- On walking, the right foot is lifted higher than the left
- There is a right-sided foot drop
- When the right foot is placed back on the ground, there is an apparent 'slap' of the sole of the foot on the floor
- The left foot appears to move normally

Focused examination of the right lower limb:

- Weakness in dorsiflexion
- Weakness of foot eversion
- Sensory signs such as loss of sensation over the dorsal and lateral aspect of the foot in the distribution of the superficial peroneal nerve

Follow with a summary of relevant negative findings

- No signs of bilateral disease
- Weakness of foot inversion would suggest an L5 radiculopathy and the sensory loss would not correspond to that of the superficial peroneal nerve
- Absence of any scars around the head of the fibula

State the most likely diagnosis on the basis of these findings

'This patient has a unilateral high-stepping gait as a sign of common peroneal nerve palsy.'

Offer relevant differential diagnoses

The causes of common peroneal nerve palsy include:

- Trauma – the course of the peroneal nerve, wrapping around the lateral side of the fibula head, leaves in vulnerable to injury. Compression or transection caused by the impact of a car in road traffic accidents is common
- Any cause of a mononeuropathy affecting this nerve – diabetes mellitus, mononeuritis multiplex commonly as the result of vasculitis

Demonstrate the importance of clinical context – suggest relevant questions that would be taken in a patient history

Rule out trauma and enquire as to recent immobilisation in a below or above knee cast which may in of itself result in compression.

Demonstrate an understanding of the value of further investigation

Nerve conduction studies will provide supportive evidence of the diagnosis demonstrating superficial peroneal nerve conduction block.

Other investigations may include blood tests to rule out causes of mono-neuropathies including HbA1c, ESR, and auto-antibodies (ANCA, dsDNA).

Always offer a management plan

In the absence of underlying diseases such as diabetes, management is supportive in the context of a multi-disciplinary team. Many patients with a foot drop and high-stepping gait will have no objective problems with mobility and will require no active management at all.

Case 62: Spastic hemi-paretic gait

Instruction to the candidate

Examine the gait of this 75-year-old woman.

Begin with a summary of positive findings

Gait examination

The patient has an obvious unilateral gait disturbance. The left leg is held in full knee extension with the foot pointed towards the ground. The left leg, instead of being lifted upwards in the course of forward movement, is swung in an arc (circumducted) without much vertical movement. The right leg moves in a grossly normal way.

Further examination

Increased tone in the left lower limb with a pyramidal distribution of weakness. Brisk reflexes and an extensor plantar response.

The left upper limb is held in flexion at the elbow.

Follow with a summary of relevant negative findings

Focus upon evidence of underlying aetiologies, principally atrial fibrillation with an irregular pulse and signs of anticoagulation, murmurs or carotid bruits.

State the most likely diagnosis on the basis of these findings

'This patient has a hemiparetic gait in the context of signs of left-sided upper motor neuron weakness. The most likely cause for these signs would be a right middle cerebral artery stroke which may be either ischaemic or haemorrhagic in origin.'

Offer relevant differential diagnoses

Infarction can be considered ischaemic or haemorrhagic. Causative lesions leading to ischaemia can be due to:

- Embolism arising from the heart, aorta or proximal vessels
- Atherosclerotic plaques affecting the extracranial or intracranial arteries
- Carotid artery dissection (commonest cause of ischaemic stroke in patients under 40 years of age)
- Hypercoagulability and diseases that cause thrombosis of small vessels

Other causes of upper motor neuron weakness include:

- Space occupying lesions
- Trauma
- Degenerative disease such as motor neuron disease (should only be mentioned in the complete absence of sensory signs) or demyelinating conditions

Demonstrate the importance of clinical context – suggest relevant questions that would be taken in a patient history

- Speed of onset – sudden (stroke) versus gradual (motor neuron disease)
- Assess functional impairment
- Screen for cardiovascular risk:
  - Smoking
  - Hypertension
  - Hypercholesterolaemia
  - Diabetes

Identify symptoms consistent with previous transient ischaemic attacks.

Demonstrate an understanding of the value of further investigation

Acute stroke demands urgent CT head with subsequent consideration of thrombolysis and transfer to a stroke centre. Aside from imaging, the investigations required will depend on the likely underlying cause.

Ischaemic stroke:

- Blood tests to assess cardiovascular risk, including HbA1c and lipid profile
- A 12-lead electrocardiogram to ensure to rule out atrial fibrillation. Other, less common pieces of useful information would include the presence of sustained ST elevation post-MI which may be suggestive of left ventricular aneurysm formation which can predispose to left ventricular mural clot formation
- A trans-thoracic echocardiogram will identify any structural abnormalities of the heart and, in the setting of atrial fibrillation, give information about the size of the left atrium, which is important for consideration of cardioversion
- A 24-hour tape will potentially identify any underlying arrhythmias
- Carotid Doppler will identify any carotid stenosis. It is worthwhile reviewing the indications for carotid endarterectomy in the setting of cerebrovascular events

MRI with contrast should be considered where signs of raised intracranial pressure suggest a space-occupying lesion.

Always offer a management plan

In the first instance recommend evaluation of potential for thrombolysis in acute stroke. Then consider, secondary stroke prevention – anti-hypertensive, anti-platelets, anti-coagulation, statin therapy, and attending to reversible causes of thromboembolism including anticoagulation and/or rhythm control of atrial fibrillation or endarterectomy for critical carotid disease.

Functional impairment is often significant, with rehabilitation and recovery dependent upon a multi-disciplinary team.

Consider treatment options for neoplastic disease, including palliative management.

Case 63: Waddling gait

Instruction to the candidate

Please examine this 50-year-old woman's gait having presented complaining of increasing difficulty climbing the stairs in recent months.

Begin with a summary of positive findings

On walking, the patient appears unsteady and displays a waddling gait, with excessive hip swing. When asked to rise from a seated position with arms crossed, the patient has insufficient strength to stand. Upper limb proximal weakness may be suggested by an inability to raise arms above the head.

Candidates should be alert to signs of underlying causes on general inspection:

- Centripedal obesity, purple striae, characteristic facial appearance – Cushingoid
- Heliotrope rash and Gottron's papules.

Muscles may be painful –dermatomyositis
- Scleroderma/SLE
- Irregular pulse of atrial fibrillation, profuse sweating, in a thin patient – thyrotoxicosis
- Ptosis and fatiguability – myasthenia gravis

Follow with a summary of relevant negative findings

Signs consistent with upper motor neuron pathology – mixed upper and lower motor neuron signs would be highly suggestive of motor neuron disease.

There is no associated sensory loss, which would favour peripheral nerve pathology.

State the most likely diagnosis on the basis of these findings

'This patient has a waddling gait, consistent with proximal myopathy.' For discussion in relation to differential diagnosis, history, investigation and management see *Proximal myopathy* (p. 101).

Case 64: Cauda equina syndrome

Instruction to the candidate

A 36-year-old man presents with a 2-week history of progressive bilateral sciatica, lower limb weakness, and sensory loss in a peri-anal distribution. Please examine the lower limbs.

Begin with a summary of positive findings

Examination findings include:

- Diminished straight leg raising (with or without positive sciatic stretch test)
- Bilateral (may be asymmetrical) global lower motor neuron weakness (flexors and extensors affected) including foot drop
- Decreased or absent lower limb reflexes with flexor plantar responses

- Sensory impairment in saddle/peri-anal (S2–5) distribution. Highlighting the importance of a comprehensive assessment of sensation that includes the posterior aspects of the thighs which will allude to this deficit
- Decreased anal sphincter tone should be suspected and an assessment offered – the examiner is likely to be content with identification of sensory disturbance and expect only a discussion in this respect

Follow with a summary of relevant negative findings

UMN signs – pyramidal weakness, brisk reflexes, and extensor plantars would suggest conus medullaris syndrome.

Signs suggestive of underlying causes:

- Vesicular rash over the lumbar spine to suggest HSV-1/2 or varicella
- Erythema nodosum to suggest sarcoid, TB or Behçet's
- Inguinal lymphadenopathy to suggest lymphoproliferative or 'atypical' infectious disorder

State the most likely diagnosis on the basis of these findings

'This patient has localisation of all his physical signs to the lower sacral roots with motor, sensory and sphincter involvement. There are no upper motor neuron signs. The abnormality is in the cauda equina only.'

Offer relevant differential diagnoses

Causes of cauda equina syndrome include:

- Neoplastic – carcinoma especially breast, ovarian, and lymphoproliferative disease including myeloma
- Infection – herpetic, varicella, CMV, Lyme, TB, Brucellosis
- Inflammatory – sarcoid, vasculitides including Behçet's and Wegener's
- Auto-immune – acute inflammatory demyelinating polyneuropathy (AIDP) (GBS), chronic inflammatory demyelinating polyneuropathy (CIDP)
- Congenital – neural tube defects including spina bifida
- Central disc bulge with compression of lower sacral roots

Demonstrate the importance of clinical context – suggest relevant questions that would be taken in a patient history

Seek to elicit onset of pain in the buttocks radiating to the lower limbs and/or difficulty walking.

Incontinence of urine or faeces represent red flag symptoms and as such must be emphasised both in the history and by making a clear assessment of sensation on the back of the legs and perineal region with or without examination of anal tone. If only the distal region of the cauda is compressed, incontinence may present in the absence of lower limb weakness.

Demonstrate an understanding of the value of further investigation

Confirming the lesion

Neurophysiology – nerve conduction velocities and denervation changes on EMG can differentiate demyelinating from axonal pathology.

Identifying a cause

- Urgent MRI lumbo-sacral spine ensuring that the field goes high enough to include the entirety of the cauda equina
- Blood tests – ESR, CRP, serum electrophoresis, blood cultures, TB Elispot, ACE, bacterial/viral serological testing, immune screen
- CSF analysis – white cell count, protein, ACE levels, oligoclonal studies, cytology, culture, PCR testing, CSF serology

Always offer a management plan

This is considered a neuro-surgical emergency, particularly with sphincter involvement.

Imaging should differentiate structural or compressive (disc/tumour) lesion requiring urgent neurosurgery, from medical (infection/inflammation) requiring anti-microbials/steroid treatments.

Case 65: Absent ankle jerks with extensor plantar reflexes – sub-acute degeneration of the cord

Instruction to the candidate

This 40-year-old man presents having experienced difficulty with co-ordination, poor balance and an unsteady gait. Please examine the lower limbs.

Begin with a summary of positive findings

Examination of the lower limbs reveals:

- Stocking distribution of sensory deficit with impaired proprioception and vibration sense
- Weakness with spasticity
- Absent ankle reflexes in the context of normal knee reflexes
- The plantar reflexes exhibit an extensor response bilaterally

Additional findings associated with B12 deficiency:

- On general inspection – aged appearance, with greying of hair and a red swollen tongue
- Gait assessment – as suggested by the vignette, cerebellar pathology with broad based ataxic gait Romberg positive
- Mild cognitive impairment

Follow with a summary of relevant negative findings

The patient does not have pes cavus. In the absence of cerebellar signs, and the setting of absent ankle jerks and extensor plantars, pes cavus would suggest a diagnosis of Friedreich's ataxia and 'rarer' spinocerebellar ataxias.

No evidence of aortic regurgitation, which could support a diagnosis of treponemal infection.

State the most likely diagnosis on the basis of these findings

'This patient has absent ankle jerks and extensor plantar reflexes in the context of peripheral neuropathy, spasticity, and a suspicion of cerebellar pathology. Deficits at multiple levels of the nervous system strongly suggest a unifying diagnosis of sub-acute degeneration of the cord as the result of vitamin B12 deficiency.'

Offer relevant differential diagnoses

Differential diagnosis of B12 deficiency

- Pernicious anaemia
- Conditions affecting the terminal ileum – commonly Crohn's disease, also coeliac's disease
- Dietary deficiency or malnutrition often in the context of alcohol dependence

Differential diagnosis of absent ankle jerks and extensor plantar response

This combination of signs is most commonly caused by dual pathology such as an upper motor neuron lesion causing extensor plantars (cervical myelopathy – spondylosis of spine) in combination with a peripheral neuropathy (diabetes) causing absent ankle jerks.

Single disease entities that can cause this combination of signs include:

- Subacute combined degeneration of the cord due to vitamin B12 deficiency
- Friedreich's ataxia
- Quaternary syphilis (tabo paresis). Candidates should note that it is better to refer to tabes or treponemal infection rather than syphilis
- Amyotrophic lateral sclerosis (ALS) – motor neurone disease
- Certain forms of hereditary spastic paraplegia
- Copper deficiency as a mimic of subacute combined degeneration of the cord

Demonstrate the importance of clinical context – suggest relevant questions that would be taken in a patient history

Look to identify triggers such as alcohol dependency or autoimmune disorders including pernicious anaemia and diabetes. Interestingly, metformin can further compound vitamin B12 deficiency.

Demonstrate an understanding of the value of further investigation

Blood testing – B12 levels. Folate levels are routinely checked however folate deficiency, while mimicking the haematolgical manifestations, do not cause neurological deficit. Often cases with significant neurological deficit are not associated with a megaloblastic anaemia, as would be expected.

Schilling test where pernicious anaemia suspected.

Where the aetiology is unclear, in addition to the above consider neurophysiological testing and cross-sectional imaging to assess for central lesions in view of spastic paraparesis.

Always offer a management plan

Intramuscular B12. Initially weekly to restore levels to normal, with monthly regimes thereafter as maintenance. Treatment reverses or halts progression of most, if not all, sequelae of B12 deficiency.

Chapter 3

Respiratory system (station 1)

Case 66: Pulmonary fibrosis

Instruction to the candidate

Please examine this 64-year-old man who has been complaining of exertional breathlessness. When you have finished, please present your findings to the examiner.

Begin with a summary of positive findings

Positive findings on examination of the chest will include:

- Bilateral decreased expansion
- Bibasal dullness to percussion
- Auscultation reveals fine, end-inspiratory crepitations bibasally with increased vocal fremitus
- There may be signs of associated pulmonary hypertension – raised JVP, parasternal heave and loud P2 on auscultation

Note that findings may be restricted to one hemithorax (e.g. in radiotherapy-related fibrosis), and might be either apical (e.g. ankylosing spondylitis, tuberculosis) or basal (e.g. fibrosing alveolitis).

See **Table 3.1** for a summary of signs that may be seen in a patient with pulmonary fibrosis, including those that may point to an underlying cause for the fibrotic process.

Follow with a summary of relevant negative findings

Important relevant negatives include:

- The absence of breathlessness at rest
- The absence of cyanosis
- The absence of signs suggestive of an underlying cause

State the most likely diagnosis on the basis of these findings

'This patient has signs consistent with a diagnosis of pulmonary fibrosis.'

Pulmonary fibrosis nomenclature

Pulmonary fibrosis has a number of alternative names: interstitial lung disease (ILD); diffuse parenchymal lung disease (DPLD). In common clinical practice these terms are used interchangeably and candidates should not worry about using either term. ILD is the nomenclature used in the BTS guidelines. The terms idiopathic pulmonary fibrosis and cryptogenic fibrosing alveolitis specifically describe fibrosis without an identifiable underlying cause, and are not alternative terms for ILD.

Table 3.1 Clinical signs that may be seen in pulmonary fibrosis		
Type of sign	Sign	Potential underlying cause of fibrosis
General	Finger clubbing	–
	Bruising (steroid use)	–
Hand	Symmetrical deforming polyarthropathy	Rheumatoid arthritis
	Sclerodactyly	Systemic sclerosis
Facial	Microstomia, 'beaked' nose	Systemic sclerosis
	Lupus pernio	Sarcoidosis
Skin	Grey discolouration	Amiodarone
	India ink tattoo Well demarcated erythema and telangiectasia	External beam radiotherapy
Posture	'Question-mark spine'	Ankylosing spondylitis

Offer relevant differential diagnoses

The differential diagnosis can be considered in relation to the clinical sign, that of crepitations, and relating to the aetiology of interstitial lung disease itself.

The differential diagnosis of lung crepitations includes:

- Consolidation
- Bronchiectasis
- Pulmonary oedema – congestive cardiac failure

The causes of interstitial lung disease can be classified by underlying cause:

- Idiopathic/cryptogenic
- Dusts:
  - Organic: bird droppings, *Aspergillus fumigatus*, *Micropolyspora faeni*
  - Inorganic: asbestos, coal dust, silica
- Drugs:
  - Common: nitrofurantoin
  - Anti-rheumatic: methotrexate
  - Anti-cancer: bleomycin
  - Anti-arrhythmics: amiodarone
- Rheumatological disease/systemic disease:
  - Rheumatoid arthritis
  - Systemic sclerosis
  - Ankylosing spondylitis
  - Sarcoidosis
- Radiotherapy
- Infection: tuberculosis

Demonstrate the importance of clinical context – suggest relevant questions that would be taken in a patient history

Relevant questions would include:

- Drug history to identify use of a medication known to cause ILD
- Past medical history
- Occupation: may elicit exposure to organic and inorganic dusts
- Exercise tolerance and other functional aspects

Demonstrate an understanding of the value of further investigation

Suspicion of fibrosis in a breathless or hypoxic patient can be supported by findings on a plain chest radiograph and to a large extent confirmed by demonstrating a restrictive pattern on spirometry. High resolution CT is diagnostic and allows classification based on pattern which is further supported by an array of laboratory tests, biopsies, and lavage where indicated.

Peripheral oxygen saturations are typically low, with hypoxia and hypocapnia due to tachypnoea on arterial blood gases.

Plain chest radiograph

Reticulonodular shadowing in the distribution of the crepitations on clinical examination, with a 'honeycombing' pattern indicative of more advanced disease. Remember also that the plain film may also demonstrate signs pointing towards an underlying secondary cause for the fibrosis, such as peri-hilar lymphadenopathy in pulmonary sarcoidosis or pleural plaques from asbestos exposure.

Spirometry and lung function tests

These demonstrate a restrictive pattern, with a reduction in gas transfer factor. Note that, in addition to providing supporting evidence towards a diagnosis of ILD, lung function tests also provide prognostic evidence. A reduction in FVC of 10% or more and/or a reduction in TLCO of 15% or more in the first 6–12 months from diagnosis indicates a higher risk of mortality.

6 minute walk test:

This is useful to quantify exercise and functional capacity, and has adverse prognostic implications in idiopathic pulmonary fibrosis if post-test peripheral oxygen saturations fall to less than 88% on air.

Laboratory blood tests

This will include ANA, ANCA, ESR and rheumatoid factor as part of a vasculitic screen. In addition, if clinically indicated based on the history, serum IgG to organic dusts are useful in confirming a diagnosis of hypersensitivity pneumonitis (also known as 'extrinsic allergic alveolitis').

High-resolution CT of the thorax

This will confirm the extent of fibrosis and will also allow classification of the fibrosis according to the radiological pattern.

Lung biopsy

With the advent of high-resolution CT scanning, histological evidence is not always necessary.

Bronchoalveolar lavage (BAL)

This is not necessary for diagnosis, but may be supportive and has particular utility in ruling out alternative diagnoses. BAL fluid composition typically includes neutrophils, a poor prognostic marker, and less commonly eosinophils. The absence of lymphocytes is indicative of idiopathic rather than nonidiopathic pulmonary fibrosis.

Always offer a management plan

Important points:

Management of pulmonary fibrosis depends upon the underlying cause. Many PACES discussions will centre upon the management of idiopathic disease in particular. In the absence of clinical signs pointing towards a secondary cause, it is perfectly reasonable to tell the examiner 'the management of idiopathic pulmonary fibrosis includes…' where a reversible or removable secondary cause has been identified, this should be treated or removed where possible. Smoking cessation should be actively promoted.

No treatment strategy has been shown to improve outcomes in idiopathic disease.

There is ongoing research into triple therapy with steroids, azathioprine and N-acetylcysteine. Interim analysis from the PANTHER (Prednisolone, Azathioprine and N-acetylcysteine: A Study That Evaluates Response in IPF) trial revealed that triple therapy was associated with greater mortality, more hospitalisations and more serious adverse events than the placebo. Therefore, the triple therapy arm of the trial was stopped. Note that neither steroid monotherapy, nor a steroid and azathioprine combination, are advocated in the BTS guidelines.

Oxygen therapy for symptomatic treatment of significant hypoxaemia.

Lung transplantation is a possibility in those <65 years old and without significant comorbidity. The indications for this are:

- TLCO <40% of predicted
- Progressive decline in FVC by 15% or more over 6 months

The BTS guidelines stress the importance of a multi-disciplinary approach to ILD and you should in turn demonstrate to the examiner that you too promote this approach.

Case 67: Consolidation

Instruction to the candidate

A 56-year-old man presented during the acute medical take with a productive cough and fever. Please examiner his respiratory system and present your findings to the examiner.

Begin with a summary of positive findings

The diagnosis is made based upon the results of chest examination, with additional findings providing further information.

Findings on chest examination, in this case indicating consolidation at the right base, include:

- Decreased expansion at the right base
- Dullness to percussion at the right base
- On auscultation, right basal coarse inspiratory crepitations with bronchial breathing and increased vocal fremitus
- Additionally, the patient may have localise pleural rubs (arising from pleural irritation) and/or a small parapneumonic effusion

Possible additional findings in the patient with consolidation include a sputum pot by the bedside, with purulent sputum and possibly haemoptysis. Herpetic lesion on the lips may be noted in the patient with streptococcal pneumonia.

Follow with a summary of relevant negative findings

If absent, comment on the lack of:

- Signs of respiratory distress
- Tar staining of the fingers (usually unilaterally as smokers tend to hold their cigarettes in the same hand each time)

State the most likely diagnosis on the basis of these findings

'This patient has signs consistent with a diagnosis of consolidation at the right lung base.'

Offer relevant differential diagnoses

Other causes of crepitations include congestive cardiac failure, interstitial lung disease and bronchiectasis.

The differential diagnosis of underlying causes for consolidation include an infective process (most commonly bacterial pneumonia), pulmonary malignancy or pulmonary infarction.

The differential diagnosis of common bacteria causing lung consolidation includes:

- *Streptococcus pneumoniae*
- *Haemophilus influenzae*
- *Staphylococcus* – can cause cavitations
- *Moraxella*

Legionella and *Chlamydia psittaci* are the most common causes of an atypical pneumonia, with constitutional signs and symptoms disproportionate to the radiographic evidence of pulmonary involvement.

Demonstrate the importance of clinical context – suggest relevant questions that would be taken in a patient history

Appropriate questioning is aimed to elicit the nature, duration and acute onset of the patient's symptoms:

- Cough, sputum, haemoptysis
- Fever, rigors, general malaise
- Breathlessness
- Effect on daily life and function

Screen for a history of recurrent pneumonia or conditions that predispose to recurrent and/ or severe infection. If elderly, enquire as to compliance with annual vaccination.

Demonstrate an understanding of the value of further investigation

Appropriate investigations in a patient with consolidation include:

- Oxygen saturations. These may be low and in the absence of underlying chronic obstructive airways disease, supplementary oxygen is given, aiming for saturations of 94–98%
- Laboratory tests: A raised white blood cell count and acute phase markers (CRP). Atypical organism serology and blood cultures. *Legionella* urinary antigen test, sputum microscopy, culture and sensitivities
- Plain chest radiograph: Expected to demonstrate a localised area of opacification in a lobar distribution with air bronchograms. Complications visible on the radiograph may include parapneumonic effusion or abscess formation

BTS guidelines advise that a chest radiograph should be repeated at 6 weeks if there is persistence of clinical symptoms or signs despite treatment, or in individuals who are at higher risk of an underlying neoplastic process (especially individuals over 50 years of age and in those with a significant smoking history).

Always offer a management plan

A general summary of the management of a patient with pneumonia would include:

- Oxygen therapy in accordance with the BTS guideline for emergency oxygen use in adult patients, noting to the examiner an awareness of safe oxygen administration in patients with concomitant COPD
- Antibiotics. 'Specific antibiotic choice would depend on local antibiotic guidelines' is a perfectly valid statement, but the examiner will expect you to have a good knowledge of the standard antibiotic choices according to the causative organism and nature and severity of illness (such as whether it is community-acquired, hospital-acquired or aspiration in aetiology
- Intravenous fluids for hypovolaemia, thromboembolic prophylaxis with low molecular heparin and TEDS, and adequate nutritional support should constitute part of the holistic in-patient care of pneumonia
- Chest physiotherapy in individuals with difficulty expectorating or with underlying comorbid chest pathology
- Ongoing monitoring includes aspects such as intravenous to oral antibiotic conversion and vaccination (influenza, parainfluenza and pneumococcus) of at-risk groups

Severity grading – the CURB65 score

The CURB65 score is a validated scoring system to help grade the severity of pneumonia and therefore stratify higher mortality risk. One point is attributed to each of the following:

- **C**onfusion: Generally applied to a AMTS of less than 8
- **U**rea: Greater than 7 mmol/L
- **R**espiratory rate: 30 respirations per minute or greater
- **B**lood pressure: Systolic <90 mmHg, diastolic 60 mmHg or less
- Age **65** or over

A CURB65 score of 2 suggests moderate severity, usually necessitating a short in-patient course of treatment. A score of 3 and above is managed as high severity. This system aids to risk stratification, used to identify a likely pathway of care, but should be applied in conjunction with and not replace clinical judgment.
Other features increasing the risk of mortality are:
- Coexisting disease
- Bilateral or multilobar involvement
- $PaO_2 < 8$ kPa or $SaO_2 < 92\%$

The appropriate management of patients with consolidation includes monitoring for development of possible complications. These include:

- Parapneumonic effusion and empyema (see *Pleural effusion*, p. 122). Exudative effusions predominate, and development of an effusion with persistent high fever and raised inflammatory markers should trigger a high clinical suspicion of empyema. Prompt thoracocentesis and, if the diagnosis is confirmed (e.g by a sample pH of <7.2), complete drainage of the effusion. Prolonged (up to 6 weeks) courses of antibiotics, and in some cases surgical drainage, may be required
- Cavity formation. Several bacteria, such as *Staphylococcus* and *Klebsiella* have a tendency to form lung cavities
- Respiratory failure. The role of non-invasive (and subsequently invasive) ventilation should be discussed in patients who develop respiratory failure.
- Disseminated sepsis and septic shock.

In a straightforward case such as consolidation, add to the standard management by bringing in concepts such as the Society of Critical Care Medicine's 'Surviving Sepsis' guidelines or the use of community acquired pneumonia care bundles.

Further reading

Lim WS, van der Eerden MM, Laing R, et al. Defining community acquired pneumonia severity on presentation to hospital: an international derivation and validation study. Thorax 2003; 58: 377–382.
Lim WS, Baudouin SV, George RC, et al. BTS guidelines for the management of community acquired pneumonia in adults: update 2009. Thorax 2009; 64:iii1–55.

Case 68: Bronchiectasis

Instruction to the candidate

This 54-year-old man complains of a chronic productive cough. Please examine his respiratory system.

Begin with a summary of positive findings

The patient is cachectic. There is evidence of clubbing in both the hands and feet. On auscultation, positive findings include bilateral widespread coarse inspiratory crepitations with associated inspiratory clicks.

The key clinical signs in bronchiectasis are: **C**lubbing, **C**repitations, and **C**licks. The presence of a sputum pot containing copious quantities of purulent sputum is a key clue in differentiating bronchiectasis from other respiratory cases.

Follow with a summary of relevant negative findings

Important relevant negative findings to comment on if absent include; resting tachypnoea, cyanosis and kyphoscoliosis.

State the most likely diagnosis on the basis of these findings

'This patient has signs consistent with a diagnosis of bronchiectasis.'

Offer relevant differential diagnoses

The differential diagnosis for crepitations includes consolidation, congestive heart failure, and interstitial lung disease.

Bronchiectasis can be congential or acquired

Congenital causes for bronchiectasis include:

- Cystic fibrosis
- Kartagener's syndrome (primary ciliary dyskinesia or immotile ciliary syndrome, characterised by bronchiectasis, infertility and situs inversus)
- Immunodeficiency due to hypogammaglobulinaemia (may be congenital or acquired)
- Congenital kyphoscoliosis

Acquired causes of bronchiectasis can be due to:

- Infection:
  - Viral: measles
  - Bacterial: pertussis, tuberculosis (the commonest cause worldwide)
  - Fungal: aspergillosis, ABPA

- Mechanical bronchial obstruction, either by a foreign body or by a mass (e.g. tumour or lymph node) causing external compression
- In association with autoimmune disorders such as rheumatoid arthritis and inflammatory bowel disease
- Recurrent aspiration in gastro-oesophageal reflux disease, in alcoholics
- Yellow nail syndrome

Additionally, the distribution of bronchiectasis can vary according to the underlying cause (**Table 3.2**).

Demonstrate the importance of clinical context – suggest relevant questions that would be taken in a patient history

Important questions in a clinical history of a patient with bronchiectasis would include:

Identifying the underlying cause

- Is there a known diagnosis of relevant conditions?
- Is there any history of childhood infections?
- Is there a history of recurrent chest infections? If there is, note the number of infective exacerbations and courses of antibiotics per year.

Establishing the patient's current symptoms and functional status

- Chronic cough with large volume, purulent sputum on a daily basis
- Haemoptysis
- Fevers, night sweats and constitutional symptoms
- Weight loss or inability to gain weight

Table 3.2 Localisation of bronchiectasis according to underlying cause	
Location	Cause
Apical	Tuberculosis
Lobar distribution	Mechanical obstruction, e.g. tumour or foreign body
Proximal	ABPA
ABPA, allergic bronchopulmonary aspergillosis.	

The functional status alludes to exercise tolerance and effect on activities of daily living.

Demonstrate an understanding of the value of further investigation

Imaging modalities include:

- Plain chest radiograph, which would show ring shadows and tramlines
- High resolution CT to clearly delineate the distribution of disease and potentially identify a secondary cause

Sputum analysis is used to identify infective organisms and antibiotic susceptibility. Patients with bronchiectasis are often colonised with multiple bacteria, which may be resistant to multiple antibiotics as a consequence of multiple acute infectious episodes, multiple antibiotic courses and nosocomial exposure to pathogens.

On formal spirometry a pattern consistent with obstructive airway disease with limited reversibility would be expected.

Investigations to identify underlying cause would include:

- CF sweat test and genetic testing
- TB elispot
- Serum immunoglobulins, electrophoresis, *Aspergillus* precipitins, rheumatoid factor
- Bronchoscopy to exclude bronchial obstruction if suggested by history (weight loss, haemoptysis, or history of foreign object inhalation) or by imaging (HRCT suggesting a bronchial malignancy). Bronchoscopy may also be indicated in sputum negative cases in which atypical mycobacterial infection is suspected.

Always offer a management plan

The management of individual cases depends on the underlying cause of the bronchiectasis.

General principles of management include:

- Physiotherapy and postural drainage on a daily basis is key
- Saline nebulisers may aid sputum expectoration
- Antibiotic therapy for acute exacerbations tailored to the patient's sputum analysis, and long-term antibiotics in cases of three or more exacerbations per annum
- Inhaled bronchodilators to reduce airway obstruction
- Orally administered mucolytics may be considered in complex cases

Other therapeutic options include control of localised disease to prevent complications including surgical removal of affected tissue, or embolisation in the setting of severe or recurrent haemoptysis.

Complications of bronchiectasis include pleural effusions, pneumothorax, cerebral abscesses and secondary amyloidosis. Cor pulmonale can also occur in the long term.

The importance of childhood vaccinations to prevent diseases such as measles, known to cause bronchiectasis, should be emphasised to demonstrate importance of disease prevention.

Further reading

Pasteur MC, Bilton D, Hill AT. British Thoracic Society guideline for non-CF bronchiectasis. Thorax 2010; 65:i1–58.I

Case 69: Pleural effusion

Instruction to the candidate

This 75-year-old woman has been complaining of worsening exertional breathlessness. Please examine her respiratory system and present your findings to the examiner.

Begin with a summary of positive findings

In a case of a right-sided, unilateral pleural effusion, the positive chest findings would be:

- Decreased expansion on the right
- A stony dull percussion note at the right base
- Decreased breath sounds and decreased vocal fremitus at the right base on auscultation

Associated findings to look for include scars. Such scars could be from chest drain insertion, biopsies (including lymph node incisions) and surgical interventions. If the patient in the station has a chest drain in situ, the candidate should comment on its contents and whether it appears to be swinging with respiration or bubbling, often elicited with a short sharp cough.

Follow with a summary of relevant negative findings

If the following signs are not present, comment on their absence:

- Tachypnoea
- Oxygen supplementation
- Cachexia
- Cervical lymphadenopathy

State the most likely diagnosis on the basis of these findings

'This patient has signs consistent with a right-sided unilateral pleural effusion.'

Offer relevant differential diagnoses

The differential diagnosis can be considered either as that of dullness to percussion, or of the underlying cause of the pleural effusion. The differential diagnosis of dullness to percussion on chest examination is:

- Lobar collapse
- Consolidation
- Pleural thickening
- Raised right hemi-diaphragm

The differential diagnosis can also be considered in the context of the cause of the effusion. Effusions can be classified as transudates or exudates. When the protein content of an effusion exceeds 30 mg/dL it is classed as an exudate, of which the most common underlying causes are pneumonia and malignancy. When the protein content is less than 25 mg/dL, the effusion is a transudate, of which the most common causes are cardiac failure, liver failure and renal failure. When the protein content is between 25 and 30 mg/dL then Light's criteria should be applied to determine its classification.

Light's criteria state that an effusion is likely to be an exudate when:

- Fluid:serum protein ratio >0.5
- Fluid:serum LDH ratio >0.6
- Fluid LDH greater than 2/3 the normal serum LDH level

Transudative pleural effusions are commonly bilateral in nature. The likely underlying process in a patient with a unilateral effusion is exudative.

Where there is no evidence of an infective process, infarction, inflammation and malignancy should be considered. Common malignancies that invade the pleura and give rise to a pleural effusion include primary lung adenocarcinoma, mesothelioma, and secondary metastases.

Demonstrate the importance of clinical context – suggest relevant questions that would be taken in a patient history

Important questions in a clinical history from a patient with a pleural effusion would include:

- Questions to elicit symptoms from the effusion including breathlessness on exertion and resultant functional deficit
- Questions to identify symptoms suggestive of an infective cause. Screen for fevers, prurulent sputum, and a history of TB exposure/risk
- Screen for malignancy. Is there weight loss, a new or persistent cough, haemoptysis or voice change in the context of a significant smoking history? Be sure to establish history of previous malignancy
- Is there a recent history of cardiac surgery, which would raise the possibility of a chylothorax?

Demonstrate an understanding of the value of further investigation

Principles of investigation of a pleural effusion include imaging and fluid analysis.

Imaging modalities include

- Plain chest radiograph to confirm the presence of an effusion. May also demonstrate evidence of consolidation, collapse, areas of cavitation or pleural plaques, all of which would give supporting evidence towards an underlying diagnosis
- Ultrasound to accurately assess the size of the effusion and comment on the degree of loculation. It is important to obtain an ultrasound if drainage is being considered

Effusion analysis

Most patients will undergo a diagnostic aspiration to allow fluid analysis, with the removal of approximately 20–40 ml of fluid. Therapeutic aspiration is only performed in the presence of cardiorespiratory compromise. Aspiration is not performed in the context of a bilateral pleural effusion unless there are atypical features or there is a failure to respond to treatment.

Fluid is sent for:

- Biochemistry: protein, LDH,
- Microscopy, culture and sensitivity
- Cytology
- pH analysis. A pH of <7.2 is suggestive of an empyema

Always offer a management plan

The management can be considered in relation to that of the effusion itself and of any underlying cause.

When fluid analysis suggests empyema, the effusion should be drained to dryness. Antibiotics for parapneumonic effusions and empyema should take note of culture results and follow local guidelines.

In the absence of underlying infection, the most likely cause of a unilateral pleural effusion is a neoplastic cause. This can lead to a discussion with the examiner of the principles of diagnosis and management of lung malignancies. This involves confirming the diagnosis through cross-sectional imaging and tissue biopsy, followed by staging. Appropriate management is decided in a multi-disciplinary setting, with treatment options including chemotherapy, radiotherapy and surgical excision, with curative or palliative intent.

Case 70: Collapse

Instruction to the candidate

This 55-year-old woman complains of chronic breathlessness. Please examine her respiratory system.

Begin with a summary of positive findings

Positive findings on respiratory examination include:

- Tracheal deviation towards the affected side
- Unilateral decreased expansion
- Ipsilateral dullness to percussion
- Ispilateral diminished breath sounds
- Ipsilateral increased vocal fremitus

Follow with a summary of relevant negative findings

Important negative findings include:

- Tachypnoea
- Evidence of bronchogenic malignancy – tar staining, clubbing, cachexia

State the most likely diagnosis on the basis of these findings

'This patient has signs consistent with a diagnosis of lung collapse [stating the location].'

> ### Collapse
>
> Collapse is essentially a differential for a chest with decreased breath sounds and dullness to percussion. That said, if the exact constellation of clinical signs does arise, the PACES candidate would be expected to arrive upon the exact diagnosis. Collapse can be differentiated from consolidation by the presence of tracheal deviation towards the affected side, and the absence of bronchial breathing.

Offer relevant differential diagnoses

A sensible differential diagnosis of the elicited signs should be given. For example, 'the differential diagnosis for dullness to percussion includes consolidation and a pleural effusion. The percussion note in a pleural effusion would be stony dull, rather than dull and as such the findings are more suggestive of consolidation'.

Commonly lung collapse is found as a complication of pneumonia or as the result of a mass lesion. Mass lesions include:

- External compression – enlarged lymph node (tuberculosis, malignancy)
- Within the airway wall – malignant endobronchial lesion
- Within the airway lumen – inhaled foreign body, mucus plugs

Demonstrate the importance of clinical context – suggest relevant questions that would be taken in a patient history

Important aspects in a clinical history of a patient with lung collapse include establishing current symptoms:

- Cough, haemoptysis
- Sudden, acute onset dyspnoea
- Concomitant infection with purulent sputum, fevers, and general malaise

Establish a smoking history and screen for features such as weight loss, cachexia, and haemoptysis suggestive of malignancy.

Identifying any past medical history of TB or TB exposure, or a previous diagnosis of asthma or ABPA.

Demonstrate an understanding of the value of further investigation

Laboratory blood tests would include quantification of inflammatory markers to assess for active infection – it is common to find pneumonia distal to collapses. Malignancy may be suggested by an anaemic picture, evident on testing of haemoglobin.

Imaging would include a plain chest radiograph with or without cross-sectional imaging. On a plain chest radiograph, expect to see a degree of opacification of the affected lung field with a degree of tracheal deviation towards the affected lung. The 'Sail sign' refers to a specific radiological finding in left lower lobe collapse where the collapsed lobe causes the appearance of a double left heart border. One of the borders is the opacity produced by the collapsed lobe. For persistent collapse, a CT of the chest would be indicated to assess for an endobronchial lesion causing the collapse.

Bronchoscopy may be indicated. As with CT, the possibility of an endobronchial lesion leading to the collapse is the main reason for this investigation. It has the added advantage of the capability to take bronchial washings and biopsies at the time of the investigation.

Always offer a management plan

The management plan depends on underlying cause of the collapse. Present yourself as a safe doctor by impressing upon the examiner the importance of cross-sectional imaging and ultimately bronchoscopy in the patient with collapse to ensure early diagnosis of possible malignancies.

Case 71: Chronic obstructive pulmonary disease

Instruction to the candidate

This 68-year-old man has presented with breathlessness and a productive cough. Please examine his respiratory system and present your findings.

Begin with a summary of positive findings

There are tar stains on the fingers. The chest is hyperexpanded with a reduced sterno-cricoid distance. Expansion is symmetrically decreased with hyper-resonant percussion. Breath

sounds are decreased globally with expiratory wheeze and a prolonged expiratory phase on auscultation. Vocal fremitus is reduced.

Follow with a summary of relevant negative findings

Important relevant negative findings to identify include:

- Signs of respiratory distress such as a resting tachypnea, the use of accessory muscles or the presence of tracheal deviation (this may be indicative of an associated tension pneumothoeax albeit not expected to arise in

the exam setting). Additionally, central and/or peripheral cyanosis, or the use of oxygen
- Signs of previous steroid use for recurrent exacerbations, with fragile thin skin and bruising
- Lymphadenopathy, a marker of possible infection or associated malignancy
- Signs of associated pulmonary hypertension – raised JVP, parasternal heave and loud P2 on auscultation
- Signs of active infective exacerbation – scattered crepitations, presence of a sputum pot containing purulent sputum
- Peripheral oedema that may be a feature of cor pulmonale, hypoalbuminaemia (malnourished patients with chronic disease and increased protein catabolism in recurrent infective exacerbations), or reflect fluid retention due to steroid administration

State the most likely diagnosis on the basis of these findings

'This patient has signs consistent with a clinical diagnosis of chronic obstructive pulmonary disease.'

Bronchitis and emphysema

Bronchitis is a clinical diagnosis that may be made when a patient has a cough productive of sputum on most days for a minimum of three consecutive months per year over a 2-year period. Emphysema is a histological diagnosis demonstrating dilatation of the airways distal to the terminal bronchioles. This can however be suggested by imaging studies.

Offer relevant differential diagnoses

The differential diagnosis for wheeze includes both respiratory (COPD, asthma) and cardiac (heart failure) causes. Strictly speaking, wheeze is an expiratory sound caused by intrathoracic airways obstruction.

Note the importance of age in that the same set of clinical signs (with the exception of the tar staining) in a younger patient could be consistent with a diagnosis of asthma. Patients with severe, difficult-to-control asthma will often have received prolonged courses of oral steroids, and therefore may have a Cushingoid appearance. In the less common scenario of a young patient with signs of COPD but without

tar staining, the diagnosis of α_1-antitrypsin deficiency must also be considered.

Demonstrate the importance of clinical context – suggest relevant questions that would be taken in a patient history

Screen for symptoms, including:

- Dyspnoea: quantify breathlessness by the MRC dyspnoea scale and the impact upon activities of daily living (i.e. a function assessment)
- Cough and sputum production
- Wheeze
- Weight loss

Establish frequency of exacerbations, the number of A&E attendances and hospital admissions in the past year, and the total number of ITU admissions requiring ventilation. Review current treatment and possible use of long-term-oxygen-therapy.

Obtain a smoking history. Smoking and the effect of cessation on retarding the natural progression of the disease should be discussed both in the history and management sections of your presentation respectively. Notwithstanding the fact that it is relevant to both sections, its importance in the management of COPD cannot be overemphasised.

Demonstrate an understanding of the value of further investigation

The investigations required to assess a patient with COPD include:

- Laboratory blood tests: full blood count is useful in demonstrating active infection and secondary polycythaemia. CRP will be raised in active infection
- A plain chest radiograph may show hyperexpanded lung fields with flattened hemi-diaphragms. Bullae may be identified, with a consequent risk of secondary pneumothoraces. Coexisting chest pathology should also be sought, and further investigated by CT
- Lung function tests demonstrate an obstructive deficit with an FEV1 <80% predicted and a post-bronchodilator FEV1:FVC ratio <70%. Note that unlike in asthma, in COPD the obstruction to airflow is not fully reversible

- Arterial blood gases are required in the evaluation for the need of long-term oxygen therapy (LTOT), see below

Always offer a management plan

Whilst COPD is a common case in clinical practice, in PACES the discussion of management is a complex one with key points that must be succinctly stated. A suggested approach might be to tell the examiner that: 'the management of COPD is multi-disciplinary in nature and involves encouragement of smoking cessation at every patient contact. Medical therapy is by a step-wise approach using; short- and long-acting bronchodilators; steroids (inhaled for maintenance therapy and oral for acute exacerbations); theophylline-based drugs are an adjunctive therapy once inhaled therapies have been instituted; mucolytics can be considered for patients with chronic productive cough. Long-term oxygen therapy is used in specific indications to provide a prognostic benefit. Surgical options are less common, but include bullectomy and lung volume reduction surgery'.

As per NICE guidelines, management of COPD should be patient-centred and adopt a multi-disciplinary approach.

Actively encourage smoking cessation. A key phrase from the NICE guidelines of 2010 states that all patients should be 'encouraged to stop, and offered help to do so at every opportunity'. Candidates may examiners by presenting themselves as a proactive doctor in this respect.

Medical therapy in COPD involves a cumulative, step-wise progression of treatment initiation:

- Inhaled therapy guided by spirometry: Bronchodilators include short- and long-acting β_2-agonists and muscarinic antagonists. Inhaled steroids are considered in individuals with FEV1 < 50% or with persistent exacerbations.
- Oral therapy: Oral corticosteroids in acute exacerbations and theophyllines for patients who require a step-up in treatment once established on inhaled therapy.
- Pulmonary rehabilitation
- Oxygen therapy: Both controlled oxygen therapy in acute exacerbations to treat hypoxia whilst avoiding hypercapnia; and LTOT in appropriately selected patients, which is the only treatment shown to improve prognosis in COPD

Long term oxygen therapy

The importance of LTOT is in the prognostic benefit it provides.

Criteria for use:
- The patient must have stopped smoking
- The patient must not have an acute exacerbation
- $PaO_2 < 7.3$kPa

OR

- PaO_2 7.3–8 and one of the following:
  - Secondary polycythaemia
  - Nocturnal hypoxaemia
  - Peripheral oedema
  - Pulmonary hypertension

Oxygen therapy should be maintained for at least 15 hours per day.

It is worth commenting that theophyllines are particularly prone to drug interactions (especially with some antibiotics, such as macrolides, that might also be prescribed in the acute setting). Furthermore, arrhythmia is particularly common given the pro-arrhythmic effects of certain medications (theophyllines, β-agonists), electrolyte depletion and in the presence of sepsis. Therefore, cardiac monitoring and careful management of electrolytes and polypharmacy should not be underestimated.

Non-invasive ventilation (NIV) is used in the acute setting where COPD is complicated by type 2 respiratory failure. Criteria include:

- Hypoxia $PaO_2 < 8$
- Hypercapnia $PaCO_2 > 6$
- Acidosis   pH 7.25–7.35

Many patients with COPD with a pH of less than 7.25 will still be instituted on NIV. This reflects the fact that many patients with COPD are considered unsuitable for endotracheal intubation and invasive ventilation, and NIV is thus an appropriate ceiling of acute treatment.

Pulmonary rehabilitation is an evidence-based programme that is recommended by NICE to reduce hospital admissions and possibly mortality in patients with a recent COPD exacerbation. It entails a programme of education and gym based regimes to increase exercise tolerance.

Further reading

National Institute for Health and Clinical Excellence (NICE), NHS Evidence. Chronic obstructive pulmonary disease: evidence update February 2012. Manchester; NICE, 2012.

Case 72: Lobectomy

Instruction to the candidate

This 73-year-old man is undergoing follow-up from the respiratory physicians. Please examine his respiratory system and present your findings to the examiner.

Begin with a summary of positive findings

The patient is comfortable at rest. The most obvious abnormality on inspection is a well-healed right-sided thoracic scar with underlying chest wall deformity. Chest signs included equal expansion bilaterally, but with dull percussion and decreased breath sounds in the right upper zone when auscultated anteriorly.

> ### Lobectomy scars
>
> Unlike the sternotomy, laparotomy, or appendicectomy scars, all of which are difficult to miss, the lobectomy scar can be very subtle. It runs parallel with the ribs and can therefore 'hide' in the natural skin crease. You must therefore actively look for a lobectomy or pneumonectomy scar, rather than simply expecting to see it on general inspection.

Follow with a summary of relevant negative findings

Important negative findings include:

- Signs of respiratory compromise
- Signs of tar staining which would indicate heavy tobacco smoking
- Signs of abnormal wound healing such as a relatively wide or disorganised scar, or keloid scarring

State the most likely diagnosis on the basis of these findings

'This patient has signs consistent with a right upper lobectomy.'

Offer relevant differential diagnoses

Table 3.3 outlines the differential diagnoses of the indications (and contraindications) for a lobectomy.

Demonstrate the importance of clinical context – suggest relevant questions that would be taken in a patient history

Questions eliciting the history of the operation should focus upon eliciting the timing and indication for lobectomy. In the context of malignancy, establish the pre-operative and post-operative oncological history.

Screen for current symptoms, particularly in relation to shortness of breath and exercise tolerance.

Demonstrate an understanding of the value of further investigation

It is reasonable to tell the examiner that, assuming the patient has been stable since his operation (especially if the procedure was many years ago) then no routine investigations are warranted. Take care to consider what the candidate information card said; if it suggests and acute presentation then give a reasonable account of relevant investigations.

Table 3.3 Lobectomy: indications and contraindications	
Indications	**Contraindications**
Lung malignancy	Poor lung function
Solitary pulmonary nodule	Operative risk
Bronchiectasis: either localised disease or massive pulmonary haemorrhage unresolved by arterial embolisation	
Pulmonary tuberculosis	

If asked, a plain chest radiograph will show absence of the resected lobe with volume loss, altered rib anatomy and tracheal shift towards the resection side.

Always offer a management plan

Given that the definitive management, the lobectomy, has already happened, it is best to use the management part of the presentation as an opportunity to discuss with the examiner the indications, complications and contraindications of thoracic surgery.

Case 73: Pneumonectomy

Instruction to the candidate

Please examine this patient's respiratory system and present your findings.

Begin with a summary of positive findings

The following positive findings assume a right-sided pneumonectomy:

- Inspection: a thoracotomy scar, running from x to y (describe exactly the anatomical site of the scar). There is deformity of the right side of the thoracic cage
- Palapation: there is decreased expansion on the right, with deviation of the trachea to the right
- Percussion: dullness to percussion on the right
- Ausculatation: decreased breath sounds throughout the whole right lung field, apart from in the apex where there is bronchial breathing (this corresponds with air flow through the deviated trachea). Vocal fremitus is decreased on the right

Follow with a summary of relevant negative findings

Relevant negative findings include:

- Signs of respiratory compromise
- Signs of tobacco use
- Signs of abnormal wound healing

State the most likely diagnosis on the basis of these findings

'This patient has signs consistent with a right-sided pneumonectomy.'

> **Pneumonectomy**
>
> In a pneumonectomy, the whole lung is taken out, rather than a single lobe. While the indications remain broadly the same, given the extent of lung involvement, they – and the complications – tend to be much more severe.

Offer relevant differential diagnoses

Give a differential for underlying respiratory conditions leading to the pneumonectomy, with lung malignancy at the top of the list. While the indications for pneumectomy versus lobectomy remain broadly the same, the symptoms and complications tend to be more severe given the extent of lung involvement.

Demonstrate the importance of clinical context – suggest relevant questions that would be taken in a patient history

As with the lobectomy case, history should focus on both the initial symptoms and diagnosis that led to the initial surgery, and also on the patient's current symptoms, questions, and concerns about their condition.

Demonstrate an understanding of the value of further investigation

Again, the investigations would be the same as with the lobectomy case:

- Plain chest radiograph

- Spirometry would demonstrate a much larger deficit in lung function in keeping with the much larger portion of lung removed

You would also mention to the examiner that you might also perform relevant investigations for the underlying respiratory pathology, especially if it is one that could also affect the contralateral lung.

Always offer a management plan

As with the previous case (*Lobectomy*, p. 128), given that the definitive management has already happened, it is best to use the management part of the presentation as an opportunity to discuss with the examiner the indications, complications and contraindications of thoracic surgery.

Case 74: Lung transplantation

Instruction to the candidate

This 50-year-old woman has previously had a cardiothoracic intervention. Please examine her respiratory system and present your findings.

Begin with a summary of positive findings

Positive findings can be divided into the following three categories:

- Signs of the lung transplantation – midline sternotomy
- Signs of an underlying respiratory condition. Note that these may be completely absent
- Signs that indicate immunosuppressant use

Follow with a summary of relevant negative findings

Important relevant negative findings include:

- Signs of respiratory compromise
- Tar staining to indicate tobacco use – Note that current smoking is a contraindication to lung transplantation

State the most likely diagnosis on the basis of these findings

'This patient has signs consistent with previous lung transplantation.'

Offer relevant differential diagnoses

The differential diagnosis for the operative scars includes a joint heart and lung transplant.

The differential diagnosis for indications for lung transplantations includes:

- Diffuse parenchymal lung disease
- Cystic fibrosis
- Bronchiectasis
- α_1-antitrypsin deficiency (the strong candidate will examine for a liver edge in a young patient)
- Pulmonary vascular disease – idiopathic pulmonary hypertension
- Rare diseases – Langerhans cell granulomatosis

Demonstrate the importance of clinical context – suggest relevant questions that would be taken in a patient history

Tell the examiner that you would ask the patient about the underlying respiratory disease that led to the transplant, any complications following the transplant, and any current symptoms.

Demonstrate an understanding of the value of further investigation

In the post-transplant patient, routine investigations may include:

- Laboratory blood tests – inflammatory markers looking for active infection and drug levels of relevant immunosuppressants
- Spirometry looking for obstructive deficit which may suggest bronchiolitis obliterans syndrome (see below).

Always offer a management plan

A management discussion may focus on indication for transplantation and patient selection. NICE states that 'lung transplants are performed in patients with non-malignant pulmonary disease that is unresponsive or minimally responsive to treatment and who have a life expectancy of less than 1 year. The underlying causes include cystic fibrosis, severe pulmonary fibrosis, pulmonary hypertension and obliterative bronchiolitis.'

Contraindications to lung transplantation include:

From the history

- Blood-borne viral infection (hepatitis B or C, HIV)
- Current tobacco use
- Unsuitable psychological profile

From investigations

- Organ dysfunction other than respiratory system

- Concommitant unresolved malignant disease
- Active pulmonary infection

Be prepared to discuss the complications of lung transplantation:

- Acute rejection
- Complications from immunosuppression
- Bronchiolitis obliterans syndrome (BOS) is a form of chronic rejection which involves a progressive obstructive lung defect. It is a process that affects most lung transplants

Further reading

National Institute for Health and Care Excellence (NICE). Living donor lung transplantation for end-stage lung disease, IPG170. London; NICE, 2006.
Todd JL, Palmer SM. Bronchiolitis obliterans syndrome: the final frontier for lung transplantation. Chest 2011; 140:502–508.

Case 75: Plethoric face and dilated chest veins – superior vena cava obstruction

Instruction to the candidate

This 45-year-old man with a significant past medical history has been referred to the acute medical team from oncology clinic. Please examine his respiratory system and comment on your findings.

Begin with a summary of positive findings

On general inspection the patient is plethoric, with rubor of the face, neck and upper chest (**Figure 3.1**). The face and arms are oedematous. On closer inspection of the neck, the patient's neck veins are dilated, with no visible waveform variation in the raised jugular venous pressure. The face is oedematous and the eyes display chemosis.

Remember Pemberton's sign: The development of facial flushing, disteneded head and neck veins, inspiratory stridor and raised JVP on raising both of the patient's arms above their head.

Follow with a summary of relevant negative findings

Things to comment on if absent:

- Signs of respiratory distress: Such signs can be due either to an underlying lung malignancy or as a direct consequence of the obstruction
- Signs suggestive of an underlying primary oncological diagnosis
- Cervical or axillary lymphadenopathy
- Evidence of tobacco use (tar staining of the fingers)

State the most likely diagnosis on the basis of these findings

'This patient has signs consistent with a diagnosis of superior vena cava obstruction, likely secondary to an underlying neoplastic process.'

Offer relevant differential diagnoses

The differential diagnosis for prominent neck veins and breathlessness includes congestive cardiac failure and cardiac tamponade.

See Table 3.4 for secondary causes of SVCO.

Demonstrate the importance of clinical context – suggest relevant questions that would be taken in a patient history

Questions relating to the symptoms of SVC obstruction

- Onset of symptoms. If chronic, suggests that the underlying process may be of gradual compression of the SVC. If acute, can suggest acute thrombosis within the SVC
- Do the symptoms get worse on lying down or stooping?
- Is the patient experiencing headaches?

Questions relating to the underlying diagnosis

- Symptoms of lung cancers (cough, haemoptysis) and general symptoms of malignancy (weight loss, malaise, anaemia symptoms)
- Given that lung cancers are the most common causes of SVC obstruction, an exact and thorough smoking history is vital
- Does the patient already have a primary oncological diagnosis or is this the first presentation of a new cancer? If they already have a diagnosis, what is it, what investigations and management have they had, and when are they next due to see an oncologist
- Any recent central line insertion?
- Any history of non-malignant diseases known to cause SVC obstruction, e.g. Bechet's? Any use of medications known to cause SVC obstruction?

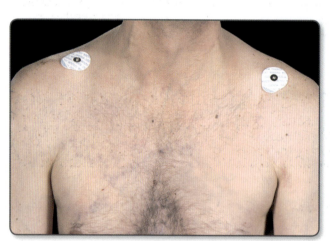

Figure 3.1 Superior vena cava obstruction (SVCO). Dilated veins can be seen over the praecordium and upper arms and the jugular veins are prominent. A plethoric appearance of the neck, although subtle, is evident with a more pronounced finding expected in the face. Oedema of the face, neck (collar of Stokes) and arms may also be seen.

Table 3.4 Secondary causes of superior vena cava obstruction	
Malignant (~90% of causes)	**Non-malignant**
Lung cancer (non-small cell most common, followed by small cell carcinoma) Lymphoma	Indwelling central venous catheter Infection, including tuberculosis Granulomata Mediastinal fibrosis

Demonstrate an understanding of the value of further investigation

A plain chest radiograph may show widening of the mediastinum. Any causative mass compressing the SVC, may be visible on the radiograph as a ring lesion. A unilateral pleural effusion is also another indicator of underlying lung malignancy.

A CT of the chest with contrast will give information on both:

- The SVC, its patency, and whether the obstruction is mechanical from external compression, or from thrombus within the vein (or both)
- Any causative mass, whether a lung malignancy, or pathologically enlarged lymph nodes

Further investigations may include diagnostic investigations aimed at obtaining tissue samples of suspected primary malignancies.

Always offer a management plan

Patients with SVC obstruction should be referred to an oncologist for urgent investigation and MDT driven management.

The good candidate will remind the examiner that SVC obstruction is an oncological emergency, with immediate attention to the patient's airway, breathing and circulation. Initial therapy usually involves the use of corticosteroids, most commonly dexamethasone. Note though, that in cases of possible high-grade lymphoma, steroids cause a decrease in the histological yield and carry the risk of precipitating tumour lysis syndrome. Other treatment options include SVC stent insertion, chemotherapy, and radiotherapy

Discussing malignancy

Traditionally, one of the biggest concerns medical students have as they approach clinical examinations is how to discuss possible cancer with patients without actually using the 'c-word' itself. Despite 2–3 years of clinical practice, this fear is often prevalent in PACES candidates also. It is important to remember that the patient has been fully prepared for the scenario by the examiners and is unlikely to flinch at the mention of cancer. That said most candidates will choose to use slightly more technical terms such as 'malignant process' or 'neoplastic cause'. Either way, one shouldn't worry about it, because neither the patient nor the examiner will.

Further reading

Kanada DJ, Jung RC, Ishihara S. Superior vena cava syndrome due to a retained central venous pressure catheter. Chest 1979; 75:734–735.

Case 76: Horner's syndrome: Pancoast's tumour

Instruction to the candidate

Please examine the respiratory system of this 82-year-old man who has presented with weight loss and haemoptysis.

Begin with a summary of positive findings

On respiratory examination, there is a localised area of consolidation in the left upper lobe, as demonstrated by dullness to percussion and bronchial breathing in that area. On further examination, the patient is noted to have ptosis and miosis of the left eye. There is also noted to be wasting of the intrinsic muscles of the left hand.

Other possible positive findings include:

- Cachexia
- Cervical lymphadenopathy
- More complex neurological signs in the ipsilateral upper limb due to brachial plexus involvement

Follow with a summary of relevant negative findings

Important relevant negative findings include:

- Respiratory compromise
- Other cranial nerve pathology

State the most likely diagnosis on the basis of these findings

'This patient has signs consistent with left upper lobe consolidation in the context of Horner's syndrome suggestive of a Pancoast's tumour.'

Pancoast's tumour

Pancoast's tumour is an apical lung tumour which, in addition to the local lung disease and local signs/symptoms directly attributable to the tumour, also causes non-respiratory symptoms, namely:

- Hand signs: wasting of the intrinsic muscles of the hands
- Eye signs: Horner's syndrome with ptosis, miosis, anhidrosis, enophthalmos

The very reason that hand and eye signs are involved in Pancoast's makes it an ideal case, not just for the respiratory station, but also for neurology or station five.

Offer relevant differential diagnoses

It would be appropriate to give a differential diagnosis of consolidation, adjusting your list to start with causes of apical consolidation:

- Pulmonary tuberculosis
- Other causes of bacterial consolidation

Demonstrate the importance of clinical context – suggest relevant questions that would be taken in a patient history

Appropriate questions would include those aimed at eliciting symptoms consistent with the clinical signs:

- Progressive weight loss, chronic cough, haemoptysis

- Pain and weakness of the hands
- Hemi-facial anhidrosis

In addition, tell the examiner you would elicit a history consistent with risk factors for lung malignancy, namely a strong smoking history.

Demonstrate an understanding of the value of further investigation

Principles of investigation would include radiographic confirmation of a tumour, followed by tissue sampling and histological confirmation of tumour type. In addition, radiographic staging will identify any tumour metastasis.

Specific investigations would include:

- Sputum cytology for malignant cells
- Plain chest radiography to identify a ring lesion in the apex corresponding to the palpable mass on examination
- Spirometry to assess further fitness for surgery
- CT chest, abdomen and pelvis. The chest portion of this scan will give further information on the tumour itself, local spread, and any metastatic mediastinal lymphadenopathy. The abdominal and pelvic slices will help to stage the patient by identifying any distant metastases
- Histological sampling in a peripheral lesion such as this would likely be by a CT-guided biopsy

Always offer a management plan

Specific management strategies depend on a range of factors, including:

- Histological subtypes. Small cell lung cancer, due to its high cell turnover rate, is highly susceptible to chemotherapy
- The patient's performance status
- Lung function testing
- The localisation of tumour and the tumour staging

All patients are managed by the local lung cancer multi-disciplinary team to decide on appropriate interventions. There may also be further input by both Macmillan nurses and palliative care teams.

Case 77: Cushingoid appearance

Instruction to the candidate

This 30-year-old woman has experienced weight gain over the past 4 months. Please examine her respiratory system.

Begin with a summary of positive findings

Positive findings can be divided into signs suggestive of a diagnosis of Cushing's syndrome and signs suggestive of an underlying diagnosis that requires long-term steroid therapy.

Signs pointing toward a diagnosis of Cushing's syndrome include:

- Cushingoid facies
- Centripedal obesity
- Intrascapular fat pad
- Abdominal striae
- Easy bruising

Signs pointing towards an underlying respiratory diagnosis necessitating long-term steroid therapy include:

- Barrel chest with wheeze on auscultation (in the young patient, think of difficult-to-control asthma, whereas in the older patient be mindful of COPD)
- If the patient has fine, end-inspiratory crepitations, think of fibrosis
- Scars, such as those related to a lung transplant

Follow with a summary of relevant negative findings

Important relevant negative findings include signs of respiratory distress and signs of chronic tobacco use.

State the most likely diagnosis on the basis of these findings

'This patient has signs consistent with a diagnosis of Cushing's syndrome, which is likely iatrogenic and secondary to their underlying respiratory disease.'

Offer relevant differential diagnoses

In this case, it is sensible to not give a differential for Cushing's syndrome, but rather to give a differential of underlying respiratory diseases which warrant steroid therapy and are therefore prone to iatrogenic Cushing's, such as:

- Asthma
- COPD
- Fibrosis
- Lung transplantation

At that stage, you may want to comment on the difference between Cushing's syndrome and Cushing's disease and the individual causes.

Demonstrate the importance of clinical context – suggest relevant questions that would be taken in a patient history

Screen past medical history and medication, current and historical.

Demonstrate an understanding of the value of further investigation

A two-pronged investigative approach would include, investigations regarding the underlying respiratory diagnosis and those to confirm Cushing's syndrome and iatrogenic steroid administration as the cause.

- A plain chest radiograph would show hyper-expanded lung fields in COPD and difficult-to-control asthma, or reticulonodular shadowing if the underlying disease process is pulmonary fibrosis
- Peak expiratory flow rate

Always offer a management plan

Assuming confirmation of iatrogenic steroid administration as a cause of the Cushing's, the management discussion would centre on trying to reduce the need for steroid through use of steroid-sparing agents. Strong candidates will also discuss management of cardiovascular risk including screening for diabetes, good glycaemic control in those with steroid-induced diabetes, addressing hypertension and lipid management.

Case 78: Abnormal nails with pleural effusions and lymphadenopathy – yellow nail syndrome

Instruction to the candidate

This patient, presenting with shortness of breath, has been referred to the respiratory clinic for assessment. Please examine her respiratory system and comment on your findings.

Begin with a summary of positive findings

On examination of this middle-aged person, positive findings include:

- On general inspection there is swelling of the lower limbs
- On inspection of the hands, there is discolouration and deformation of the nails of the hand and feet, with yellowing and abnormal curvature associated with cuticle loss (**Figure 3.2**)
- On examination of the chest, there is bilaterally decreased expansion, stony dull percussion note and absent breath sounds at the bases, with associated decreased vocal fremitus

> **Yellow nail syndrome**
>
> Yellow nail syndrome is based on the triad of:
> - Abnormal nails with a yellow/green discolouration, which display slow growth
> - Lymphoedema, most commonly of the limbs
> - Respiratory disease, classically pleural effusions, but including bronchiectasis

Follow with a summary of relevant negative findings

Important negative findings include:

- There are no signs of respiratory compromise
- There is no lymphadenopathy
- The JVP is not raised, there are no murmurs and the apex beat is not displaced

State the most likely diagnosis on the basis of these findings

'The triad of yellow nails, peripheral oedema and respiratory signs is consistent with a diagnosis of the rare condition, yellow nail syndrome.'

Emphasising the rarity of the condition at the outset is a sensible approach. As a general rule, any mention of rare diseases should be put in context and be the subsequent differential diagnosis should include a list of less likely, but more common diseases.

Offer relevant differential diagnoses

Yellow nail syndrome is essentially a spot-diagnosis, with no true differential diagnoses. Therefore, various alternative differential diagnoses can be offered, such as:

The differential diagnosis of a pleural effusion:

- Transudates: cardiac, liver or renal failure
- Exudates: infection (parapneumonic), malignancy (primary or secondary)

The differential diagnosis of lymphoedema:

- Congenital: familial lymphoedema
- Acquired: infection (filiariasis), pelvic mass, iatrogenic (surgical removal of lymphatics)

Alternative diagnoses of discoloured and deformed nails, such as fungal infection with concomitant but unrelated respiratory pathology.

Demonstrate the importance of clinical context – suggest relevant questions that would be taken in a patient history

History questions to elicit the clinical features include:

- Questions regarding nail changes, specifically a slow rate of nail growth
- Assessing the time of disease onset. In one study, the mean age of onset was 56 years, but with a range of 27–69 years
- Questions seeking to elicit any underlying disease associations. Although rare, yellow nail syndrome has been associated with other respiratory tract involvement such as rhinosinusitis or bronchiectasis, autoimmune conditions, and malignancy
- Family history – familial disease has been described

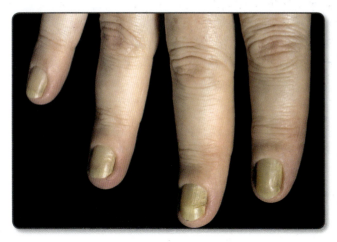

Figure 3.2 Yellow nails. Yellow discoloration with thickening and deformity of the nails, and associated swelling and loss of cuticles evident. Similar findings would be expected on examination of the toes.

Demonstrate an understanding of the value of further investigation

Yellow nail syndrome is a clinical diagnosis, however a patient presenting with any or all of the signs of yellow nail syndrome would receive an extensive investigative work-up.

Investigation of pleural effusion should form the predominant focus of discussion. Pleural effusion analysis in yellow nail syndrome classically shows a clear fluid, with a lymphocytosis, rich in protein and LDH.

Investigation of limb swelling: Note that although yellow nail syndrome describes lymphoedema rather than peripheral oedema, it is appropriate to include investigations relating to the more common causes of limb swelling:

- Uninalysis and urinary protein:creatinine ratio for heavy proteinuria
- Simple blood tests including albumin, liver function tests and renal function
- Cardiological tests, including a 12-lead electrocardiogram and an echocardiogram, to rule out a primary diagnosis of heart failure, which could easily be the cause of peripheral oedema and pleural effusions
- Ultrasound of the abdomen would provide information on liver echotexture, thus ruling out liver cirrhosis as a cause of lymphoedema and in the case of lower limb swelling, provide information on any pelvic masses causing lymphatic obstruction

- Lymphatic investigations. Given that specific lymphatic investigations are the remit of vascular surgery, the candidate may choose to tell the examiner that 'a referral to a vascular surgeon would be indicated for investigations of primary lymphoedema'

Finally, indicate the possibility of ruling out alternative nail pathology given its prominence in making a clinical diagnosis. Nail investigations would centre upon nail scrapings to rule out fungal infection.

Always offer a management plan

Given the rarity of yellow nail syndrome, it is acceptable for the candidate to tell the examiner that a referral to a specialist with expertise in this condition would be made. Of course, in the respiratory station, it would be perfectly appropriate to mention the above and then focus on the management of a pleural effusion.

Further reading

Hoque SR, Mansour S, Mortimer PS. Yellow nail syndrome: not a genetic disorder? Eleven new cases and a review of the literature. Br J Dermatol 2007; 156:1230–1204.

Norkild P, Kroman-Andersen H, Struve-Christensen E. Yellow nail syndrome – the triad of yellow nails, lymphedema and pleural effusion. A review of the literature and a case report. Acta Med Scand 1986; 219:221–227.

Case 79: Signs of right-sided heart failure – cor pulmonale

Instruction to the candidate

This 70-year-old man has frequent chest infections and has noted progressive shortness of breath on exertion. Please examine his respiratory system and present your findings to the examiner.

Begin with a summary of positive findings

On examination of the respiratory system, positive findings include:

- On inspection, the patient has a hyperexpanded chest with reduced sternohyoid distance. The patient may be either cachectic ('pink-puffer') or with increased BMI ('blue-bloater'). If the patient has significant disease such that they are in the exam, will likely be short of breath at rest.
- On expansion, there is equal but bilaterally reduced chest excursion
- There is a globally resonant or hyper-resonant percussion note
- On auscultation, as with uncomplicated COPD, the range of clinical signs on auscultation may range from globally reduced breath sounds, to scattered wheeze and crepitations

The patient with cor pulmonale will have additional signs on examination. In the setting of COPD, noting any of the following clinical signs should lead the candidate to seek to elicit them all:

- Loud second heart sound (P2), representing forceful closure of the pulmonary valve
- Raised jugular venous pressure
- Peripheral oedema

Follow with a summary of relevant negative findings

In addition to the standard negative findings for the respiratory examination, comment on the absence of clinical signs suggestive of acute exacerbation or active infection.

Additionally, in the case of cor pulmonale, it is important to identify the absence of pulmonary oedema. This is a key finding because it differentiates between right-sided heart failure and congestive heart failure suggested by the triad of raised JVP, bibasal crepitations, and peripheral oedema.

State the most likely diagnosis on the basis of these findings

'This patient has signs consistent with a diagnosis of chronic obstructive pulmonary disease complicated by cor pulmonale.'

Offer relevant differential diagnoses

Cor pulmonale is simply right heart failure due to raised pulmonary pressures reflected from a primary chronic pulmonary disorder. It is a sequela of many chronic respiratory diseases, including COPD, interstitial lung disease and chronic thromboembolic disease. Such irreversible, chronic and progressive conditions are ideal substrates for consequent increases in pulmonary pressures, with the development of right heart dilatation and dysfunction.

Demonstrate the importance of clinical context – suggest relevant questions that would be taken in a patient history

Relevant history questions should focus on eliciting current symptoms, importantly exertional breathlessness with exact quantification of current exercise tolerance and any change over time.

Screen for symptoms suggestive of an underlying cause for the cor pulmonale:

- Heavy smoking history: likely in this case as the clinical scenario is of advanced COPD. In COPD also assess severity and level of current treatment including use of long-term oxygen and non-invasive ventilation
- Other chronic lung disease, such a pulmonary fibrosis or bronchiectasis
- A history and/or symptoms of thromboembolic disease

As always, assess the effect of symptoms on the patient's daily life and offer to address the patient's ideas, concerns, and expectations in relation to their condition.

Demonstrate an understanding of the value of further investigation

Patients with cor pulmonale will undergo a wide range of tests, possibly fewer if the patient is known to have long-standing COPD and therefore the likely underlying diagnosis is known.

Imaging with high-resolution CT scan will identify the underlying pulmonary pathology and a CT pulmonary angiogram, with or without a ventilation-perfusion scan, will elicit any chronic thromboembolic disease.

Patients will also need spirometry and echocardiography to assess lung and cardiac function respectively, and many will require right and left heart catheterisation to measure the pulmonary pressures.

Always offer a management plan

It is important to communicate to the examiner that you realise that, in the context of COPD, cor pulmonale represents an advanced state of pathology in an irreversible clinical state.

Chapter 4

Abdominal system
(station 1)

Case 80: The syndrome of chronic liver disease

Instruction to the candidate

You are the registrar in the gastroenterology clinic. A 53-year-old man has been referred by his GP after a recent finding of abnormal liver function tests. Please examine the patient's abdominal system and report your findings to the examiner.

Begin with a summary of positive findings

Seek to identify not only signs suggestive of a diagnosis of chronic liver disease, but also signs which would suggest an underlying cause.

Signs of chronic liver disease

- On general inspection – cachexia with muscle wasting, scratch marks
- In the hands – clubbing (**Figures 4.1** and **4.2**), leukonychia (**Figure 4.3**), palmar erythema
- In the face – scleral icterus
- On the praecordium – spider naevi (**Figure 4.4**), paucity of body hair, gynaecomastia
- In the abdomen – jaundice, ascites, collaterals and caput medusae (all of which are suggestive of advanced or decompensated disease)

Additional signs suggestive of an underlying cause

- Alcoholic liver disease:
  - Facial telangiectasia – non-specific but common in alcohol excess
  - Dupuytren's contracture – predominantly idiopathic but with a recognised association with alcoholic liver disease
  - Bilateral swollen parotid glands
  - Neurological signs of alcoholism – including peripheral neuropathy, proximal myopathy and cerebellar syndrome
- Signs suggestive of viral hepatitis:
  - Tatoos
  - Track marks suggestive of intravenous drug use
- Primary biliary cirrhosis:
  - Periorbital xanthelasma, commonly with jaundice
- Haemachromatosis:
  - Slate grey skin pigmentation

The character of the liver edge can also be of use in forming a differential. A cirrhotic liver will either be impalpable, or shrunken, hard and irregular. In fatty liver disease or active hepatitis, the liver may be tender, smooth and enlarged. Non-tender hepatomegaly is suggestive of a range of causes, but if craggy should direct investigations towards hepatocellular carcinoma.

Follow with a summary of relevant negative findings

Advanced liver disease progresses towards cirrhosis with implications both on portal venous pressure and reduced functional reserve with eventual loss of liver function. The clinical manifestations of portal hypertension should not be missed, not least as they serve as a useful indicator of the severity of disease and alert to the likelihood of varices. Eliciting the features of hepatic failure and establishing decompensated disease is fundamental to a basic evaluation where liver disease is suspected and must be commented upon.

Patients with portal hypertension may have some or all of: splenomegaly, a venous hum on auscultation, abdominal collateral vessels (and caput medusa) and/or ascites.

Decompensated hepatic failure can presents with a constellation of the following signs:

- Asterixis
- Jaundice
- Coagulopathy. On clinical examination this may present as bruising and/or active bleeding
- Ascites
- Hepatic encephalopathy. If encephalopathy is present, seek to grade its severity

State the most likely diagnosis on the basis of these findings

'This patient has clinical signs consistent with compensated chronic liver disease with no evidence of portal hypertension.'

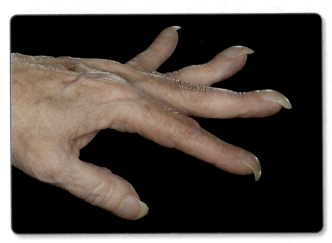

Figure 5.1 Clubbing of the fingers. Loss of the normal angle between the nail bed and cuticle/skin is evident; normally approximately 160 degrees, in clubbing the angle is commonly greater than 180 degrees. There is an exaggerated convexity of the nail fold. Thickening of the distal portions of the fingers is appreciable and sponginess would be expected with softening and fluctuation of the nail bed. The skin is also taught and has a shiny quality.

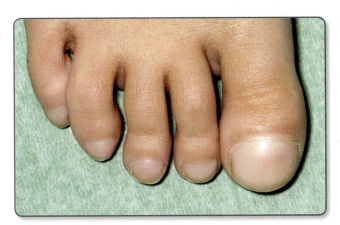

Figure 5.2 Clubbing of the toes. The clinical findings are identical to that described in Figure 5.1. The process is indiscriminate, affecting toes and fingers alike.

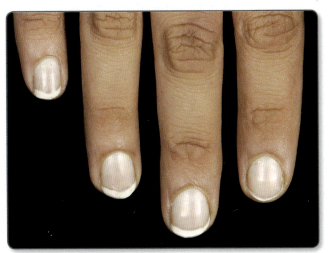

Figure 5.3 Leukonychia. Whitening of the entire nail (leukonychia totalis) reflects hypoalbuminaemia. This should not be confused with partial leukonychia secondary to illness (Mee's lines) or nail bed injury, where white lines or spots can be observed in an otherwise normal nail.

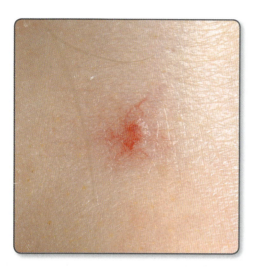

Figure 5.4 Spider naevus. Telangiectasia which blanch and subsequently refill centrally when pressure is applied; they are found within the distribution of the superior vena cava.

Offer relevant differential diagnoses

From the examination findings it may be possible to offer and justify a likely underlying aetiology for the evident liver disease, as outlined above, followed by a differential. Where this is not possible, proceed directly to a sensible differential:

- Common causes:
  - Alcoholic liver disease
  - Non-alcoholic fatty liver disease
  - Chronic hepatitis C infection
- Less common:
  - Chronic hepatitis B
  - Autoimmune hepatitis
  - Primary biliary cirrhosis
- Rare:
  - Primary sclerosing cholangitis
  - Wilson's disease
  - Haemachromatosis

Demonstrate the importance of clinical context – suggest relevant questions that would be taken in a patient history

Screening for risk factors associated with commonly recognised underlying aetiologies.

Where alcoholic liver disease is suspected screening for dependency and establishing current level of consumption is paramount. Risk factors for hepatitis B and C include blood transfusions; intravenous drug use; tattoos; and high-risk sexual intercourse. It is important to enquire about medication use, such as methyldopa, amiodarone and methotrexate.

Establishing a history of previous episodes of decompensation requiring admission and/or treatment, particularly in the high dependency or intensive care setting, gives important context for the potential for deterioration. Ask specifically about previous episodes of ascites, and where there is a history of varcies, haemorrhage.

Demonstrate an understanding of the value of further investigation

A sensible approach to investigation of a patient with chronic liver disease would include simple blood testing and imaging tests, with further investigations as appropriate. The two key aims of investigation are to assess liver function (importantly including synthetic function) and to identify the underlying cause if possible.

Blood tests

Appropriate blood testing to assess liver function would include:

- Liver function tests (LFTs), including bilirubin (conjugated and unconjugated), transaminases and alkaline phosphatase. An AST:ALT ratio of greater than two suggests alcoholic liver disease. This is due to chronic alcohol consumption causing a lack of vitamin B6, which is required for ALT function. A ratio of less than one suggests non-alcoholic liver disease. An elevated alkaline phosphatase is suggestive of cholestasis
- Markers of synthetic function include the prothrombin time, serum albumin and platelets. Impaired synthetic function is suggested by a prolonged prothrombin time and/or a reduced serum albumin and/or a reduced platelet count

Blood tests to identify the aetiology of the chronic liver disease would include:

- Serological testing to identify viral infections such as:
  - Hepatitis A, B, or C
  - CMV
  - EBV
- Auto-antibody testing:
  - Primary biliary cirrhosis – positive anti-mitiochondrial antibodies in 95%
  - Autoimmune hepatitis – positive ANA, anti-smooth muscle antibody
  - Primary sclerosing cholangitis – positive ANCA in 80%
- Other tests for miscellaneous causes such as:
  - Ferritin as a screen for haemachromatosis
  - Caeruloplasmin for Wilson's disease
  - Alpha-1-antitrypsin levels
  - Tumour markers if appropriate

Imaging

In the acute setting it is prudent to consider arranging simple imaging with ultrasound to rule out an obstructive cause before embarking upon expensive laboratory investigations.

Abdominal ultrasound is the first line imaging modality of the liver. It provides information about the liver echotexture (cirrhosis, fatty infiltration) and can identify masses. Additionally, ultrasound allows a Doppler assessment of portal blood flow and will provide information on the presence or absence of splenomegaly. If ascites is present, this can be identified, quantified and marked for drainage.

Biopsy may be considered for diagnostic purposes where the aetiology is unclear with equivocal or unexplained laboratory results, or where there is suspicion of multiple causes of liver disease such as alcohol and viral hepatitis.

Importantly, where biopsy is proposed, ensure clotting is not significantly deranged.

Always offer a management plan

A discussion on the management of chronic liver disease should involve discussion not only of general aspects of management, but also of the management of the underlying cause, assuming one has been identified through clinical examination.

General management aspects include:

- Dietary and lifestyle advice with B vitamin supplementation in patients with chronic alcohol consumption, and a low salt and high protein diet in those with ascites
- Endoscopic surveillance for varices
- Screening ultrasound and α-fetoprotein levels 6 monthly for hepatocellular carcinoma
- Need for early referral to high-dependency/intensive care (if appropriate) in the deteriorating liver patient.
- Medication prescribing in the liver patient

Management dependent upon the underlying cause:

- Alcohol – abstinence
- Viral hepatitis (B/C) – interferon, ribavirin, protease inhibitors such as telapravir and beceprivir
- Autoimmune hepatitis – prednisolone, azathioprine
- Haemochromatosis – therapeutic phlebotomy (usually to maintain a ferritin of 20–50 ng/mL) and chelation
- Primary biliary cirrhosis – ursodeoxycholic acid
- Wilson's disease – trientine and zinc

Case 81: Organomegaly – isolated hepatomegaly

Instruction to the candidate

This 45-year-old man has been referred to the gastroenterology clinic following a routine medical examination. Please examine his abdominal system.

Begin with a summary of positive findings

Hepatomegaly is suggested by a palpable mass below the right costophrenic margin which moves towards the right iliac fossa on inspiration, and is dull to percussion. Further characteristics of the hepatomegaly to identify include:

- Is it smooth or craggy?
- Is it firm/hard?
- Is it tender or non-tender?

Associated findings to look for include any scars to indicate previous biopsy or paracentesis.

Follow with a summary of relevant negative findings

In patients with isolated hepatomegaly it is important to report the absence of signs to suggest chronic liver disease or hepatic decompensation. Additionally, comment on the absence of:

- Concurrent splenomegaly
- Lymphadenopathy: if present, lymphadenopathy may suggest an infective cause, but the presence of hepatosplenomegaly and lymphadenopathy would raise suspicion of a lymphoproliferative disorder
- Features of congestive cardiac failure or tricuspid regurgitation. Tricuspid regurgitation classically presents with a pulsatile liver edge

State the most likely diagnosis on the basis of these findings

'This patient has signs consistent with isolated hepatomegaly.'

Offer relevant differential diagnoses

There is a wide range of causes of hepatomegaly and these can be classified in various ways.

Congenital causes of hepatomegaly include Riedel's lobe and polycystic disease.

Acquired causes include:

- Infections, such as the viral hepatitides, CMV, EBV, amoebiasis, toxoplasmosis, malaria
- Drugs, such as alcohol, amiodarone, methotrexate
- Metabolic and Infiltrative causes, such as NASH, haemachromatosis, Wilson's disease, amyloidosis, Gaucher's
- Autoimmune conditions such as autoimmune hepatitis, primary biliary cirrhosis, primary sclerosing cholangitis
- Neoplastic disease, in which you would expect to find irregular firm hepatomegaly on clinical examination. Secondary liver metastasis are more common than primary hepatic neoplasms
- Passive venous congestion due to right heart failure with resistance to right ventricular filling:
  - Tricuspid regurgitation: classically pulsatile hepatomegaly. Examination of the JVP can be useful in this regard, as giant V waves would be virtually pathognomonic
  - Constrictive pericarditis
  - Restrictive cardiomyopathy
- Vascular causes such as Budd–Chiari or sickle cell disease

In view of the extensive differential, to avoid the potential of listing and appearing prescriptive it is useful to consider the differential diagnosis of isolated hepatomegaly in relation to the additional features sought on examination. It is paramount that the presentation of positive and negative findings be comprehensive and clear enabling the candidate to proceed with a narrowed differential.

Demonstrate the importance of clinical context – suggest relevant questions that would be taken in a patient history

A suitable clinical history would include questions to screen for known risk factors of liver disease, including:

- Alcohol: ask about average usage, including episodes of bingeing
- Recent travel: has the patient been to any areas known to increase risk for certain underlying causes?
- Risk factors for viral hepatitis such as blood transfusions, intravenous drug use, tattoos, or unprotected or high risk sexual intercourse

Demonstrate an understanding of the value of further investigation

Blood testing would include inflammatory markers, liver function tests and liver disease screen.

Ultrasound of the liver would be the first line imaging modality to confirm clinical findings of hepatic enlargement and assess presence of fatty infiltrate, masses, cysts or abscesses. It can also rule out biliary duct dilatation to help distinguish parenchymal liver disease from extrahepatic bililary obstruction.

Further imaging such as CT or magnetic resonance cholangiopancreatography should be considered where ultrasound scanning fails to provide adequate assessment, is limited by obesity or poor views or where a malignant process is suspected.

Needle aspiration or biopsy, as appropriate, for evaluation of lesions suggestive of an infectious process, a cystic mass or neoplastic disease.

Always offer a management plan

Directed to the cause. The focus will vary greatly from case to case and may inevitably be guided by the examiner.

Case 82: The distended abdomen – ascites

Instruction to the candidate

This 57-year-old woman has presented complaining of abdominal swelling. Please examine her abdominal system and present your findings to the examiner.

Begin with a summary of positive findings

On clinical examination, the abdomen is distended – and may be tense – but soft and non-tender to palpation, with demonstrable shifting dullness. Abdominal herniae may be prominent or be suggested by a flattened or everted umbilicus.

Additional associated signs include:

- Hepatomegaly, which is often difficult to elicit in the distended abdomen but may indicate non-alcoholic fatty liver, early

  cirrhosis with fatty infiltration or chronic cirrhosis with hepatocellular carcinoma
- Peripheral oedema: ascites caused by liver disease is usually isolated or disproportionate to peripheral oedema whereas the reverse is true where the cause is generalised fluid retention attributable to congestive heart failure
- Signs of an underlying cause of liver disease

Follow with a summary of relevant negative findings

Important relevant negative findings to consider include:

- Signs of portal hypertension: splenomegaly, venous hum, caput medusa
- Other signs of hepatic decompensation, importantly encephalopathy, asterixis, jaundice

- Signs of sepsis, which if present would raise the possibility of spontaneous bacterial peritonitis (SBP)

State the most likely diagnosis on the basis of these findings

'This patient has ascites, of which the most common cause is cirrhosis with portal hypertension.'

Offer relevant differential diagnoses

The differential diagnosis of ascites can be divided into hepatic and non-hepatic causes.

Hepatic causes include portal hypertension due to cirrhosis. This is the underlying cause inapproximately 90% of all cases. Such patients demonstrate the stigmata of chronic liver disease. An additional hepatic cause would include severe alcoholic hepatitis (without cirrhosis).

Non-hepatic causes of ascites would include:

- Peritoneal malignancy
- Intra-abdominal tuberculosis
- Fluid retention due to congestive cardiac failure, which on clinical examination would reveal peripheral oedema and a raised JVP (note comparison with portal hypertension where, as a result of venous dilatation, the cardiac filling pressure is low with a JVP typically difficult to elicit)
- The nephrotic syndrome and generalised hypoalbuminaemia will also give the picture of generalised oedema and fluid overload
- An important vascular cause is that of hepatic vein thrombosis, known as Budd–Chiari syndrome
- Less common causes include, pancreatitis, SLE, hypothyroidism, Meig's syndrome and chylous ascites

Demonstrate the importance of clinical context – suggest relevant questions that would be taken in a patient history

Questions identifying risk factors for, and symptoms of, the conditions listed below:

- Cirrhosis and portal hypertension
- Cardiac disease
- Malignancy
- TB

It would also be important to ask about fevers and abdominal pain, which would lead to consideration of SBP.

Demonstrate an understanding of the value of further investigation

Investigations should include an assessment of the ascitic fluid. This will aid both the identification of the underlying cause of the ascites and allow exclusion (or confirmation) of spontaneous bacterial peritonitis.

A diagnostic paracentesis should be performed with appropriate analysis of the fluid according to the following parameters:

- Colour and appearance: is it blood stained, chylous, turbid, or straw coloured?
- White cell count: if the polymorph count is >250 this is indicative of spontaneous bacterial peritonitis: Further microscopy, culture and sensitivity will allow identification of the causative organism
- Fluid biochemistry: the protein level differentiates transudate versus exudate. Additionally, the serum albumin to ascites albumin gradient (SAAG) differentiates portal hypertensive ascites (SAAG > 11g/L) from non-portal hypertensive ascites
- Cytological assessment allows for identification of malignant cells in the ascitic fluid

---

Serum-to-ascites albumin gradient

Assessment of the ascitic fluid will include comparison of the albumin content in the ascites with the serum albumin content to give the serum to ascites albumin gradient (SAAG). Measuring SAAG enables the classification of portal hypertensive (SAAG >11 g/L) versus non-portal hypertensive (SAAG < 11 g/L) causes of ascites. This is calculated by subtracting the ascitic fluid albumin value from the serum albumin value, from samples obtained at the same time. The value correlates with portal pressure. While typically absolute protein levels, transudates and exudates are rarely applied to ascitic fluid, the protein level in conjunction with SAAG can be useful. An elevated SAAG and a high protein level are observed in most cases of ascites due to hepatic congestion. However, the combination of a low SAAG and a high protein level is characteristic of malignant ascites.

Where there is clinical suspicion of non-cirrhotic aetiology, consider the following:

- Cardiac investigations should include ECG and echocardiogram
- For malignancy consider appropriate imaging and serum tumour markers
- For pancreatic pathology assess ascitic amylase
- Thyroid function tests

Always offer a management plan

In portal hypertensive ascites, initial management should include bed rest and salt restriction. Salt restriction represents the best conservative approach, aiming for <2 g/day. Fluid restriction should be applied where hyponatraemia exists. Diuresis with spironolactone should be considered if salt and fluid restriction unsuccessful. Ideally, weight loss of 0.5 kg per day should be achieved. Where more weight is lost, it is likely to represent diuresis from the intravascular compartment, not peritoneal, and can result in complications including renal dysfunction and worsening electrolyte derangement.

Management options for refractory ascites include:

- Therapeutic paracentesis: ascitic drains should remain in situ for no longer than 6–8 hours and should not be clamped. 100 mL of 20% albumin should be administered for every 2 litres drained. Transjugular intrahepatic porto-systemic shunting (TIPS) is utilised in ascites resistant to other treatment or where rapid reaccumulation occurs with haemodynamic compromise. An invasive technique not without its complications one must ensure against a coagulopathy, and thereafter be alert to the potential for porto-systemic encephalopathy and worsening of hepatic disease.
- Transplantation

Non-portal hypertensive ascites is largely unresponsive to diuretics and requires recurrent paracentesis.

Where SPB is suspected, it should be treated as a medical emergency with broad spectrum antibiotics, in line with local guidance. Where possible, obtain ascitic, blood, and urine cultures prior to initiation of antibiotics. Diagnostic paracentesis should not delay the start of treatment where there is strong clinical suspicion. Culture yield is traditionally poor from ascitic fluid but diagnosis can be made in the first instance on the presence of greater than 250 neutrophils per micro-litre. Antibiotic prophylaxis may be considered for those patients at high risk of developing SBP with advanced cirrhosis and significant ascites, subsequent to successful treatment, and in those admitted with acute variceal bleeding.

Case 83: Portal hypertension

Instruction to the candidate

This 69-year-old man has a history of excess alcohol consumption. Please examine his abdomen and present your findings to the examiner.

Begin with a summary of positive findings

Portal hypertension, a process heralding cirrhosis in the context of chronic liver disease, is manifest as:

- Splenomegaly

- Porto-systemic anastomoses such as caput medusae and oesophageal varices
- Ascites
- A venous hum on auscultation

Additional findings to identify include those of chronic liver disease

Follow with a summary of relevant negative findings

Important relevant negative findings would include:

- Evidence of confusion caused by porto-systemic encephalopathy

- Evidence of decompensated liver disease, particularly coagulopathy given the propensity for gastrointestinal bleeding from varices

State the most likely diagnosis on the basis of these findings

'This patient has clinical signs suggestive of portal hypertension.'

Offer relevant differential diagnoses

The most common cause of portal hypertension in developed countries is liver cirrhosis.

Causes of non-cirrhotic portal hypertension include:

- Schistosomiasis (in travellers from endemic areas) and HIV are important infective causes
- Increased resistance to right ventricular filling – constrictive pericarditis, restrictive cardiomyopathy and tricuspid regurgitation
- Hepatic vascular aetiologies such as Budd–Chiari causing a post hepatic obstruction
- Increased portal venous flow – although rare, this may occur in arteriovenous malformation or as the result of massive splenomegaly caused by a primary haematological disorder (see *Splenomegaly*, p. 163).

Demonstrate the importance of clinical context – suggest relevant questions that would be taken in a patient history

In a clinical history, the patient should be asked regarding whether varices have been identified and also whether there has been any previous gastrointestinal bleeding and/or intervention. The risk factor profile for liver disease should be explored, specifically asking about alcohol and – where suspected – other precipitants including infection and heart disease.

Demonstrate an understanding of the value of further investigation

A diagnosis of portal hypertension is inferred in patients with evidence of cirrhosis by clinical examination. Direct measurement of the portal pressure with transjugular catheter is rarely performed due to the incumbent risks involved. Thus, the diagnosis is confirmed with ultrasound or CT demonstrating engorged intra-abdominal collaterals and with Doppler to assess portal vein patency and flow.

Endoscopy with direct visualisation of oesophageal and gastric fundus varices confirms the diagnosis and allows intervention as appropriate.

Where no clear precipitant for liver disease has been identified, the patient should be investigated with a full liver screen. Suspected cirrhosis, most commonly due to alcohol with a clear history, should be investigated to assess severity with blood tests and imaging ensuring no signs of decompensation.

Always offer a management plan

Prevention of bleeding is key. Acute variceal bleeds carry mortality rates upwards of 50%, and are associated with high rates of re-bleeding in survivors.

All patients diagnosed with cirhosis should undergo an endoscopy to screen for varices. Primary prophylaxis is with beta-blockade (typically propranolol or carvedilol) to reduce portal blood flow. The dose is titrated up to maintain a resting heart rate of <55 beats/min. In addition to reducing the likelihood of a variceal bleed, if successful in reducing portal pressure, beta-blockers may also reduce chronic bleeding from gastric mucosal vascular congestion (portal hypertensive gastropathy). Patients who respond poorly to medical therapy may be considered for TIPS or porto-caval shunting. Liver transplantation may be considered depending on the clinical picture.

Splenomegaly rarely causes complications in the context of portal hypertension and thus splenectomy is avoided as a general rule.

The patient should be educated on avoidance of causative/contributory factors.

> ### Prognosis
>
> In the presence of cirrhosis, clinical examination and the results of laboratory information can be combined to provide a prognostic score, as in the Child–Pugh score (**Table 4.1**). A CPT score greater than 10 carries a 50% 1 year mortality in those with advanced cirrhosis. The Model for End-stage Liver Disease (MELD) scoring system has become increasingly favoured over the CPT classification in predicting mortality although the modified-CPT which takes into consideration creatinine levels has been shown to be as useful as MELD in predicting short and medium term mortality and is significantly simpler in execution. Reference: Papatheodoridis et al. MELD vs Child–Pugh and creatinine-modified Child–Pugh score for predicting survival in patients with decompensated cirrhosis.

Table 4.1 Child–Pugh score for prognosis in liver cirrhosis			
Clinical variable	1 point	2 points	3 points
Encephalopathy	None	Grade 1–2	Grade 3–4
Ascites	Absent	Slight	Moderate/large
Bilirubin mg/dL	<34	34–50	>50
Albumin g/L	>35	35–28	<28
INR	<1.7	1.7–2.3	>2.3

INR, international normalised ratio
Child–Pugh classification serves as a measure of the severity of liver disease. The grades correlate with one and two year patient survival as follows. Grade A (5–6 points): 100% and 85%; Grade B (7–9 points): 80% and 60%; Grade C (10–15 points): 45% and 35%

Further reading

Papatheodoridis GV, Cholongitas E, Dimitriadou E, et al. MELD vs Child-Pugh and creatinine-modified

Child-Pugh score for predicting survival in patients with decompensated cirrhosis. World J Gastroenterol 2005; 11:3099–3104.

Case 84: Abnormal skin pigmentation – jaundice

Instruction to the candidate

This 47-year-old man has presented with abnormal skin discolouration. Please examine and present your findings to the examiner.

Begin with a summary of positive findings

Jaundice is demonstrated by yellow pigmentation of the sclera, skin and mucosa (**Figures 4.5, 4.6,** and **4.7**).

Associated findings which can help form a suitable differential diagnosis include:

- Signs of chronic liver disease and portal hypertension (see *Portal* h*ypertension* p. 149)) If these signs are present, signs suggesting an underlying cause of the liver disease should be sought
- Signs suggestive of acute onset liver disease – tender hepatomegaly, abdominal discomfort
- Tattoos or needle track marks which would suggest an increased risk of viral hepatitis

Follow with a summary of relevant negative findings

Important relevant negatives include:

- Signs of liver failure, such as confusion and encephalopathy. Jaundice as the result of acute on chronic liver disease, in a cirrhotic liver, may be associated with other signs of decompensation, importantly hepatic encephalopathy. Indeed, jaundice and encephalopathy serve as sensitive indicators of both severity and decompensation in chronic disease. In the context of ascites or portal hypertension one should consider jaundice as decompensation and be prepared to discuss the CPT score with the examiner (see *The syndrome of chronic liver disease,* p. 142)
- The absence of a palpable gallbladder. This mainly concerns 'surgical' jaundice but one should bear in mind Courvoisier's law which states that in the presence of a palpable gallbladder, painless jaundice is unlikely to

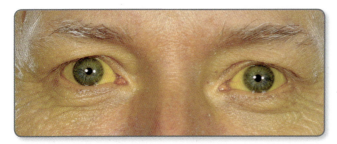

Figure 4.5 Jaundice. The normally white sclerae are noticeably discoloured with a yellow hue, scleral icterus, consistent with jaundice. There is also visible yellowing of the peri-orbital skin.

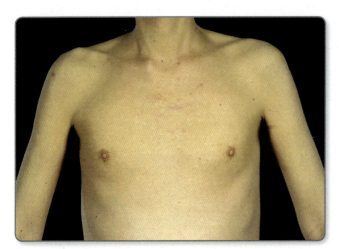

Figure 4.6 Jaundice. Gross yellowing of the skin is evident. There is also praecordial spider naevi and the paucity of body hair consistent with underlying liver disease.

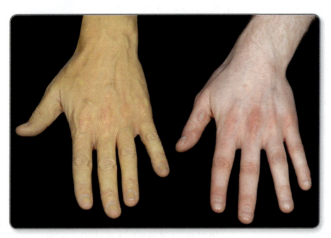

Figure 4.7 Jaundice. Jaundice may be appreciable on general inspection of the hands prior to examination of the torso and abdomen.

be due to cholelithiasis. The implication is that the clinical picture is more likely to be due to pancreatic malignancy

- Lymphadenopathy: where jaundice exists in the context of diffuse lymphadenopathy, it is important to consider viral causes and haematological malignancy

State the most likely diagnosis on the basis of these findings

A possible presentation to the examiner in the case of jaundice could be: 'This patient appears grossly jaundiced. There are no clinical signs suggestive of a clearly identifiable cause and thus I would like to take a full history and investigate further to establish an underlying diagnosis on which to base my management.'

In a jaundiced patient always attempt to identify the underlying cause and present it to the examiner accordingly. If the patient clearly exhibits clinical signs consistent with chronic liver disease the candidate may choose to discuss predominantly liver disease with jaundice as a manifestation and consideration of exacerbating or decompensating factors. Alternatively, acknowledge the finding of jaundice in the presence of chronic liver disease and thereafter consider the differential diagnoses of jaundice itself. There will inevitably be overlap between the two approaches but the candidate should be clear on the distinction and commit to one or other to avoid confusion.

Offer relevant differential diagnoses

The differential diagnosis of jaundice includes:

Jaundice with unconjugated bilirubinaemia

- Increased turn over commonly due to haemolysis or ineffective erythropoeisis (sickle cell disease). Less commonly due to resorption of large haematomas
- Hepatic congestion with decreased uptake. Seen in congestive cardiac failure, post-imaging with contrast, iatrogenic including rifampicin
- Impaired conjugation seen most commonly in Gilbert's. Less commonly Crigler–Najjar syndrome and hyperthyroidism

Jaundice due to conjugated bilirubinaemia

- Hepatocellular dysfunction:
  - Viral hepatitides, CMV, and EBV
  - Alcoholic cirrhosis
  - Haemachromatosis
  - Autoimmune hepatitis
  - Wilson's disease
  - Alpha-1 antitrypsin deficiency
- Impaired hepatic excretion. Importantly, this is often associated with intractable pruritis and thus excoriations serve as a good discriminating clinical sign allowing you to narrow the differential. Possible causes include:
  - Alcoholic liver disease
  - Primary biliary cirrhosis
  - Ascending cholangitis
  - Head of pancreas carcinoma

Demonstrate the importance of clinical context – suggest relevant questions that would be taken in a patient history

Important symptoms would include:

- Pruritis – a common symptom in jaundiced patient's
- Dark urine – this often precedes icterus
- Risk factors for liver disease, past medical history and family history
- In the context of chronic liver disease, screen for triggers of decompensation

Demonstrate an understanding of the value of further investigation

Testing of the urine differentiates between conjugated and unconjugated hyperbilirubinaemia. Conjugated urine is soluble and thus causes the urine to be dark.

In a patient with jaundice, the serum bilirubin will be raised. Analysis of the conjugated and unconjugated subtypes of bilirubin will help narrow the differential diagnosis. Assessment of transaminase and alkaline phosphatase levels assists in the differentiation between cholestasis and hepatocellular dysfunction.

Where conjugated jaundice is suspected, routine blood testing is likely to reveal little with no significant derangement of liver function expected. Thus, investigation should be focused upon establishing a cause for haemolysis including: blood film/smear, electrophoresis, and Coombe's test.

Deranged liver function and a raised conjugated bilirubin in the absence of symptoms suggestive of obstructive jaundice should prompt a liver screen. (See *The syndrome of chronic liver disease*, p. 142.)

Depending on the results of urine and blood testing, a range of imaging modalities can be used.

Ultrasound of the abdomen is usually first line, providing important information about the liver and portal circulation and about the gallbladder and biliary tree (including gallstones).

Obstructive symptoms where dilatation is demonstrated with ultrasound but no gallstones are seen should lead to magnetic resonance or MRCP/ERCP. Where no dilatation is demonstrated, consider biopsy to establish the cause of infiltrative liver disease or intrahepatic cholestasis.

A CT or MRI may be considered where there is suspicion of malignancy.

Always offer a management plan

The management of jaundice can be divided into management of the symptoms of jaundice and of the underlying cause. The management of the various underlying causes can be found elsewhere.

With regard management of symptoms, obstructive jaundice may cause intractable pruritis, which can be alleviated to varying degrees dependent upon the cause, with cholestyramine. However, where the obstruction is complete, such as extrahepatic cholestasis secondary to gallstones, such medical therapy is generally unsuccessful.

Case 85: Abnormal skin pigmentation – haemachromatosis

Instruction to the candidate

This 44-year-old man has been referred to the gastroenterology clinic with deranged liver function tests. Please perform an abdominal examination and present your findings to the examiner.

Begin with a summary of positive findings

The main positive findings in a case of haemachromatosis would involve hepatomegaly in a patient with slate-grey skin pigmentation and scanty axillary hair. Additionally, there are likely to be stigmata of concurrent diabetes with abdominal lipodystrophy, bruising from subcutaneous insulin administration and finger pulp bruising from blood sugar monitoring.

Associated signs in a case of haemachromatosis include:

- Cardiovascular: displaced apex beat suggestive of concurrent cardiomyopathy
- Musculoskeletal: pseudogout usually effects the second and third metacarpophalangeal joints
- Urogenital: testicular atrophy – candidates should offer to examine for this but refrain from actually doing so

Follow with a summary of relevant negative findings

Important relevant negative findings to note and present to the examiner as such include:

- Signs of decompensated cirrhosis
- Peripheral oedema and a raised jugular venous pressure consistent with signs of decompensated cardiomyopathy

State the most likely diagnosis on the basis of these findings

'This patient has signs consistent with a diagnosis of haemachromatosis.'

Offer relevant differential diagnoses

Given its characteristic features, haemachromatosis is usually considered as a 'spot-diagnosis'. Therefore, rather than giving a differential diagnosis of the condition itself, choose a particular sign and give a differential diagnosis of that. This may involve giving a differential diagnosis of hepatomegaly (see *Organomegaly: isolated hepatomegaly*, p. 146). Alternatively, a differential diagnosis of slate-grey skin pigmentation would include iatrogenic administration of amiodarone.

Haemachromatosis is a disease of iron overload, the differential diagnosis of which includes:

- Primary (or hereditary) haemachromatosis
- Secondary iron overload in conditions such as sickle cell disease, thalassaemia, and sideroblastic anaemia. Due to a combination of increased iron absorption and iron supplementation for anaemia and in repeated transfusions

Demonstrate the importance of clinical context – suggest relevant questions that would be taken in a patient history

Screen for symptoms consistent with a diagnosis of haemachromatosis, such as lethargy, which is the most common presentation. Arthropathy and erectile dysfunction are other common symptoms.

Lethargy is the most common presentation. Haemachromatosis can be considered as either genetic, or as acquired due to iron accumulation from repeated transfusions. Demonstrate this knowledge in your differential and elicit risk factors to strengthen diagnosis including:

- Family history
- A history of regular transfusions and consider haematological disorders, commonly sickle cell disease or thalassaemia

It is prudent to include a social history to gauge alcohol intake.

Demonstrate an understanding of the value of further investigation

Investigations can be divided into those aimed at confirming the diagnosis and those aimed at assessing end-organ damage.

Tests to confirm the diagnosis include:

- Blood tests:
  - A raised serum ferritin >1000 µg/L is highly suggestive of primary haemachromatosis. Additionally, the transferrin saturation will be increased and the total iron binding capacity decreased

  - Liver function tests are often minimally affected
- Genetic testing: HFE genotyping is used but note incomplete penetrance of C282Y gene and the finding of primary haemachromatosis in C282Y -/- individuals
- Biopsy with Perl's staining remains the gold standard for diagnosis
- Imaging: MRI is effective in demonstrating iron overload

Tests to assess end-organ damage include:

- Fasting glucose, OGTT and HbA1c to confirm and assess severity of diabetes mellitus
- Assessment of pituitary function, importantly gonadotrphin secretion
- 12-lead electrocardiogram and echocardiogram are important where suspicion of cardiomyopathy exists

Always offer a management plan

Principles of management in haemachromatosis include:

- Regular venesection with measurement of Hb aiming for lower end of normal and ferritin aiming for 20–50 µg/L. Venesection required 3–6 weekly for up to 2 years initially. Where not tolerated, chelation with desferrioxamine can be considered
- Referral to endocrinology for management of diabetes and consideration of pituitary hormone replacement. Venesection will result in falsely lowered HbA1c levels
- Abstinence from alcohol is strongly advised, with acceleration of cirrhosis
- Cirrhotic patients have increased (>10%) risk of hepatocellular carcinoma so 6 monthly screening with ultrasound and α-fetoprotein advisable in advanced disease
- Family screening

Case 86: Periorbital xanthelasma – primary biliary cirrhosis

Instruction to the candidate

This 52-year-old woman has presented with pruritis. Please examine her abdominal system and present your findings to the examiner.

Begin with a summary of positive findings

Positive findings in primary biliary cirrhosis include:

- Jaundice
- Excoriations
- Peri-orbital xanthelasma (**Figure 4.8**)
- Associated signs of chronic liver disease

Follow with a summary of relevant negative findings

It is important to confirm the absence of signs of cirrhosis, portal hypertension or decompensated liver disease. Additionally, where primary biliary cirrhosis (PBC) is suspected, relevant negatives would include signs consistent with other commonly associated autoimmune disorders:

- Rheumatoid arthritis
- Sjögren's disease
- Systemic sclerosis
- Thyroid disease

State the most likely diagnosis on the basis of these findings

In a woman with signs of obstructive jaundice and xanthelasma a diagnosis of primary biliary cirrhosis should be considered until proven otherwise.

Offer relevant differential diagnoses

A range of differential diagnoses can be given.

The differential diagnosis of primary biliary cirrhosis itself includes autoimmune hepatitis and autoimmune cholangitis.

The differential diagnosis of obstructive jaundice includes biliary obstruction (e.g. secondary to gallstones) and primary sclerosing cholangitis.

The differential diagnosis of xanthelasma includes primary and secondary dyslipidaemias.

Demonstrate the importance of clinical context – suggest relevant questions that would be taken in a patient history

The classical presentation is typically that of unexplained fatigue, right upper quadrant discomfort, and jaundice with pruritis in a middle-aged woman. Questions in a clinical history would therefore be aimed at eliciting these features.

Non-specific symptoms of lethargy and malaise are common at presentation, as are those of dry eyes and mouth, and cholestasis (pruritis and steatorrhoea). Other features may include previous episodes of jaundice and/or a family history of liver disease or autoimmune disorders.

Demonstrate an understanding of the value of further investigation

PBC is the most common chronic cholestatic disease of the liver with progressive destruction of small to medium sized bile

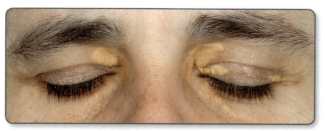

Figure 4.8 Periorbital xanthelasma. Subcutaneous deposits of lipid rich macrophages, resulting in plaques or nodules, often with well-demarcated borders and yellow/orange hue, in the peri-orbital region.

ducts. Investigation centres on establishing a cholestatic picture on liver function testing, identifying an autoimmune basis for disease and imaging the bile ducts to rule out a mechanical obstruction. Confirmation of the disease is commonly made on biopsy.

Liver function tests will typically demonstrate elevated ALP and GGT with unremarkable transaminases. Bilirubin is not normally raised in the early stages of PBC, where hyperbilirubinaemia exists it is predominantly conjugated and represents disease progression with a poorer prognosis.

Serum levels of auto-antibodies include positive antimitochondrial antibodies (95%). Anti-nuclear (ANA), anti-smooth muscle (Anti-SM) and rheumatoid factor (RF) are also commonly present.

Suitable imaging modalities include a liver ultrasound and MRI.

Liver biopsy, performed early, proves diagnostic where characteristic bile duct lesions are identified. Delayed biopsy in advanced disease may fail to differentiate more generic cirrhotic changes.

Always offer a management plan

Conservative measures, including avoiding alcohol and hepatotoxic drugs, are advised where possible.

Medical therapies include:

- Ursodeoxycholic acid (UDCA) is thought to decrease hepatocellular damage and slows progression to fibrosis but does not decrease time to transplantation
- Pruritis may be controlled with an antihistamine, cholestyramine rifampicin or UDCA however care should be taken to avoid co-administering with ursodeoxcholic acid as this will reduce absorption of the latter. Ultraviolet light is thought to be a beneficial adjuvant therapy
- In advanced disease where malabsorption is likely, vitamin replacement is advised and measures to protect against osteoporosis, including bisphosphonates, prudent.

Liver transplantation is the definitive treatment. Recurrence rates are high despite immunosuppression however the course of recurrent disease appears to be benign with promising 10-year survival rates and good quality of life. Indications for referral to a transplantation centre include worsening hyperbilirubinaemia, intractable pruritis, severe osteoporosis, hypoalbuminaemia or evidence of decompensated liver disease.

Case 87: The patient requiring renal replacement therapy

Instruction to the candidate

This 50-year-old woman has presented to the nephrology clinic. Please examine her abdomen and present your findings to the examiner.

Begin with a summary of positive findings

The patient may display clinical findings consistent with one or more mode of renal replacement therapy. Remember that many patients will, over time, undergo more than one mode of renal replacement. Such clinical signs include:

- Arteriovenous fistula in the antecubital fossa or forearm (brachiocephalic communication) are used for haemodialysis
- Indwelling catheters that may be present include Tesio lines (long-term tunnelled lines used for haemodialysis) or short-term vascaths used for haemofiltration.
- Patients with peritoneal dialysis will have abdominal scars and a Tenckhoff catheter

Additionally, the patient may display general clinical signs related to renal failure, such as:

- Anorexia
- Dry skin with excoriations

- Anaemia
- Mobility aids necessitated by bony pain secondary to renal osteodystrophy.
- Parathyroidectomy scar

It is important to look for clinical signs which may indicate an underlying cause of renal failure:

- Diabetes – fingertip echymoses, abdominal lipodystrophy, ulceration and amputation
- Hypertension – renal bruit
- Autosomal dominant polycystic kidney disease – bilateral ballotable kidneys

Follow with a summary of relevant negative findings

Pertaining to arteriovenous fistulas, it is important to palpate and auscultate for flow but be mindful that flow does not correlate with use. Examine fistulas closely for signs of recent instrumentation consistent with ongoing use. In the absence of needle marks the fistula is unlikely to represent an active site of dialysis delivery.

It is important to assess fluid status, examining for a raised JVP, bibasal crepitations, and peripheral oedema. Lack of fluid overload is an important relevant negative to record.

An additional relevant negative to note is the absence of signs of previous renal transplantation. If present, this would suggest a failed transplant requiring re-initiation of renal replacement therapy.

State the most likely diagnosis on the basis of these findings

'This patient has evidence of renal replacement therapy raising the suspicion of underlying renal disease.'

An example presentation: 'The patient has an arteriovenous fistula in the right antecubital fossa with a palpable bruit and needle marks consistent with recent instrumentation for use in haemodialysis. The need for renal replacement in this patient may be secondary to diabetic renal disease as evidenced by abdominal lipodystrophy indicative of regular subcutaneous insulin administration.'

Offer relevant differential diagnoses

Common causes of chronic kidney disease leading to a requirement for renal replacement therapy include:

- Diabetes
- Hypertension
- APKD

Demonstrate the importance of clinical context – suggest relevant questions that would be taken in a patient history

In a history it would be important to identify whether the patient has symptoms of renal failure, and to assess risk factors for renal disease.

Symptoms of renal failure include lethargy, nocturia, and pruritis.

Risk factors for renal disease:

- Diabetes
- Hypertension
- Family history

Demonstrate an understanding of the value of further investigation

Investigations can be focused on those that evaluate the renal dysfunction and its severity, and those which assess for the severity and systemic complications of the underlying cause(s) of the renal dysfunction.

Investigations directed towards assessing the renal dysfunction itself include:

- Urine: dip for haematuria and proteinuria. Protein:creatinine ratio to quantify proteinuria
- Blood tests: renal function, eGFR, electrolytes, haemoglobin, bicarbonate, calcium, phosphate
- Imaging: ultrasound

Investigations to assess underlying causes include:

- Diabetes: HbA1c.
- Hypertension: 12-lead electrocardiogram and chest radiograph assessing cardiomegaly, left ventricular hypertrophy and where appropriate echocardiogram to investigate cardiomyopathy

Always offer a management plan

Renal replacement therapy is utilised to treat both acute kidney injury (AKI) and end stage chronic kidney disease (ESCKD). The use of renal replacement therapy in AKI, where a rapid reduction in kidney function results in a failure to maintain fluid, electrolyte and acid–base homoeostasis, represents a holding measure to allow reversal of the underlying pathology with restoration of renal function.

Indications for renal replacement therapy in AKI include:

- Clinical features of uraemia – pericarditis, hypothermia, encephaolpathy
- Fluid retention with pulmonary oedema refractory to diuresis
- Hyperkalaemia >6.5 mmol/L refractory to medical management
- Sodium >155 mmol/L or <120 mmol/L
- Metabolic acidosis pH <7.0
- Severe renal failure – urea >30 mmol/L, creatinine >500 mmol/L

Indications for dialysis in ESCKD are less clear, but centre around the measured fall in glomerular filtration rate with generally accepted implementation at <10 mL/minute or <15 mL/minute on a background of diabetes. Consideration should be given to conservative management where appropriate e.g. view of mortality and quality of life.

Also consider:

- Erythropoietin
- Vitamin D
- Anti-pruritics

Case 88: Bilateral ballotable kidneys

Instruction to the candidate

This 29-year-old man has been complaining of abdominal pain. Please examine his abdomen and report your findings to the examiner.

Begin with a summary of positive findings

Positive findings include: Bilateral, ballotable, flank masses together with a palpable irregular, non-tender, hepatomegaly with a relative paucity of other clinical signs.

Follow with a summary of relevant negative findings

Important relevant negative findings to note include:

- A lack of fluid overload and/or clinical evidence of uraemia to suggest renal dysfunction
- A lack of evidence of current and/or previous renal replacement therapy or evidence of transplantation
- A lack of evidence of chronic liver disease (in view of the hepatomegaly)

State the most likely diagnosis on the basis of these findings

'Adult polycystic kidney disease.'

Offer relevant differential diagnoses

Various differential diagnoses can be given. The differential diagnosis of bilateral palpable kidneys includes:

- Polycystic kidney disease
- Bilateral multiple simple cysts
- Bilateral hydronephrosis
- Bilateral renal cell carcinoma (rare)
- Amyloidosis

The differential diagnosis of bilateral cystic kidneys, where neither or only one kidney may be palpable on examination includes:

- Polycystic kidney disease
- Multiple simple cysts
- von Hippel–Lindau syndrome
- Tuberous sclerosis
- Laurence–Moon–Biedl syndrome
- Meckel–Gruber syndrome

Demonstrate the importance of clinical context – suggest relevant questions that would be taken in a patient history

Appropriate questioning would include those aimed at eliciting common symptoms preceding diagnosis, such as:

- Abdominal fullness or pain
- Haematuria
- Nocturia
- Treatment of hypertension

Additionally, it is appropriate to include in a history questions regarding complications of the condition, such as:

- A history of subarachnoid haemorrhage
- A family history of the disease
- Any history and/or treatment of hypertension

Demonstrate an understanding of the value of further investigation

Bedside tests include an assessment of the blood pressure, which may be raised, and a urine dipstick to look for haematuria.

Blood tests are rarely of diagnostic benefit. Anaemia or polycythaemia are possible. Renal function should be monitored for disease progression. Liver dysfunction is uncommon even in presence of cysts.

Ultrasound confirms diagnosis, assesses severity and investigates for involvement of liver, pancreas, and spleen. An MRI brain allows assessment of aneurysms predisposing to subarachnoid haemorrhage

Always offer a management plan

Important aspects of management include:

- Close control of blood pressure, minimising systemic effects of hypertension where possible. ACE inhibitors have a recognised role
- Pain management
- Early referral for consideration of renal replacement therapy and transplantation. Nephrectomy may be considered at time of transplantation
- Screening of relatives:
  - Genetic screening
  - Ultrasound scanning from the age of 20 years
  - MRI of the brain

Case 89: Iliac fossa scar with a palpable mass – renal transplant

Instruction to the candidate

This 39-year-old woman is under follow up in the renal clinic. Please examine her abdomen.

Begin with a summary of positive findings

There is fullness of the abdomen with a scar in the right iliac fossa on general inspection. There is a palpable, discrete, firm mass, which is non-tender with no fluctuance and is non-tender to percussion which is dull in note.

There is associated evidence of previous renal replacement therapy, notably an arteriovenous fistula in the antecubital fossa with a palpable bruit but no recent instrumentation marks.

Follow with a summary of relevant negative findings

Important relevant negative findings in a renal transplant case include:

- Signs of renal failure:
  - Fluid balance
  - Uraemia: confusion, fasciculations, skin pigmentation
  - Signs of current active renal replacement therapy such as recent needle marks in an AV fistula, or the presence of a tunnelled dialysis catheter
- Signs of possible rejection such as a tender graft
- Signs related to immunosuppression:

- Steroids – cushingoid features
- Ciclosporin – gum hypertrophy
- Tacrolimus – excoriations from pruritis
- Skin infections and malignancies

State the most likely diagnosis on the basis of these findings

'A mass below a scar in the right iliac fossa, consistent with a renal transplant which appears to functioning in view of no evidence of active renal replacement therapy. There is/is not evidence of the side effects of immunosuppression. A preliminary skin survey does/does not reveal pathology.'

Offer relevant differential diagnoses

The differential diagnosis of a right iliac fossa mass includes:

- Terminal ileal disease – Crohn's, infection, TB, lymphadenopathy
- Ovarian pathology

The differential diagnosis of the underlying aetiology of renal disease necessitating transplantation (along with appropriate clinical findings) includes:

- Diabetes – lipodystrophy, finger pulp ecchymoses, offer ophthalmoscopy. Note that people with type 1 diabetes are often considered for dual kidney-pancreas transplantation or pancreas after kidney transplant – mention any additional scars
- Hypertension – renal artery stenosis with audible bruit, offer ophthalmoscopy
- Polycystic kidney disease – ballotable kidneys or associated nephrectomy scar

Demonstrate the importance of clinical context – suggest relevant questions that would be taken in a patient history

Appropriate questioning would include questions regarding:

- Symptoms of renal insufficiency – nocturia, fluid status and exercise tolerance
- Previous history of renal replacement therapy
- Past medical history, specifically an underlying cause

- Full drug history including current immunosuppression and potentially nephrotoxic drugs

Demonstrate an understanding of the value of further investigation

Investigations to evaluate transplant and renal function:

- Blood tests: renal function, inflammatory markers, immunosuppressant levels
- Urine: dip for blood and protein. Protein:creatinine to quantify proteinuria
- Imaging: ultrasound scanning and Doppler evaluation of transplanted vessels to ensure patency and flow

Basic investigations to elicit common underlying causes:

- Blood pressure – hypertension.
- HbA1c – poor glycaemic control
- Renal ultrasound for cystic disease

Always offer a management plan

Important aspects of management include:

- Titration of calcineurin targeted immunosuppression post transplantation balancing risk of rejection against that of nephrotoxicity under corticosteroid cover
- Tight glycaemic control and blood pressure in patients with diabetes and hypertension respectively
- Surveillance for rejection or infection:
  - Rejection most commonly occurs within 4 months of transplantation. Living-donor grafts are more successful than deceased-donor grafts. Of those patients who survive 1 year post transplantation, half die of other causes with a functioning graft, while the other half will suffer chronic allograft nephropathy with graft failure within 1–5 years
  - Intensified immunosuppression with pulsed high dose corticosteroids usually reverses accelerated or acute rejection but where unsuccessful haemodialysis is required. In a rejected graft, nephrectomy may be required if infection suspected on cessation of immunosuppression
  - Surveillance is best achieved through serial measurement of serum creatinine plotted over time with some benefit from ultrasound assessment of patency and flow in transplanted vessels

Case 90: Flank scar – nephrectomy

Instruction to the candidate

This 82-year-old man has been experiencing weight loss. Please examine his abdomen and present your findings.

Begin with a summary of positive findings

Cachectic elderly patient with a flank scar but relative paucity of other clinical signs.

Follow with a summary of relevant negative findings

It is important to note the absence of:

- Renal replacement therapy
- A renal transplant
- Contralateral kidney pathology, where polycystic is suspected ensure no hepatomegaly

State the most likely diagnosis on the basis of these findings

Summary of the findings and the pertinent negatives with a discussion of the differential diagnosis before committing to a discussion on renal cell carcinoma.

Offer relevant differential diagnoses

Of the flank scar – access to the retroperitoneal space:

- Lattisimus dorsi flap – look for evidence of breast reconstruction
- Adrenalectomy – look for a medical alert bracelet
- Retroperitoneal abdominal aortic aneurysm repair – arteriopathic patient, look for evidence of peripheral circulation, venous harvesting, bypass scars and amputations
- Abscess incision and drainage
- Skin lesion excision

Of the need for nephrectomy:

- Renal cell carcinoma (radical or partial nephrectomy – see below). Also, transitional cell carcinoma, Wilms' tumours and sarcoma
- Polycystic kidneys due to compression of surrounding structures or symptom relief
- Irreversible symptomatic kidney damage secondary to infection, trauma, parenchymal disease or obstruction due to significant calcinosis

Demonstrate the importance of clinical context – suggest relevant questions that would be taken in a patient history

Symptoms consistent with renal cell carcinoma, which would be included in a history, include:

- Painless haematuria
- Abdominal discomfort and bloating
- Weight loss, cachexia, lethargy
- Venous dilatation, lower limb oedema, and in men the presence of varicoceles

A screen for risk factors for renal cell carcinoma would include:

- Family history, including von Hippel–Lindau disease
- Occupational history and carcinogen exposure
- Smoking history

Demonstrate an understanding of the value of further investigation

Investigation of suspected renal cell carcinoma (RCC) after onset of symptoms and prior to nephrectomy:

- Imaging. CT with contrast or MRI – the diagnosis is often made as an incidental finding on imaging performed for other reasons. There is minimal role for needle biopsy. Where the diagnosis is not made radiographically it will usually be confirmed at surgery.
- Chest radiograph, where cannon ball metastases suspected, further imaging with CT warranted.
- Blood tests: Where ALP or calcium raised, bone scanning is indicated. Renal function is not normally deranged unless there is bilateral renal involvement. Polycythaemia is possible secondary to increased erythropoeitin production, more commonly patients are anaemic.

Post nephrectomy investigations include surveillance with appropriate radiology and monitoring of residual renal function, full blood count and bone profile.

Always offer a management plan

Management of RCC depends on the disease staging (TMN).

Early RCC – surgical intervention:

- Radical nephrectomy (removal of kidney, adrenal gland, perirenal adipose tissue and Gerots' fascia) – indicated for isolated local disease with curative intent
- Partial nephrectomy – nephron sparing, for small tumours or where bilateral disease exists

Late RCC – palliative therapies with or without surgery:

- Tumour embolisation
- Nephrectomy, debulking, or resection of metastases considered
- Radiotherapy typically used for bone metastases and pain. RCC and non-bony metastases are relatively radiotherapy resistant and thus this is no longer used as standard adjuvant therapy
- Interferon α and new, targeted biological therapies have shown promise and may be used increasingly as adjuvants to nephrectomy with curative intent

Case 91: Splenomegaly

Instruction to the candidate

This 47-year-old woman has presented with abdominal pain. Please examine her abdomen.

Begin with a summary of positive findings

Middle aged patient with a fullness of the abdomen and a mass on palpation extending to the right iliac fossa, with palpable notch, moving with inspiration and dull to percussion consistent with splenomegaly. The patient may be cachectic with signs of anaemia and plethoric facies.

Associated findings commonly include hepatomegaly. Where splenomegaly is encountered, given its strong correlation with liver disease it is important to exclude the manifestation of portal hypertension heralding cirrhosis. Where no signs of chronic liver disease are found, paradoxically splenomegaly will then more often than not be associated with hepatomegaly and lymphadenopathy and represent a haematological disorder or infectious disease. Jaundice in the absence of liver disease may occur as the result of haemolysis.

Follow with a summary of relevant negative findings

As mentioned above, important relevant negatives include:

- Hepatomegaly and/or signs of chronic liver disease. Remember that, in the absence of liver disease, jaundice may occur as a result of haemolysis
- Signs of portal hypertension
- Lymphadenopathy

State the most likely diagnosis on the basis of these findings

The patient has signs consistent with isolated splenomegaly.

Offer relevant differential diagnoses

With regard its various causes, splenomegaly and the differential diagnosis can be categorised according to size.

Massive splenomegaly

- Chronic myelocytic leukaemia – less commonly associated with hepatomegaly or lymphadenopathy
- Myelofibrosis – more commonly associated with hepatomegaly
- Less commonly in temperate climates but more common in the tropics and worldwide, malaria and leishmaniasis (kala-azar)

Moderate splenomegaly

- Portal hypertension
- Lymphoproliferative disorder – more commonly associated with hepatomegaly and lymphadenopathy such as non-Hodgkins lymphoma or chronic lymphocytic leukaemia
- Haemoglobinopathies, including thalassaemias, and sickle cell disease (although commonly associated with autoinfarction unless early in disease)

Mild splenomegaly

- Myeloproliferative disorders, although generally considered as causes of only mild splenomegaly, are worth mentioning to demonstrate an appreciation for the spectrum of disease:
  - Polycythaemia rubra vera
  - Essential thrombocythaemia

Infiltrative, connective tissue disease and storage disorders should also be considered in the differential however given the prevalence of haematological and infectious causes it is sensible to clearly and comprehensively deal with these before offering a brief synopsis of these rarer causes:

- Infiltrative/inflammatory: sarcoidosis, amyloidosis
- Connective tissue: SLE, Felty's syndrome
- Storage disorders: Gaucher's, Langerhans cell histiocytosis

Demonstrate the importance of clinical context – suggest relevant questions that would be taken in a patient history

Screen for constitutional symptoms of anaemia, infection or malignancy (B-symptoms) including weight loss, lethargy, night sweats and recent travel. Consider retroviral status and risk factors for liver disease.

In considering haematological disorders, enquire as to evidence of marrow failure, including bruising and fatigue associated with thrombocytopaenia and anaemia respectively. Bone pain may be secondary to increased haematopoiesis or marrow infiltration, whilst joint pain may result from hypeuricaemia.

A family history of haematological disorders, autoimmune conditions or transplantation with immunosuppression should be considered.

Demonstrate an understanding of the value of further investigation

Appropriate investigations include:

- Blood tests. Exclude pancytopaenia secondary to the cellular sequestration associated with hypersplenism. This predisposes to anaemia, infection and bleeding. Thus, a basic check of haemoglobin, platelets, white cell differential, inflammatory markers, and clotting is essential
- Imaging. Ultrasound will serve to confirm splenomegaly and assess the liver for hepatomegaly and allow duplex of portal venous flow. Thereafter, CT or PET scanning may be required to assess degree of associated lymphadenopathy. MRI may be necessary to identify portal or splenic thromboses

Other investigations:

- Thick and thin blood films if clinical suspicion of malaria
- Blood film with or without progression to bone marrow biopsy
- Lymph node biopsy if concomitant lymphadenopathy

Always offer a management plan

In the case of 'isolated splenomegaly' the discussion with the examiner on management may be directed towards a number of possible underlying diagnoses. For example, the examiner may direct the conversation towards myeloproliferative disorders, particularly CML.

Case 92: Felty's syndrome

Instruction to the candidate

This 45-year-old woman has been referred from the rheumatology clinic, where she was being assessed for painful hands. Please examine their abdomen.

Begin with a summary of positive findings

A patient with Felty's syndrome will have signs both in the hands and in the abdomen:

- In the hands: severe, symmetrical, deforming polyarthropathy, associated with extra-articular manifestations of rheumatoid arthritis, e.g. rheumatoid nodules
- In the abdomen: splenomegaly

Follow with a summary of relevant negative findings

It is important to exclude signs of current infection (this is important due to the finding of neutropaenia in Felty's syndrome).

State the most likely diagnosis on the basis of these findings

In a patient with extensive RA and palpable spleen, a diagnosis of Felty's syndrome should be considered and confirmed by a finding of neutropenia.

Offer relevant differential diagnoses

Of splenomegaly:

- Portal hypertension
- Haematological
- Infectious
- Infiltrative/inflammatory
- Connective tissue disease
- Storage disorders

Demonstrate the importance of clinical context – suggest relevant questions that would be taken in a patient history

Pertinent questions to consider include:

- Symptoms of a long preceding period of aggressive and poorly controlled RA
- Weight loss is common

Demonstrate an understanding of the value of further investigation

Felty's syndrome is characterised by the triad of RA, splenomegaly and granulocytopaenia with resultant susceptibility to overwhelming, often fatal, infections. Investigation should be directed to confirm splenomegaly, assess the rheumatoid arthritis and importantly establish the immune status of the patient.

- Blood tests:
  - Full blood count and inflammatory markers with white cell count differential to assess the severity of granulocytopaenia. Anaemia and thrombocytopaenia are common due to hypersplenism. ESR will be raised
  - Anti-CCP and rheumatoid factor
  - Anti-GCSF. Felty's syndrome has been linked to the presence of these auto-antibodies, possibly playing a role in the pathology of granulocytopaenia together with splenic sequestration
- Imaging:
  - USS and CT to confirm splenomegaly and assess hepatomegaly where present
  - Plain film radiographs of affected joints demonstrating destruction and loss of joint space
- Tissue
- Bone marrow aspirate

Always offer a management plan

Management is multi-disciplinary, involving contribution from a rheumatologist, haematologist and occasionally an infectious diseases specialist.

Focus upon achieving control of RA – (see *Symmetrical deforming polyarthropathy* p. 172).

Rituximab (anti-CD20) is establishing a role in the treatment of Felty's.

Colony-stimulating factors, G-CSF and GM-CSF are increasingly used where management of RA is poor and recurrent infections fail to respond to antibiotics.

Splenectomy in cases refractory to improvement with medical treatment or experiencing recurrent infections. 25% of patients after splenectomy experience further relapses of granulocytopaenia.

Case 93: Multiple abdominal scars

Instruction to the candidate

Please examine the abdomen of this 22-year-old woman who has had surgery in the past.

Begin with a summary of positive findings

Multiple abdominal scars, of varying age, in a young cachectic patient should raise the possibility of inflammatory bowel disease.
Associated signs include:

- Nutritional state – growth retardation and muscle wasting (particularly pterygoids and triceps)
- Anaemia – tongue, palmar creases, conjunctival pallor. Anaemia may be present from:
  - Chronic disease
  - Iron deficiency
  - B12/folate deficiency
  - Autoimmune haemolysis
- Clubbing (**Figure 4.1** and **Figure 4.2**)
- Apthous ulceration, stomatitis, telangiectasia, pigmentation
- Erythema nodosum or pyoderma gangrenosum
- Perianal disease – abscess, fistulae, skin tags
- Metabolic bone disease with mobility aids or kyphoscoliosis from osteoporotic fracture
- Uveitis, iritis, episcleritis

Follow with a summary of relevant negative findings

Relevant negative findings include:

- Abdominal pain or discomfort consistent with active disease
- Arthropathy (seronegative)

State the most likely diagnosis on the basis of these findings

'Multiple surgical interventions for underlying inflammatory bowel disease.'

Offer relevant differential diagnoses

When considering the differential diagnosis of multiple abdominal scars it is prudent to include other medical conditions which may require extensive abdominal surgery including complications of chronic pancreatitis, end-stage liver failure with transplantation where a roof top incision is present, or with midline laparotomy emergency access for gastrointestinal perforation or vascular complications such as abdominal aortic aneurysm rupture and mesenteric ischaemia.

The differential diagnosis of inflammatory bowel disease Crohn's disease and ulcerative colitis includes:

- Microscopic colitis
- Colorectal cancer
- Coelic disease
- Gastrointestinal infections (e.g. TB, *Yersinia*, amoebiasis, CMV)
- Behçet's disease
- Ischaemic colitis
- Radiation-induced colitis
- NSAID enteropathy
- Functional bowel disorders

Demonstrate the importance of clinical context – suggest relevant questions that would be taken in a patient history

Clinical questioning would seek to elicit a history of relapsing and remitting abdominal pain, diarrhoea, with or without mucus and blood.

Additional questioning would involve joint or back pain and difficulty with mobility, which may suggest an underlying seronegative arthropathy.

Demonstrate an understanding of the value of further investigation

To support a diagnosis:

- Blood tests:
  - Full blood count for anaemia, thrombocytosis
  - Inflammatory markers (CRP and ESR)
  - Screen for electrolyte abnormalities (including U+Es, Ca^{2+}, PO_4, vitamin B_{12} and D)
  - LFTs, including albumin

- Imaging:
  - Plain radiographs of (erect) chest and abdomen
  - Barium follow-through assessing stomach, small bowel and colon with additional plain radiographs
  - MRI enterogrpaphy
- Endoscopy: sigmoidoscopy or colonoscopy with direct visualisation and biopsy
- Stool sample to exclude infective aetiology
- Faecal calprotectin

To monitor disease progression, the patient's symptoms are backed up by inflammatory markers and markers of nutrition. There is no role for imaging in routing monitoring of disease progression, however some radiological signs do indicate severe and/or long-standing disease, such as a 'lead-pipe colon' in long-standing UC.

Always offer a management plan

The treatment of Crohn's and ulcerative colitis is similar and the importance of the distinction between the two only arises from a management perspective when considering surgical intervention or experimental therapy.

Maintenance therapies include:

- 5-ASA – sulfasalazine
- Corticosteroids
- Steroid-sparing agents

The management of acute flares includes:

- Fluid balance management
- Topical +/– systemic corticosteroids
- Ciclosporin (steroid unresponsive)
- Anti-TNF – infliximab or adalumimab considered in disease refractory to standard treatment where no evidence of infection exists

Complications requiring specific intervention include:

- Obstruction treated with nasogastric tube and intravenous fluid. Surgery may be indicated, see below
- Abscess formation requiring incision and drainage or percutaneous drainage with cover of intravenous antibiotics
- Fistulae are treated with antibiotics (including anaerobic cover) and consideration of infliximab

Case 94: Rooftop incision

Instruction to the candidate

Please examine this 51-year-old man's abdominal system and comment on his abdominal scar.

Begin with a summary of positive findings

When encountering a roof-top incision in PACES it will commonly represent a liver transplant. The strong candidate will consider the alternative indications for such a surgical approach, outlined in the differential diagnosis that follows, but the focus will be placed upon establishing the aetiology of liver disease necessitating transplantation, examining for evidence of recurrence, and ruling out signs consistent with decompensation, and complications of immunosuppression.

Associated signs:

- Palpable liver edge
- Signs suggesting chronic liver disease
- Evidence of renal insufficiency, or renal replacement therapy

Follow with a summary of relevant negative findings

It is important to note the absence of signs of hepatic decompensation.

State the most likely diagnosis on the basis of these findings

Where the scar is the predominant finding, lead with this in a succinct summary of positive and negative findings. Indicate to the examiner that you believe this would be consistent with a surgical approach to the liver, of which transplantation is a possibility before discussing the differential as outlined below.

Offer relevant differential diagnoses

The differential diagnosis of the underlying indication for surgical intervention, and thus a roof top incision, include:

- Liver transplantation
- Extensive hepatic resection with curative intent for neoplastic disease
- Gastrectomy
- Oesophageal cancer – Ivor-Lewis oesophagectomy, usually an abdominal and right thoracic approach
- Whipple's procedure

Having established liver transplantation as your principle diagnosis, consider the common causes of liver failure necessitating transplantation in attempting to offer a likely cause in this case followed by a differential.

An example of an acute cause is fulminant hepatic necrosis, which may be due to:

- Viral hepatitis
- Toxins – death cap mushroom
- Over-the-counter and recreational drugs – paracetamol, ecstasy

Chronic causes include:

- Cirrhosis
- Primary biliary cirrhosis
- Autoimmune hepatitis
- Primary sclerosing cholangitis
- Metabolic disease: haemachromatosis, Wilson's disease, storage disorders
- Hepatocellular carcinoma – Milan criteria: single tumour less than 5 cm or up to three tumours each less than 3 cm
- Biliary atresia in children

Demonstrate the importance of clinical context – suggest relevant questions that would be taken in a patient history

Review past medical history of liver disease, symptoms and disease progression necessitating transplantation. Screen for evidence of disease recurrence or transplant failure, enquire specifically with regard hepatitis C. Enquire as to medication regimen and compliance.

Demonstrate an understanding of the value of further investigation

Investigation may focus on establishing the indications for transplantation, discussed below in management, or on the post-transplant patient.

To assess the function of the graft, routine liver function including synthetic function with albumin and clotting. Formally assess for signs of encephalopathy.

Inflammatory markers including white cell count and differential, particularly in view of immunosuppression. Emphasise the potential for renal insufficiency, with the need for routine testing of renal function.

Where there is doubt with regard to the diagnosis, a CT would better evaluate the abdominal anatomy and where there was suspicion of post-operative complications such as infection, collection, anastamotic leak, or stricture, the threshold for performing such imaging would be low.

> ### Indication for liver transplantation - King's College criteria
>
> The King's College criteria determine prognosis in acute liver failure and stratify patients based on early parameters to identify those in whom a liver transplant would be beneficial or inevitable.
> Non-acetaminophen induced:
> - INR >6.5, or
>
> Three of:
> - Age less than 11 years or greater than 40 years
> - Serum bilirubin >300 µmol/L
> - Time from onset of jaundice to development of coma – more than 7 days
> - INR >3.5
> - Drug toxicity, regardless of whether it was the cause of acute liver failure
>
> Liver transplantation in chronic liver disease is generally considered where there is evidence of end stage cirrhosis.

Always offer a management plan

This may involve discussion of treatment options, prior to transplantation, of the underlying cause.

In the transplant patient, there is a need for immunosuppression. Commonly, one or combination of:

- Calcineurin inhibitor
- Mycophenilate mofetil
- Corticosteroids

Regular review and surveillance for rejection with tapering of immunosuppression where possible.

Be prepared to discuss the indications for transplantation, both for acute and chronic liver failure.

Important absolute contraindications to liver transplantation include:

- Raised intracranial pressure or low cerebral perfusion pressure
- Severe cardiopulmonary disease including pulmonary hypertension
- Extrahepatic malignancy
- AIDS (HIV infection is a relative contraindication)
- Non-compliance with medication

Case 95: Obesity with evidence of laparoscopic procedure

Instruction to the candidate

This 44-year-old woman has had abdominal surgery. Please examine her abdomen and comment on her abdominal scars.

Begin with a summary of positive findings

Obese patient, abdominal striae with increased sweat and skin secretions. Excess skin folds indicative of rapid weight loss. Scars consistent with laparoscopic port insertion, looking closely in the peri-umbilical area and flanks.

Follow with a summary of relevant negative findings

Conditions commonly related to obesity:

- Evidence of diabetes – finger pulp ecchymoses, abdominal bruising and lipodystrophy.
- Ischaemic heart disease – scars consistent with coronary bypass grafting.Thoracotomy with or without venous harvesting
- Hepatomegaly – where examination and palpation not limited by habitus, think of fatty liver
- Signs of excess lipids – xanthelasma

State the most likely diagnosis on the basis of these findings

Obesity – commenting on distribution, evidence of weight loss and with scars of previous laparoscopic surgery consistent with possible bariatric intervention.

Offer relevant differential diagnoses

Of obesity, centripetal, or abdominal fullness:

- Cushingoid
- Hypothyroidism
- Ascites

  Of the laparoscopic procedure:

- Cholecystectomy
- Bariatric surgery – restrictive procedure (gastric banding or sleeve gastrectomy) or bypass procedure (Roux-en-Y gastric bypass)
- Nissen's fundoplication

Demonstrate the importance of clinical context – suggest relevant questions that would be taken in a patient history

Past medical history including childhood obesity and specifically diseases related to obesity including cardiac disease, diabetes and depression or mental ill health.

- Enquire about reflux symptoms and biliary colic
- Rule out recent pregnancy associated weight gain and rapid loss
- Full drug history screening for medication with weight gain as side effect:
  - Corticosteroids

– Antidepressants
– Antipsychotics

Demonstrate an understanding of the value of further investigation

Body mass index (BMI) weight in kilograms divided by the square of height in metres.

Waist circumference: It is prudent to investigate the possibility of metabolic syndrome; a clustering of risk factors for the development of severe ischaemic cardiac disease and type 2 diabetes:

- Insulin resistance – measure fasting glucose
- Dyslipidaemia with elevated triglycerides, low HDL and increased intra-abdominal adiposity
- Hypertension

In unexplained obesity consider the need to rule out rare causes of weight gain including:

- Hyperinsulinism due to pancreatic cancer
- Craniopharyngioma

Always offer a management plan

Of obesity:
- Dietary and exercise advice
- Medication – orlistat, GLP-1 receptor agonists in those with diabetes
- Cognitive behavioural therapy
- Bariatric surgery

Most bariatric surgery is performed laparoscopically. It is generally indicated where all reasonable efforts have been made to exhaust alternative methods of weight loss and where there are no concerns about compliance with subsequent dietary requirements, mental health concerns or substance misuse. A BMI > 40, or >35 with a serious complication such as diabetes or ischaemic heart disease, represents objective indications.

Metabolic risk factors should be treated aggressively with diet and exercise advice, metformin where appropriate and optimisation of modifiable cardiac risk factors with hypertension control and a low threshold for statin use.

Chapter 5

Station 5

Case 96: Rheumatoid arthritis

Instruction to the candidate

This 70-year-old patient has been experiencing increasingly painful hands over the last 2 years. Please take a short history and perform a relevant focused examination. Summarise your findings to the patient and explain your investigation and management plan. A discussion with the examiner will then follow.

Take a focused history

Utilise open questioning to ascertain the nature of the problem in the patient's own words. Leading with a statement such as 'I understand you have been experiencing some problems with your hands? Can you tell me some more about that...' while open, will keep the patient on track with a focused approach and avoid initial deviation from the station instruction.

Specific, closed questioning should cover both a review of hand symptoms and include relevant systemic features of rheumatological disease, ensuring to consider the importance of any co-morbidity.

In the hands, consider:

- Nature of the pain
- Timing and duration of stiffness
- Pattern of joint involvement
- Associated skin changes

Look to specifically consider systemic features of rheumatological disease:

- Eye involvement – dry eyes, change in appearance (the red eye), or changes in visual acuity
- Lung disease – shortness of breath, cough, and haemoptysis
- Renal involvement – manifesting as lower limb oedema or potential changes in frequency of urination or qualitative changes to the urine itself (foamy or frothy)

Evidence in the past medical and family history of a tendency towards autoimmune disorders offers important context to the case and should not be overlooked. Thereafter screen medication, specifically the use of non-steroidals in the first instance. Finally, assess the effect on the patient's daily life being alert to the likelihood of depression in view of the chronic nature of the symptoms.

Positive findings of a focused examination

Always consider the benefit of initiating the examination during the history to maximise the consultation. During the history be confident in asking to examine the hands and encourage the patient to keep talking as you do so.

When examining the hands, assess for both deformity and for a deficit in function.

Deformity

Positive findings (**Figure 5.1**) include symmetrical MCP and PIP involvement. Tender joints, with subluxation and ulnar deviation. Boutonniere and swan neck deformity are clearly demonstrable. Z-shaping of the thumb with 1st and 2nd MCP most markedly involved. There are rheumatoid nodules at the elbows.

Function

Examine for difficulty unbuttoning their shirt, removing their watch and/or picking up a coin from a flat surface.

Consider further examination:

- To assess the extent of joint involvement – large joint examination and gait examination
- To evaluate systemic disease/complications of treatment such as fibrosis – respiratory examination
- To exclude known associations such as Felty's syndrome with splenomegaly – abdominal examination

---

Key clinical findings in rheumatoid arthritis

History:
- Multiple joints
- Morning stiffness
- Duration >6 weeks
- Effect on daily life

Examination:
- Bilateral joint involvement
- MCP subluxation
- Ulnar deviation
- Rheumatoid nodules

Relevant negatives

See **Table 5.1** for a summary of relevant negative findings to elicit in a case of rheumatoid arthritis. It will be important to be seen to consider alternative aetiologies, such as osteoarthritis, psoriatic arthropathy, and gout.

What to tell the patient

Consider the following approach:

'The pain and stiffness you describe and the changes to the joints in your hands suggest that you have a condition called rheumatoid arthritis. To confirm this, we will need to do some blood tests and imaging (X-rays) of the affected joints. Rheumatoid arthritis is usually treated with medications both to relieve pain and to stop further progression of the disease.

'I would like to bring you back to clinic in 6 weeks with the results of these investigations.

In the meantime, I will prescribe you tablets for pain relief.

'I will be writing to your GP to inform them of your visit today, asking them to refer you to the physiotherapist and occupational therapy team who can assess your needs further.

'Do you have any further concerns of questions I can address today?'

What to tell the examiner – state the most likely diagnosis on the basis of the history and clinical findings

'This patient describes early morning stiffness and pain affecting predominantly the knees and hands. Examination confirmed a symmetrical deforming polyarthropathy consistent with a diagnosis of rheumatoid arthritis.'

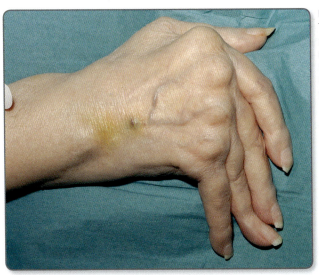

Figure 5.1 Rheumatoid hands.
The right hand of a patient with rheumatoid arthritis showing ulnar deviation with subluxation of the metacarpophalangeal joints. There is a Boutonierre deformity of the ring finger. ·

Table 5.1 Relevant negative findings in rheumatoid arthritis. The findings in the joints, skin and nails are important as they might indicate an alternate diagnosis		
Joints	**Skin and nails**	**Extra-articular**
DIP joint involvement (OA)	Erythema (psoriasis)	Dry eyes/mouth (Sjogren's)
Tophi (gout)	Psoriatic plaques (psoriasis)	Lung fibrosis (extra-articular disease or adverse effect of treatment for RA - methotrexate)
Telescoping (psoriasis)	Nail pitting (psoriasis)	Splenomegaly (Felty's)
DIP, distal interphalangeal.		

British Society for Rheumatology guidelines

'A diagnosis of RA should be made as early as possible, on the basis of persistent joint inflammation affecting at least three joint areas, involvement of the metacarpophalangeal or metatarsophalangeal joints or early morning stiffness of at least 30 minutes' duration.'

Offer relevant differential diagnoses

Of a symmetrical deforming polyarthropathy:

- Rheumatoid arthritis
- Psoriatic arthropathy, which would be suggested by nail pitting and psoriatic plaques
- Jaccoud's arthropathy, which is suggested when, despite deformity, the patient is able to make a fist, reflecting a lack of true joint destruction

Demonstrate an understanding of the value of further investigation

Investigations should seek to reinforce the clinical findings and support a diagnosis of rheumatoid arthritis. Diagnostic criteria are available, but these are primarily for research purposes.

Blood tests

- Serology: rheumatoid factor; anti-CCP antibodies
- Full blood count: anaemia is common. The strong candidate should recognise that there is a multitude of causes of anaemia in RA. The patient may have anaemia of chronic disease due to the RA itself. Alternatively, they may have a macrocytic anaemia due to methotrexate use, or a microcytic anaemia due to iron-deficiency secondary to NSAID use. Further, in Felty's syndrome, they may have anaemia due to splenic sequestration
- Inflammatory markers: ESR, CRP

Imaging

Plain radiographs of all affected joints should be obtained looking for loss of joint space and periarticular erosions.

Always offer a management plan

The management of rheumatoid arthritis involves symptom control, arresting disease progression, and continual disease monitoring.

Symptom control:

- Analgesia, NSAIDs

Arrest disease progression:

- Early initiation of DMARD combination therapy
- Corticosteroids for flares
- Biologics in active disease with disease activity score (DAS-28) >3.2 after a trial of two or more DMARDs (including methotrexate unless contraindicated)

Disease monitoring: DAS-28 to monitor response to treatment.

Thereafter, offer management plans for any functional impairment the patient may have:

- Involve physiotherapy and occupational therapy early to help the patient adapt to any disability and maintain as much function as is possible
- Surgical intervention – release of tendon strictures

Further reading

Luqmani R, Hennell S, Estrach C, et al. British Society for Rheumatology and British Health Professionals in Rheumatology guideline for the management of rheumatoid arthritis (after the first 2 years). Rheumatology (Oxford) 2009; 48:436–439.

National Institute for Health and Care Excellence (NICE). CG79, Rheumatoid arthritis: NICE guideline. London; NICE, 2009.

Deighton C, Hyrich K, Ding T, et al. BSR and BHPR rheumatoid arthritis guidelines on eligibility criteria for the first biological therapy. Rheumatology (Oxford) 2010; 49:1197–1199.

Case 97: Symmetrical deforming polyarthropathy–psoriatic arthritis

Instruction to the candidate

This 40-year-old man has presented with pain and deformity in his hands. Please take a brief history and perform a focused examination. When you have finished your assessment, inform the patient of your findings and suggest a suitable management plan.

Take a focused history

A brief history should include both specific questions regarding hand symptoms and also discriminative questions to distinguish between the possibility of rheumatoid and psoriatic arthropathy. Thus, in addition to asking questions focussing on hand symptoms such as pain, stiffness and reduced mobility, also enquire about:

- The presence of a rash, including its appearance and distribution. If the patient does not have psoriatic plaques currently, is there a past medical history of psoriasis?
- Is there nail deformity?
- Is there a family history of either rheumatoid arthritis or psoriasis?
- Is there a history of spondyloarthropathy or systemic disease such as inflammatory bowel disease? Psoriatic arthropathy is one of the seronegative spondyloarthropathies. The others are: ankylosing spondylitis, Reiter's syndrome, enteropathic arthritis

During the brief history, ensure to ascertain function and the effect of the patient's symptoms on their daily life. Enquire about common daily activities such as opening the front door, opening jars of food, dressing. What can the patient not do because of their condition? What effect is this having on their daily life?

Positive findings of a focused examination

Hand examination and assessment of skin - when examining the hands, assess for both deformity and for a functional deficit:

- Deformity: positive findings may include asymmetrical oligoarticular arthritis, symmetrical polyarthritis (commonest type and similar to rheumatoid arthritis), distal interphalangeal involvement, or arthritis mutilans with subluxation and ulnar deviation at the MCP joints. Dactylitis with 'sausage' digits is another possible clinical feature of this condition
- Function: assess function by asking the patient to unbutton their shirt or to pick a coin off a flat surface

Consider further examination for additional features such as:

- Enthesitis: achilles tendon attachment or plantar fascia to the calcaneus
- Skin rash: symmetrical pink scaly plaques on extensor surfaces of elbows or knees (**Figure 5.2**)
- Nail signs: marked pitting of the nails affecting both hands or feet and pale pink discolouration of the nail beds. Onycholysis or oil spots (pathognomonic).

Relevant negatives

Although the diagnosis of psoriatic arthropathy may be obvious in the setting of symmetrical deforming polyarthropathy and psoriatic plaques, seek to exclude findings suggestive of alternative diagnoses such as rheumatoid nodules or gouty tophi.

What to tell the patient

'The pattern of joint disease in the hands and the plaques on your elbows suggest you have a condition called psoriatic arthropathy. We will need to carry out some investigations such as X-rays of the hands and some blood tests. This is not a dangerous condition, and there are many strategies we can implement to help you maximise hand function.'

Following this, ask the patient if they have any further questions or concerns that you can address. Tell them that you will see them again in clinic after an appropriate interval.

What to tell the examiner – state the most likely diagnosis on the basis of the history and clinical findings

'A diagnosis of psoriatic arthropathy is suggested by symmetrical joint involvement, dactylitis, the absence of rheumatoid nodules, and DIP

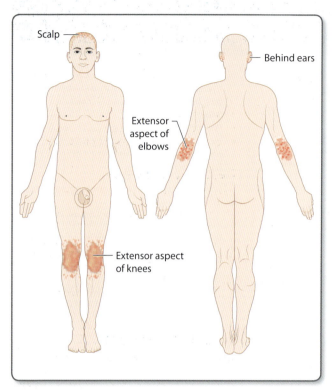

Figure 5.2 Sites of plaques in psoriasis. The main sites of plaques found in chronic plauque psoriasis, namely the extensor aspects of the elbows and knees, the scalp and behind the ears.

Labels on figure: Scalp; Behind ears; Extensor aspect of elbows; Extensor aspect of knees

involvement in the absence of osteoarthritis. This is most consistent with a symmetrical deforming polyarthropathy; however, alternative presentations of psoriatic arthropathy also include:

- Arthritis mutilans
- Predominance for DIPS
- Large joint oligoarthropathy (asymmetrical)
- Spondyloarthropathy'

Offer relevant differential diagnoses

The differential diagnosis of a symmetrical deforming polyarthropathy includes rheumatoid arthritis, psoriatic arthropathy and Jaccoud's arthropathy.

   Psoriatic arthropathy can also present as an asymmetrical arthropathy, the differential diagnosis of which includes gout and osteoarthritis.

Demonstrate an understanding of the value of further investigation

No specific diagnostic tests are available.

Clinical and radiological criteria are normally used. In blood testing, inflammatory markers such as ESR and CRP may be raised. Rheumatoid factor is usually negative although may be positive in a small number of cases. Testing for ANA is of no diagnostic benefit. Plain radiographs of the hands are used to demonstrate bony erosive disease. In contrast to rheumatoid arthritis, there is minimal juxta-articular osteopenia.

Always offer a management plan

Management of the disease itself involves symptom control, with simple analgesia and NSAIDs, and the arrest of disease progression, with DMARDs and biologic treatments. Management of associated manifestations includes topical therapies for skin disease. Offer lifestyle advice especially with regards to cardiovascular disease and diabetes which are associated with chronic psoriasis. Multi-disciplinary input is important to address any functional impairment the patient may have as a result of the condition.

Case 98: Jaccoud's arthropathy

Instruction to the candidate

A 40-year-old woman who has noticed deformity of her hands over the last 6 months. Please take a brief history and perform a focused examination. Discuss your findings and management plan with the patient.

Take a focused history

As with other cases of symmetrical polyarthropathy, screen for symptoms of pain and stiffness. The patient may have symptoms ranging from painless arthropathy to pain that is disproportionate to joint swelling. There may be associated myalgia. In addition to the small joints of the hands, there may be involvement of the wrists and knees.

Screen for systemic rheumatological disease. The tendency in a case of symmetrical deforming polyarthropathy will be to focus on rheumatoid arthritis, however this case highlights the importance of considering alternatives such as systemic lupus erythematosus (SLE). The symptoms of SLE may be vague due to the widespread nature of the disease with involvement of a range of organs/systems. Consider:

- Constitutional symptoms of fever, general malaise, weight loss
- Skin involvement with characteristic rash, either malar or discoid in distribution
- Current or past medical history of renal, neuropsychiatric, pulmonary, cardiac or gastrointestinal problems. Perhaps best achieved through a review of symptoms

Positive findings of a focused examination

Hand examination and skin assessment.

With regard to deformity, positive findings include a symmetrical polyarthropathy with PIP or MCP joint involvement. Tendonitis may be present. Look for tenderness, oedema and effusions.

A key finding is resolution of the apparent ulnar deviation on successful formation of a clenched fist. Function is usually preserved.

Additional findings:

- Skin manifestations rashes (malar eruption or butterfly rash as Jaccoud's occurs in up to 50% of patients with SLE) and history of photosensitivity
- Alopecia and livedo reticularis
- Mouth ulceration
- A cardiorespiratory examination may detect pleural or pericardial effusions if present

Relevant negatives

Important relevant negative findings include:

- The absence of rheumatoid nodules or psoriatic plaques
- A unilateral swollen joint out of proportion to others may suggest a reactive arthritis, or, in the presence of a fever, would raise suspicion of septic arthritis
- Avascular necrosis in patients taking corticosteroids

What to tell the patient

'The changes you have noticed in your hands together with the other symptoms you have mentioned suggest you have a condition called Jaccoud's arthropathy, which is often seen in the context of a systemic disease called systemic lupus erythematosis,

'To confirm this, we will need to run some tests, including blood tests and X-rays of the affected joints. Jaccoud's arthropathy is usually managed with medications to relieve pain but the underlying condition, often needs to be treated too with systemic medication,

'I would like to bring you back to clinic in 6 weeks' time with the results of the tests. In the meantime, I will prescribe you some tablets for pain relief if it is still a problem. I would advise you wear sunscreen and avoid sun exposure to limit the extent of the rash that you have,

'I will also be writing to your GP to inform him of your visit today. Do you have any questions or concerns that I can address today?'

What to tell the examiner – state the most likely diagnosis on the basis of the history and clinical findings

'This patient demonstrates symmetrical deformation of the metacarpophalangeal joints that is reversible with movement. These examination signs and history of systemic lupus erythematosus make the diagnosis that of Jaccoud's arthropathy.'

What is Jaccoud's arthropathy?

Jaccoud's arthropathy is a non-erosive, reversible deforming arthropathy with dislocation of the extensor tendons in the metacarpal fossa. In modern clinical practice it is most commonly associated with SLE however it has previously been described in a range of conditions including rheumatic heart disease. It was in patients with rheumatic heart disease that the French physician Jaccoud initially described this type of arthropathy.

Offer relevant differential diagnoses

In addition to Jaccoud's arthropathy, the differential diagnosis of a symmetrical deforming polyarthropathy includes rheumatoid arthritis and psoriatic arthropathy. When considering the key clinical differences between rheumatoid arthritis and Jaccoud's, consider that the features of rheumatoid arthritis include pain and stiffness, with an irreversible deformity and resulting functional impairment. Other joints may also be involved. Jaccoud's arthropathy, however, is often painless with no joint stiffness. There is a reversible deformity with often no functional deficit. There is no other joint involvement, but the patient may have other clinical features of SLE.

When considering the differential diagnosis of the causes of Jaccoud's arthropathy, consider that, in addition to SLE, it can also be caused by rheumatic heart disease, systemic sclerosis and sarcoidosis.

Jaccoud's arthropathy

Jaccoud's place in MRCP PACES is that of a differential of rheumatoid arthritis. It is a case that can easily catch out the PACES candidate, yet it is essentially a single clinical examination technique that will change your diagnosis from rheumatoid arthritis to Jaccoud's. The station 5 format, with elements of both history taking and clinical examination, makes the differential slightly easier because there are also marked differences in the history to help the candidate.

Demonstrate an understanding of the value of further investigation

The investigative strategy of a suspected Jaccoud's arthropathy case would focus on the following:

- Plain radiographs of the hands confirming the absence of erosive disease
- Blood tests for supportive evidence of SLE including ANA, double stranded DNA antibodies (anti-dsDNA) and complement, looking for reduced levels of C3 and C4

Always offer a management plan

The management of this case will not focus on the hands themselves, but rather on the management of the underlying SLE and its complications. Briefly, management is usually conservative and involves NSAIDs, low dose corticosteroids as well as methotrexate and antimalarials in more severe cases.

Further reading

Grahame R, Mitchell AB, Scott JT. Chronic post-rheumatic fever (Jaccoud's) arthropathy. Ann Rheum Dis 1970; 29:622–625.

Bradley JD, Pinals RS. Jaccoud's arthropathy in scleroderma. Clin Exp Rheumatol 1984; 2:337–340.

Sukenik S, Hendler N, Yerushalmi B, Buskila D, Liberman N. Jaccoud's type arthropathy: an association with sarcoidosis. J Rheumatol 1991; 18:915–917.

Case 99: Osteoarthritis

Instruction to the candidate

This 92-year-old woman has had difficulty opening jars at home. Please take a brief history and examine as appropriate.

Take a focused history

Screen for symptoms of pain and stiffness:

- Pain is usually worse with use and relieved by rest
- In osteoarthritis, the joints become stiff when rested ('gelling'). In contrast to rheumatoid arthritis, morning stiffness usually lasts less than 30 minutes

  Other important points to address include:

- Is there other joint involvement, e.g. in the knees and hips? Have they had any lower limb joint operations? How does the patient mobilise?
- What is the effect on function and daily living? Establish functional limitations such as the ability to dress independently, wash, as related to turning taps, and prepare food linked to the use of kitchen utensils. Be sure to make reference to specific functional limitations as outlined in the station instruction

Positive findings of a focused examination

Hand examination followed by assessment of large joints and/or gait.

On examination of the hands, the distal interphalangeal (DIP) joints are predominantly affected (**Figure 5.3**) with MCP sparing evident. Expect a reduced range of joint motion and crepitus. Swellings of the distal and proximal interphalangeal joints are noticeable, consistent with Heberden's and Bouchard's nodes, respectively.

Relevant negatives

Specific relevant negatives would include:

- No erythema or warmth over affected joints
- Absent inflammatory changes
- Absence of rheumatoid nodules, tophi or psoriatic plaques (unless co-existent disease)

What to tell the patient

'The symptoms you are describing today together with the changes to the joints suggest that you have a condition called osteoarthritis. This is the commonest degenerative joint condition, commonly described as 'wear and tear' of the joints. The diagnosis is usually made on a clinical basis without the need for further tests although sometimes X-rays can be helpful. The mainstay of management is through analgesia and physiotherapy. In severe cases of osteoarthritis of the knees or the hips, surgical options might be explored, in the form of joint replacement surgery.

I would like to prescribe you some tablets for pain relief and refer you to the physiotherapy department for an assessment.

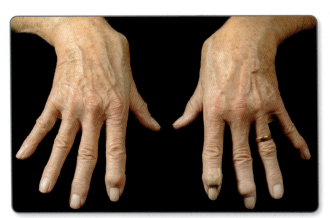

Figure 5.3 Osteoarthritis. This patient has osteoarthritis in both hands. Note the predominance of distal interphalangeal joint involvement with Heberden's nodes present on both forefingers and the middle finger of the patient's left hand.

'I would then like to bring you back in a few months' time to see how you are getting on. Do you have any questions or concerns that I can address today?'

What to tell the examiner – state the most likely diagnosis on the basis of the history and clinical findings

'This patient has symptoms and signs consistent with a diagnosis of osteoarthritis.'

Offer relevant differential diagnoses

The differential diagnosis includes the following:

- Psoriatic arthropathy (associated skin lesions)
- Rheumatoid arthritis (rarely involves DIP, prolonged morning stiffness)
- Crystal arthropathies (usually monoarticular, big toe or knee)

Demonstrate an understanding of the value of further investigation

With a good clinical diagnosis of OA, necessary investigations are limited. Plain radiographs of affected joints are needed, but little else. Radiographic features of osteoarthritis include:

- Loss of joint space
- Osteophyte formation
- Sub-chondral sclerosis
- Periosteal cysts

Always offer a management plan

Symptom control includes pain alleviation with simple analgesia, NSAIDs (but caution in using NSAIDs in older patients). A pain team referral may be necessary in severe and/or uncontrolled symptoms.

Note that although intra-articular corticosteroid injections and surgical options (arthroscopy/joint replacement) are features of the management of osteoarthritis, in practical terms they do not apply to disease affecting the joints of the hand. Therefore, if you mention them to the examiner in your discussion of management options, make sure you discuss them in the appropriate context.

Chondroitin and glucosamine supplements are commonly used by patients with the aim of alleviating symptoms in osteoarthritis. There is, however, considerable controversy surrounding their use. A recent meta-analysis of 10 clinical trials involving 3803 patients found that 'compared with placebo, glucosamine, chondroitin and their combination do not reduce joint pain or have an impact on narrowing of joint space' in osteoarthritis of the hip and knee. The MRCP PACES candidate would do well to avoid getting bogged down in the arguments. When presenting to the examiner, a simple statement such as: 'Chondroitin and glucosamine are often used in the management of osteoarthritis, however their use remains controversial' should suffice.

A multi-disciplinary approach is important to maximise functional capacity.

Further reading

Wandel S, Jüni P, Tendal B, et al. Effects of glucosamine, chondroitin, or placebo in patients with osteoarthritis of hip or knee: network meta-analysis. Br Med J 2010; 341:c4675.

Case 100: Sclerodactyly/systemic sclerosis

Instruction to the candidate

Please examine this 50-year-old woman who has noticed pain in her hands over the past year.

Take a focused history

As the patient has presented with symptoms of hand pain, start with an open question: 'I understand you have pain in your hands, can you tell me more about it?' After that (in conjunction with inspection of the hands that confirms sclerodactyly), a focused history would include:

- Symptoms of Raynaud's, including whether there is a relationship of the patient's pain to cold and whether there is a classical pattern of finger skin colour change in the cold. Is there any relationship to medications such as beta-blockers? Does the patient smoke?
- Ask about other symptoms of systemic sclerosis, such as problems with swallowing, weight loss and/or exertional breathlessness
- Does the patient have a confirmed diagnosis of systemic sclerosis and if so what organ systems are involved. What investigations have they had? Have they had any treatments in the past?

Positive findings of a focused examination

Assessment of the hands should be followed by consideration of a focused respiratory examination.

Positive findings include sclerodactyly, with shiny, tight skin on the fingers, associated calcinosis or fingertip ulceration. The skin changes may extend to the forearms but not above the elbow.

Consider further examination for:

- Nail changes – capillary infarcts
- Facial features – microstomia, facial telangiectasia characteristic nasal changes of systemic sclerosis (pinched or beak nose)
- Respiratory system – pulmonary fibrosis

Relevant negatives

As this case is clearly that of systemic sclerosis, relevant negatives should include other clinical signs and symptoms associated with systemic sclerosis that are not present. In addition, comment on potential complications of systemic sclerosis. As such, a relevant negative list may include, for instance, the absence of digital ulceration.

What to tell the patient

'The symptoms you describe together with the changes to your fingers and the rest of your skin point to the diagnosis of a condition called systemic sclerosis. This is a condition that as well as affecting the skin of the hands, can affect internal organs such as the lungs, oesophagus and kidneys. I would like to organise some tests to help confirm the diagnosis and to assess for any wider involvement of the organs I have just mentioned.'

'The management of the condition would depend on the results of the tests. There are some general measures such as wearing gloves and avoiding exposure to cold that will help with your hand symptoms. It is vital you stop smoking as it will greatly help your symptoms. Additionally, I can prescribe some tablets that can help with the pain.'

'Do you have any further concerns or questions that I can address today? I will be seeing you again with the results of the tests in 6–8 weeks' time.'

What to tell the examiner – state the most likely diagnosis on the basis of the history and clinical findings

'The patient has signs and symptoms consistent with systemic sclerosis.'

Offer relevant differential diagnoses

Given that sclerodactyly is often a 'spot diagnosis' instead of offering a differential of the diagnosis itself, offer a differential diagnosis of one of the signs or symptoms you have elicited.

Demonstrate an understanding of the value of further investigation

Investigations will include laboratory blood tests. These may be aimed at pointing to the underlying diagnosis (ANA, anti-centromere antibodies, anti-Scl70) or at the effects of the disease process (a raised creatinine indicative of renal dysfunction; a full blood count which may demonstrate anaemia or a secondary polycythaemia due to chronic hypoxia from pulmonary fibrosis).

In the presence of respiratory symptoms, investigations would include a plain chest radiograph looking for reticulonodular shadowing, followed by a high-resolution CT scan to further delineate the fibrosis. Lung function test would seek to identify a restrictive picture with raised diffusion factor.

In the presence of gastrointestinal symptoms an oesophageal-gastro-duodenoscopy (OGD) with oesophageal manometry would assess for oesophageal dysmotility.

In the presence of abnormal renal function, one would request a urine dipstick looking for proteinuria and haematuria and a full renal screen to rule out other causes of renal dysfunction.

Always offer a management plan

General lifestyle advice includes avoiding the cold and wearing gloves. The patient should avoid medications that exacerbate symptoms. Symptomatic relief includes the use of calcium channel blockers and in severe cases intravenous prostaglandins. Immunomodulatory strategies involve corticosteroids and methotrexate.

Management of complications includes:

- Other treatment modalities include ACE inhibition in renal involvement
- Oesophageal dysmotility is the main GI complication of systemic sclerosis. It usually presents with dysphagia and weight loss. Diagnosis is made by OGD and oesophageal manometry showing disordered contraction of the oesophagus. Medical management involves prokinetic agents such as metoclopramide, along with proton pump inhibitors
- Nifedipine and prostacyclin may be helpful in lung disease

Case 101: Gout

Instruction to the candidate

This 84-year-old man has been experiencing recurrent attacks of pain in his forefinger. Please take a brief history and focused examination. Report your findings to the patient and tell him about your management plan.

Take a focused history

Ask specific questions about the presenting symptom. Which joint is painful? Is there associated swelling and/or erythema? Ask about the frequency of episodes? Is there an obvious precipitant?

Take a drug history and a past medical history. Drugs that can precipitate gout include thiazide diuretics and calcineurin inhibitors. Many diseases are known to increase the risk of gout, including:

- Hypertension
- Diabetes, obesity and the metabolic syndrome
- Renal failure

- Psoriasis
- Tumour lysis syndrome

Take a focused social history asking about alcohol intake, specifically red wine, and intake of food rich in purines.

Positive findings of a focused examination

The hands are one of the less common sites for acute gout to occur. The MTP is the commonest site. It is, however, possible for gout to occur in the fingers and hands and this possibility is used here as a vehicle for discussion of gout. Perhaps more likely as a hand case is chronic tophaceous gout. This occurs when urate crystal deposits form nodules around joints. The most common sites for tophi are the ears, hands, toes and knees. Tophaceous gout is the consequence of chronic, poorly-controlled gout.

Thus, examination should proceed with an assessment of the hands followed by the knees and/or feet.

Assess for deformity and function. The metacarpo-phalangeal joint (MCP) of the forefinger of the right hand is swollen, tender and erythematous. It is warm to touch, suggesting acute inflammation. The patient has restricted range of movement of the affected joint, mainly due to pain.

Relevant negatives

Important relevant negative findings include the absence of symmetrical deformity and the absence of clinical features of sepsis (important in a patient with a hot, red joint).

What to tell the patient

'From the symptoms you describe and my examination findings, the most likely diagnosis is that of acute gout. Gout is where crystals form in the joint, causing it to become painful and inflamed. It is not a dangerous condition and the frequency of attacks can be reduced with the right treatments and avoidance of triggers. Today I am going to start you on some medications to reduce the inflammation. It is called colchicine. One of the side-effects of colchicine is that it can cause diarrhoea, so if this occurs you should stop taking it. I would like to order some investigations and I will see you in clinic again in 10 weeks.'

What to tell the examiner – state the most likely diagnosis on the basis of the history and clinical findings

'This patient has symptoms and signs consistent with a diagnosis of acute gout.'

Offer relevant differential diagnoses

The most important differential diagnosis of an acutely inflamed joint is septic arthritis.

Demonstrate an understanding of the value of further investigation

The key in any hot, swollen joint is to rule out a septic joint.

Specific investigations for gout include:

- Blood tests: inflammatory markers (expect the white cell count to be raised in addition to C-reactive protein, even in the absence of bacterial infection). Serum urate is routinely measured
- Joint aspirate: acute gout is a crystal arthropathy. The crystals can be detected using spectrophotometry examination of the joint aspirate. Positive aspirates contain needle-like crystals that display negative birefringence under polarised light. The joint aspirate will also undergo gram staining and culture to aid exclusion of a septic joint
- Plain radiographs of affected joints

Always offer a management plan

Principles of management include symptom control, followed by measures to induce remission, and subsequently maintain remission.

Symptom control is with non-steroidal anti-inflammatory agents with colchicine to reduce inflammation. Use of colchicine is often limited by diarrhoea and caution is needed in patients with renal impairment.

Allopurinol, a xanthine oxidase inhibitor, is used to maintain remission in those patients experiencing severe or recurrent bouts of disabling gout. It should not be started in an acute attack due to precipitation of soft tissue crystal stores, worsening and prolonging the acute episode. The patient should avoid foods and medications that trigger attacks.

Further reading
Roddy E, Doherty M. Epidemiology of gout. Arthritis Res Ther 2010; 12:223.

Case 102: Carpal tunnel syndrome

Instruction to the candidate

This 34-year-old woman has been experiencing tingling in her hands over a period of 6 months. Please make an assessment with a brief history and examination, as you feel appropriate. Advise the patient as to what you think the cause of her problem is.

Take a focused history

As the primary symptom is that of tingling in the hand, get a full description of the tingling. Specifically seek to obtain a history of tingling in the distribution of the median nerve. Are there any specific circumstances in which the tingling occurs or is worse? Are the symptoms unilateral or bilateral? Is there associated pain or numbness?

Take a past medical history for conditions which are all associated with carpal tunnel syndrome including: obesity, trauma, hypothyroidism, diabetes, rheumatoid arthritis, acromegaly, or pregnancy.

Take an occupational history. Is there evidence of overuse of the wrist?

Positive findings of a focused examination

Assessing for deformity, there is wasting of the muscle bulk of the thenar eminence. Explore the possibility of neurological deficit, both sensory and motor, in the distribution of the median nerve. Assessing for function, there is weakness of thumb abduction.

Utilise the following special tests to gain evidence towards a diagnosis of carpal tunnel syndrome:

- Tinel's test: reproduction of the patient's symptoms by repetitive percussion of a finger over the volar aspect of the patient's wrist
- Phalen's test: reproduction of the patient's symptoms by holding the patient's wrist in fixed flexion for a prolonged period of time (>45 seconds)

Consider further examination for clinical signs of conditions known to cause carpal tunnel syndrome. In particular:

- Visual field assessment in patients with suggestive of acromegaly on general inspection – spade-like hands, large stature and coarse facial features with prominent brow and jaw
- Neck examination where there is suspicion of thyroid disease or inspection suggests a possible goitre

Relevant negatives

Note the absence of scars to suggest previous carpal tunnel decompression.

What to tell the patient

'The symptoms you describe to me and the fact that they are reproduced when I tap on your wrist and when I hold your wrist flexed suggest that you have a condition known as carpal tunnel syndrome, where one of the nerves that run to your hand gets pressed upon as it passes through the wrist. To make a certain diagnosis, I will have to request an investigation to test the affected nerve. In the meantime it is reasonable to start conservative treatment with the use of a wrist splint and the avoidance of overuse of the wrist. It is also possible to inject steroids into the wrist. You may have heard that surgery is an option in this condition, but we normally wait to see how simple measures work first.

'Are there any other questions or concerns that I can address today?'

What to tell the examiner – state the most likely diagnosis on the basis of the history and clinical findings

'This patient has signs and symptoms consistent with carpal tunnel syndrome.'

Offer relevant differential diagnoses

Causes of carpal tunnel syndrome include:

- Idiopathic
- Obesity
- Hypothyroidism
- Diabetes mellitus
- Rheumatoid arthritis
- Pregnancy
- Acromegaly
- Post-traumatic

Demonstrate an understanding of the value of further investigation

Investigations aim to confirm pathology of the median nerve:

- Nerve conduction studies: a positive test, suggestive of median nerve pathology, will show decrease conduction velocities in the median nerve in the context of normal nerve conduction at other sites
- Imaging options include ultrasound of the carpal tunnel and MRI
- Investigations to rule out secondary causes of carpal tunnel syndrome include thyroid function tests, β-HCG if appropriate and IGF-1 for acromegaly (however, the clinical picture should be enough to confirm or refute a diagnosis of acromegaly)

Always offer a management plan

Where identified, management should be directed to the underlying cause. Specific management of the carpal tunnel syndrome can be divided into conservative and surgical.

- Conservative management involves splinting and steroid injection
- Surgical management is second line. Intervention includes decompression of the carpal tunnel by division of the transverse carpal ligament. A recent systematic review has shown that both conservative and surgical measures confer symptomatic benefit in carpal tunnel syndrome, but that surgical management was more effective

Further reading

Marshall S, Tardif G, Ashworth N. Local corticosteroid injection for carpal tunnel syndrome. Cochrane Database Syst Rev 2007:CD001554.

Shi Q, MacDermid JC. Is surgical intervention more effective than non-surgical treatment for carpal tunnel syndrome? A systematic review. J Ortho Surg Res 2011;6:17.

Case 103: Wrist drop – radial nerve lesion

Instruction to the candidate

Please examine this 52-year-old man who has been complaining of weakness and abnormal sensation in the right hand, which he noticed when he woke from sleep 3 days ago.

Take a focused history

The clinical history may vary. Ascertain the circumstances of the onset of the weakness. A common scenario involves the 'saturday night palsy' where a patient has fallen asleep, under the influence of alcohol, in an awkward position with an arm straddling a chair with resultant axillary compression. On waking, weakness of the arm is noted to persist.

Additionally screen for:

- Trauma to the neck and arm
- A history of use of crutches
- Any exposure to lead

Positive findings of a focused examination

Motor deficit includes weakness of wrist extension, known as 'wrist drop'. Sensory loss is evident on the dorsum of the hand. The area affected includes the thumb to the interphalangeal joint and the fore- and middle finger to the distal interphalangeal joint. The lateral half of the ring finger may also be affected.

Relevant negatives

Specific relevant negative findings would include:

- An absence of signs of other neurological dysfunction (therefore, this is a mononeuropathy)
- No sign of neck trauma
- No sign of trauma to the humerus
- No crutches by the bedside

What to tell the patient

'From what you have told me and from what I have found on examination, it appears that you have caused some damage to one of the nerves that supplies some of the muscles in the arm – the radial nerve. Sustained pressure on the nerve, such as from falling asleep with your arm draped over a chair, causes dysfunction of the nerve. This is why you have weakness and why the sensation on the back of the right hand is affected. In most cases when the radial nerve is damaged in this way the damage is only temporary will usually get better by itself. However, I will organise some tests to check the function of the nerves of your arm and will see you again in 4 weeks' time. Are there any other questions or concerns that I can answer for you?'

What to tell the examiner – state the most likely diagnosis on the basis of the history and clinical findings

'This patient has signs consistent with radial nerve palsy due to prolonged compression of the radial nerve.'

Offer relevant differential diagnoses

Radial nerve lesions can be caused by damage anywhere along the course of the nerve, including:

- Posterior cord of the brachial plexus
- Axilla: Persistent use of crutches
- As the nerve runs in the spiral groove of the humerus: Fractured humerus
- At the elbow: nerve entrapment
- In the forearm: fractured radius

Demonstrate an understanding of the value of further investigation

The history and examination will guide the exact investigative strategy, but tests to consider include neurophysiology, with assessment of nerve conduction.

Always offer a management plan

Management depends on the underlying cause. If the patient is suffering pain, analgesia may include gabapentin, pregabalin or amitriptyline to target the neuropathic component. Wrist splinting can be considered.

Depending on the level of disability caused, you may need to refer to occupational therapy and physiotherapy as part of a multi-disciplinary strategy to minimise the effect of the functional impairment on the patient's activities of daily living.

Case 104: Ulnar nerve lesion

Instruction to the candidate

This 68-year-old woman has presented to clinic complaining of tingling and numbness in her left hand. Please take a brief history and perform a focused examination. Inform the patient of your findings and formulate a management plan.

Take a focused history

Enquire about the type of deficit and its distribution, i.e. sensory, motor, or both. Accurately define the type of sensory disturbance. Is it tingling, numbness or pain? Is the sensory disturbance transient or continuous? Explore exacerbating or triggering factors.

Explore the past medical history:

- Is there a history of carpal tunnel syndrome, nerve entrapment or mononeuropathy?
- Is there a history of degenerative or traumatic pathology at the elbow?
- Does the patient have diabetes or hypertension?

Explore the social history:

- What is the patient's occupation? Are they a construction worker who operates vibrating tools?
- Do they, or did they smoke? Take a systematic review of weight loss, cough and haemoptysis when suspecting a Pancoast tumour
- What effect do the symptoms have on the patient's daily life?

The typical ulnar nerve lesion will present as sensory disturbance comprising of tingling and numbness, felt at the lateral aspect of the palmar surface of the hand. The 5th finger is usually the most affected.

Positive findings of a focused examination

Motor findings include muscle wasting. There is weakness of flexor carpi ulnaris and flexor digitorum profundus weakness. Check intrinsic muscle function.

In ulnar nerve palsy, there is weakness of thumb adduction. Testing for Froment's sign involves asking the patient, with their hand flat and pronated, to hold a piece of paper between the straight thumb and the medial aspect of the forefinger. The person examining then tries to pull the piece of paper out of the hand while the patient resists. A subject with normal function of adductor pollicis will be able to hold the paper while keeping the thumb straight. A subject with weakness in adductor pollicis will compensate by flexing the thumb to hold the paper in place. The latter denotes a positive Froment's sign.

Sensory deficit includes sensory loss over the palmar surface of the ulnar aspect of the palm, extending to involve the little finger and the medial aspect of the ring finger.

Consider further examination of the elbow for any deformity. Also examine the neck and shoulder. Pain on neck movement mimicking the patient's symptoms could indicate brachial plexus pathology.

Relevant negatives

Important relevant negative findings include:

- There is no clawing of the hand, which would indicate severe, long-term ulnar nerve dysfunction
- There is an absence of signs of previous trauma to the elbow
- There are no scars to indicated previous ulnar nerve decompression – see section on management

What to tell the patient

'The symptoms you describe together with my clinical findings suggest you have a problem with the ulnar nerve which supplies part of your hand and arm. Because of its anatomic position, it is subject to entrapment and injury by many causes. Because of its superficial position at the elbow it is prone to injuries by excessive pressure in this area such as leaning on the elbow during work, which I suspect is the case in your case. With the aid of physiotherapy and occupational therapy it should get better. Failing that there are surgical options we can consider for your symptomatic relief. I would like to run some nerve studies to confirm how the nerve is functioning and would like to bring you back in 6 weeks' time to discuss the results and discuss options. Are there any questions or concerns that I can address?'

What to tell the examiner – state the most likely diagnosis on the basis of the history and clinical findings

'This patient has symptoms and signs consistent with a diagnosis of ulnar nerve palsy.'

Offer relevant differential diagnoses

The most common cause of ulnar nerve palsy is due to entrapment in the cubital tunnel at the elbow. Other causes include:

- Cervical disc disease
- Brachial plexus abnormalities
- Thoracic outlet syndrome
- Pancoast tumour
- Elbow abnormalities, such as epicondylitis
- Tumours
- Wrist fractures
- Compression within Guyon's canal

Demonstrate an understanding of the value of further investigation

Nerve conduction studies will confirm nerve pathology.

Always offer a management plan

The management of ulnar nerve dysfunction due to compression at the cubital tunnel is undertaken in the context of a multi-disciplinary team setting. It includes initial conservative management with regular review and involvement of occupational therapy and physiotherapy as appropriate.

If conservative measures fail, then surgical intervention is indicated. Surgical options include:

- Cubital tunnel decompression
- Medial epicondylectomy
- Transposition of the ulnar nerve

Further reading

Cutts S. Cubital tunnel syndrome. Postgrad Med J. 2007; 83:28–31.

Case 105: Cataracts

Instruction to the candidate

This 72-year-old woman has been complaining of declining vision over the past year. Please take a short history and perform a focused examination. Summarise your findings to the patient and explain your investigation and management plan. A short discussion with the examiner will then follow.

Take a focused history

Attempt to gain more information on the nature of the visual loss. Ask about whether it is lateralised to one eye in particular. How severe is it? What has been its speed of onset (the candidate information suggests one year)? Is there associated pain (cataracts is usually painless)?

Ask regarding associated features:

- Is there any scalp tenderness or jaw claudication? If present, these symptoms would suggest giant cell arteritis

- Does the patient suffer from 'glare' particularly noticeable when driving at night?

Explore the past ophthalmic history. Has there ever been trauma to eyes, either blunt or penetrating? Is there any history of ocular inflammation? Is there a history of squint (turn in eye) or amblyopia?

Enquire about the patient's past medical history, seeking to elicit a history of diabetes mellitus or other conditions associated with cataract. Do they use medications such as corticosteroids?

Assess the effect of the visual loss on the patient's activities of daily living. Make sure to elicit the patient's occupation and driving status.

Positive findings of a focused examination

The key positive findings are of reduced visual acuity with a diminished red reflex.

Examination reveals reduced visual acuity. If possible test with Snellen chart (distance) and Near Vision chart. Ensure appropriate glasses. Using a pinhole helps to negate the effect of uncorrected refractive error.

There is a diminished red reflex – you may see generalised dimming of red reflex, spokes, flecks, dots. In advanced cataract, the lens may be seen as white or brown, obscuring the red reflex.

Relevant negatives

Important relevant negative findings include:

- Examination of pupil reactions reveals an absence of a relative afferent papillary defect (patient may have had prior mydriatic drops in which case this will not be possible)
- Visual fields to confrontation are normal
- Using the +10 dioptre setting on the direct ophthalmoscope to provide illumination and magnification , the cornea is clear and there is no obvious pupillary or iris deformity
- Fundoscopy is normal

What to tell the patient

'The reduction in vision you describe appears to be due to cataract. This is a misting of the lens in the eye that occurs over time, and is often helped with surgery.

'If you wish to consider an operation to help your vision I can ask your GP to refer you to an eye surgeon who can discuss this further with you. In the meantime it might help to attend your optometrist to check if a new pair of glasses would improve your vision.

'The RNIB might be able to offer you some practical advice and gadgets to make things easier for you at home.

'Do you have any questions or concerns?'

What to tell the examiner – state the most likely diagnosis on the basis of the history and clinical findings

'The patient has lens opacity consistent with senile cataracts.'

Offer relevant differential diagnoses

A differential diagnosis of secondary causes of cataracts includes:

- Diabetes mellitus

- Medication, such as corticosteroids
- Previous ocular trauma or intraocular surgery
- Ocular inflammation
- Chronic retinal detachment
- A posterior segment tumour

Age related macular degeneration might also cause gradual decline in vision over many years and should be considered in such a history.

Demonstrate an understanding of the value of further investigation

Cataract is a clinical diagnosis and management plans are based usually on clinical findings.

In cases where the fundus cannot be visualised due to dense lens opacity (white or brunescent cataract), B-scan ultrasonography can be used to check for the presence or absence of major posterior segment abnormalities such as retinal detachment or tumour (choroidal melanoma or choroidal metastasis).

Always offer a management plan

Early cataract may cause visual loss due to refractive change that may be amenable to a change in glasses prescription; therefore, a referral to an optometrist is necessary.

Surgical treatment of cataract is indicated when the patient's corrected visual acuity no longer meets their visual demand and they are unable to perform their activities of daily living. The lens is removed and an artificial lens implanted. Most cataract surgery in the United Kingdom is carried out as a day case under local anaesthetic. The main complication is visual loss with an incidence of 1 in 800 approximately.

Many hospitals in the United Kingdom have a liaison officer from the Royal National Institute of the Blind (RNIB) who can assist patients with visual impairment with their practical needs.

Remember that in the United Kingdom the legal visual standard for driving is to be able to read a standard number plate at 20 metres in good daylight. This translates approximately to 6/10 on the Snellen chart. If the patient does not meet this with either eye they should be advised of this.

Further reading

The Royal College of Ophthalmologists (RCOphth). Cataract Surgery Guidelines. London; RCOphth, 2010.

Driver and Vehicle Licensing Agency (DVLA). For medical practitioners. At a glance guide to the current medical standards of fitness to drive. Swansea; DVLA, 2011.

Case 106: Diabetic retinopathy

Instruction to the candidate

This 30-year-old diabetic man complains of reduced vision in his left eye. Please take a short history and perform a focused examination. Summarise your findings to the patient and explain your investigation and management plan. A short discussion with the examiner will then follow.

Take a focused history

As with all visual loss, seek to characterise it further by asking questions to elicit – its nature, laterality, severity and speed of onset. When asking about any associated pain, remember that diabetic retinopathy and vitreous haemorrhage are usually painless.

Screen for any prodromal features:

- Preceding floaters, cobwebs or a red tinge to the vision would indicate vitreous haemorrhage
- Preceding visual distortion indicates a macular pathology

Ask about a past medical history of diabetes. Characterise the sub-type of diabetes. How long is it since the patient was diagnosed? Assess blood sugar control. Ask if the patient is aware of their most recent HbA1c level. Take a medication history. Does the patient have a history of macro- and/or microvascular complications of their diabetes?

Explore the past medical history. Does the patient have a history of hypertension or hyperlipidaemia?

Take a brief social history, assessing whether or not the patient smokes. What is the effect of the visual loss on the patient's lifestyle? What is their occupation? Are they currently driving?

Positive findings of a focused examination

Anterior segment examination

Examine with +10 dioptre lens on ophthalmoscope. There may be lens opacity or rubeosis iridis (fine new vessel formation on iris – a sign of advanced proliferative disease).

Posterior segment examination

There may be any of the following:

- Microaneurysms
- Blot haemorrhages
- Hard exudates
- Cotton-wool spots
- Venous beading
- Intra-retinal microvascular abnormalities
- New vessels at the disc or elsewhere
- Vitreous haemorrhage (large dark floaters/ red haze/no view to retina at all)

State the location of any haemorrhages or hard exudates, paying particular attention to whether the macula is affected.

Relevant negatives

Check the pupillary reactions for a relative afferent papillary defect but this may not be possible if mydriatic drops have already been instilled.

What to tell the patient

'My examination today has shown a small amount of bleeding inside the eye, preventing you from seeing through it. Hopefully it will clear over the next few weeks, making the vision brighter. I will refer you to an ophthalmologist who may recommend laser treatment to prevent further bleeding and permanent loss of vision.

'This might be a good time to look at helping you to improve your blood sugars and blood pressure. I will arrange for you to see the diabetes team who can give you more advice.'

What to tell the examiner – state the most likely diagnosis on the basis of the history and clinical findings

'The patient has proliferative diabetic retinopathy with vitreous haemorrhage.'

Grading diabetic retinopathy

There are many systems for classifying diabetic retinopathy. The RCOphth guidelines recommend this simple system for clinical use:

Low risk (background), non-proliferative diabetic retinopathy is characterised by mildly dilated veins, microaneurysms, dot haemorrhages, exudates and the occasional cotton-wool spot.

High risk (pre-proliferative), non-proliferative diabetic retinopathy is characterised by intraretinal microvascular abnormalities, venous beading and loops, clusters of large 'blot' or 'blotch' haemorrhage, and multiple cotton-wool spots.

A patient with proliferative diabetic retinopathy will have new vessels at disc or elsewhere. This may be accompanied by vitreous haemorrhage and tractional retinal detachment.

See **Figures 5.4–5.8** for examples of diabetic retinopathy at various stages.

Offer relevant differential diagnoses

If vitreous haemorrhage is present, remember there are other causes apart from proliferative diabetic retinopathy:

- Retinal tear or detachment
- Proliferative retinopathy secondary to vascular occlusion or ocular ischaemic syndrome

- If loss of vision but no obvious vitreous haemorrhage, consider diabetic macular oedema
- If loss of vision but no obvious vitreous haemorrhage or macular oedema, consider cataract or ischaemic optic neuropathy

Demonstrate an understanding of the value of further investigation

- HbA1c should be measured to gauge glycaemic control
- B-scan ultrasonography can be used to exclude retinal detachment if no view to fundus
- Slit lamp biomicroscopy, OCT and/or fundus fluorescein angiography can be used to ascertain if there is any macular oedema, if it is suspected

Always offer a management plan

Offer the patient lifestyle advice. Tell the patient to avoid vigorous activity or heavy lifting to allow the vitreous haemorrhage to clear. This can take several weeks. Smoking cessation advice should be offered if necessary.

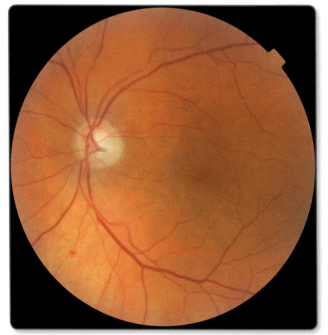

Figure 5.4 Diabetic retinopathy. The left fundus with dot and blot haemorrhages in the inferonasal quadrant.

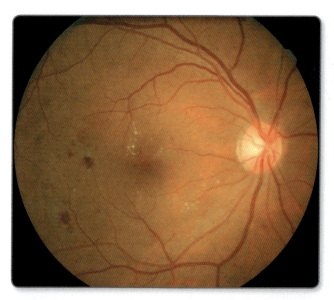

Figure 5.5 Diabetic retinopathy. The macula of the right eye showing exudates adjacent to the fovea (the darker area with no vessels at the centre of the macula). Dot and blot haemorrhages can be seen in the temporal macula.

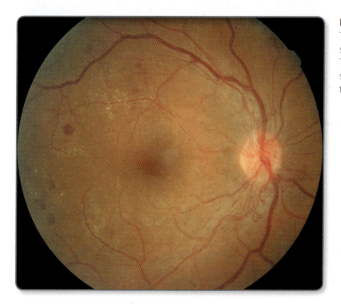

Figure 5.6 Diabetic retinopathy. The macula of the right fundus showing new vessels at the disc. There are circinate exudates surrounding blot haemorrhages in the temporal macula.

Refer the patient to an ophthalmologist for consideration of laser photocoagulation therapy (**Figure 5.8**), although laser treatment may have to wait until a clear view of the fundus is possible. Laser treatment can reduce the risk of severe visual loss over 2 years by 50–70%. Non-clearing vitreous haemorrhage or tractional detachment may require surgery (a vitrectomy). Intravitreal injections of steroid or anti-vascular endothelial growth factor agents may have a role in diabetic retinopathy treatment.

Risk factor modification is important. The patient's presentation affords an opportunity to address systemic risk factors, including blood sugar levels. Any tightening of blood sugar control should be gradual, as rapid reductions in blood sugar levels can be associated with worsening of retinopathy. Both the DCCT

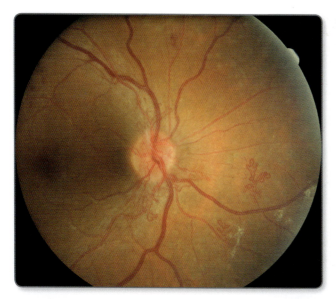

Figure 5.7 Diabetic retinopathy. Neovascularisation at the optic disc, with venous loops on the inferonasal retinal veins.

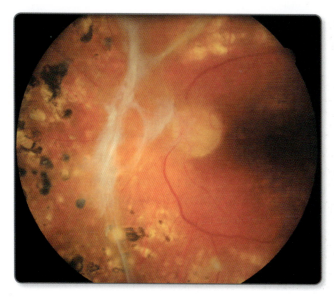

Figure 5.8 Laser treated diabetic retinopathy. The optic disc of the left eye showing treated proliferative diabetic retinopathy. There are fibrovascular bands in front of the disc and pigmented laser scars on the periphery of the retina.

and UKPDS trials have shown risk reductions associated with improved glycaemic control. Good hypertensive control and addition of a statin are indicated if appropriate.

Vitreous haemorrhage is not a contraindication to continue antiplatelet therapy if it is required for cardiovascular risk reduction.

Consider referral to low vision services or RNIB liaison officer.

Further reading

The Royal College of Ophthalmologists (RCOphth). Diabetic retinopathy guidelines. London; RCOphth, 2012.

Photocoagulation treatment of proliferative diabetic retinopathy: the second report of diabetic retinopathy study findings. Ophthalmology 1978; 85:82–106.

The effect of intensive treatment of diabetes on the development and progression of long-term complications in insulin-dependent diabetes mellitus. The Diabetes Control and Complications Trial Research Group. N Engl J Med 1993; 329:977–986.

Intensive blood-glucose control with sulphonylureas or insulin compared with conventional treatment and risk of complications in patients with type 2 diabetes (UKPDS 33). UK Prospective Diabetes Study (UKPDS) Group. Lancet 1998; 352:837–853.

Case 107: Hypertensive retinopathy

Instruction to the candidate

This 58-year-old woman with a history of hypertension complains of headaches and transiently blurred vision. Her blood pressure is 210/110 mmHg. Please take a history and perform a focused examination. Summarise your findings to the patient and explain your investigation and management plan. A short discussion with the examiner will then follow.

Take a focused history

Most patients with hypertension are asymptomatic. Worrying symptoms in this context include a headache which is worse in the morning or on lying down, associated with nausea and transient blurring of vision or visual obscurations.

Take a history of hypertension including its duration, what current medications (if any) are being used to control it, and any symptoms suggestive of a systemic cause.

Positive findings of a focused examination

Fundoscopy in hypertensive retinopathy can show a constellation of signs, including:

- Narrowed retinal arterioles
- Arteriovenous nipping
- Flame shaped haemorrhages
- Hard exudates
- Cotton wool spots
- Swollen optic discs

If possible, measure the patient's blood pressure yourself.

Relevant negatives

Relevant negative findings include the absence of signs suggestive of diabetic retinopathy, although remember that the two conditions may co-exist.

What to tell the patient

'Your blood pressure is very high today and this is causing some changes at the back of your eyes affecting your vision. I need to arrange some tests to check if there is any particular reason that your blood pressure is so high, and I will change your medication to help bring your blood pressure down. Usually there will be no lasting effects on your eyesight if your blood pressure is treated.'

What to tell the examiner – state the most likely diagnosis on the basis of the history and clinical findings

'The patient has retinal changes in keeping with hypertensive retinopathy.'

Grading hypertensive retinopathy

Hypertensive retinopathy can be classified into either mild, moderate, or malignant disease. Mild retinopathy, which carries a modest association with risk of stroke, coronary heart disease and mortality, is characterised by the presence of one or more of the following arteriolar signs:

- Generalised arteriolar narrowing
- Focal arteriolar narrowing

- Arteriovenous nipping
- Arteriolar wall opacity (silver wiring)

Moderate retinopathy, which has a strong risk of stroke, cognitive decline and cardiovascular mortality, is characterised by one or more of the following retinal signs:

- Haemorrhage (blot, dot, or flame shaped)
- Microaneurysm
- Cotton-wool spot
- Hard exudates

Malignant retinopathy denotes any patient displaying moderate retinopathy plus optic disc swelling. It has a strong association with mortality.

Offer relevant differential diagnoses

Both central retinal vein occlusion and diabetic retinopathy can present with florid haemorrhages, cotton wool spots and swollen optic discs. Bilateral ischaemic optic neuropathy presents with bilateral swollen discs, loss of vision and sectoral visual field defects without peripheral retinal vascular changes and haemorrhages.

Demonstrate an understanding of the value of further investigation

Consider a CT scan of head if any concern regarding other causes of raised intracranial pressure.

If you have not measured the patient's blood pressure as part of the focused examination, mention it as a necessary investigation.

Always offer a management plan

Acute management of patients with malignant hypertension with optic disc swelling involves urgent but controlled reduction of blood pressure, as a rapid reduction can result in end organ ischaemia. There should be screening for causes of secondary hypertension.

Ophthalmic referral is advised in cases of moderate hypertensive retinopathy or worse, or in cases where the retinal findings are out of keeping with the degree of hypertension. An ophthalmologist can examine for signs of other retinal vasculopathies. Usually observation of the fundal changes is all that is required; there is seldom any need for ophthalmic surgical intervention.

The patient will require long-term management of blood pressure and attention paid to other cardiovascular risk factors.

Further reading

Wong TY, Mitchell P. Hypertensive retinopathy. N Engl J Med 2004; 351:2310–2317.

Grosso A, Veglio F, Porta M, Grignolo FM, Wong TY. Hypertensive retinopathy revisited: some answers, more questions. Br J Ophthalmol 2005; 89:1646–1654.

Case 108: Retinitis pigmentosa

Instruction to the candidate

A 30-year-old man has been referred to you by his general practitioner. He has become increasingly clumsy and prone to bumping into things of late. There is a family history of poor vision. Please take a history and perform a focused examination. Summarise your findings to the patient and explain your investigation and management plan. A short discussion with the examiner will then follow.

Take a focused history

Ask regarding the nature of his clumsiness, including enquiring about symptoms that may suggest cerebellar or vestibular disease.

Elicit a history of poor peripheral vision and 'not seeing' the objects being bumped into. Ask regarding nyctalopia (poor night vision). In children this may manifest as fear of dark environments. Does the patient need to sleep with the light on? Do they bump into things when walking outside at night (particularly if the patient lives in the country)?

Ask about associated symptoms:

- Glare and blurred reading vision are important secondary symptoms
- History of hearing loss
- History suggestive of other developmental abnormalities

Is there a family history of visual impairment? If so, who was affected, at what age? Characterise the type of visual impairment suffered by family members. Try to go back as far as grandparents in the family history, and do ask about aunts, uncles and cousins. Beware, some family trees can be complicated! Try to draw out a family tree if possible, and mark on it the affected individuals to ascertain the mode of inheritance.

Take a social history, including the patient's employment and driving status.

Positive findings of a focused examination

Test visual acuity if facilities available – central acuity may be normal though.

Visual fields to confrontation show reduced peripheral visual field in a concentric and symmetrical pattern.

Fundoscopy shows a pale disc, attenuated retinal blood vessels, and pigment spicules in peripheries **(Figure 5.9)**.

There may be cataract – diminished red reflex, speckles/spots in red reflex.

Relevant negatives

Important relevant negative findings include:

- The absence of a relative afferent papillary defect
- The absence of nystagmus
- Normal colour vision (tested using Ishihara plates if available)

What to tell the patient

'It is possible that you have a condition called retinitis pigmentosa, meaning that the retina does not work as well as it should do. This can cause your eyesight to fail over time, particularly at the edges of your vision or when it is dark. Sometimes this runs in families, and sometimes it can be passed on to any children you might have. Sometimes it is made worse by treatable things such as cataract and fluid accumulating in the retina and so I will refer you to an eye doctor.'

What to tell the examiner – state the most likely diagnosis on the basis of the history and clinical findings

'The patient has signs in keeping with retinitis pigmentosa, an inherited rod dystrophy.'

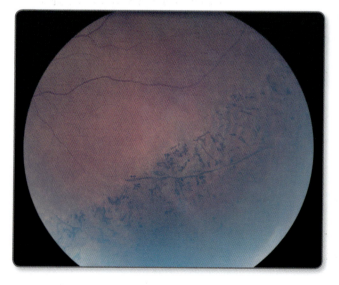

Figure 5.9 Retinitis pigmentosa. Characteristic pigmented spicules in the peripheral retina.

Offer relevant differential diagnoses

There are a number of conditions which have retinitis pigmentosa as a feature, including:

- Usher's syndrome – retinitis pigmentosa associated with hearing loss
- Laurence–Moon–Bardet–Biedl syndrome – retinitis pigmentosa associated with truncal obesity, short stature and polydactyly

Diabetic retinopathy with heavy laser photocoagulation treatment can look similar to retinitis pigmentosa, and peripheral fields and night vision can be affected in a similar way.

Demonstrate an understanding of the value of further investigation

Automated visual field testing can more accurately plot and quantify peripheral field loss, and provide a baseline measure.

If central acuity is poor, both fundus fluorescein angiography (FFA) and optical coherence tomography (OCT) can be used to identify the presence of cystoid macular oedema.

Always offer a management plan

If cataract or macular oedema suspected, refer to ophthalmologist for consideration of further medical or surgical management.

If the patient has younger siblings, or is considering starting a family, a referral to a geneticist for counselling is advised.

Consider referral to low vision services or RNIB liaison officer.

Consider eligibility to hold a driving license if applicable. The patient should be advised to inform the licensing authority of their condition.

Case 109: CMV retinitis

Instruction to the candidate

This 46-year-old man is an inpatient on the infectious diseases ward. He has been complaining of blurred vision. Please take a history and perform a focused examination. Summarise your findings to the patient and explain your investigation and management plan. A short discussion with the examiner will then follow.

Take a focused history

Characterise the nature and duration of visual loss. Is there a painful or red eye?

Assess the general health of the patient. Why are they in the infectious diseases ward? Is there a history of immunocompromise or immunosuppression? What current medications are they taking?

Positive findings of a focused examination

Test the visual acuity if facilities are available. It will likely be reduced.

Fundoscopy shows creamy retinal infiltrates with scattered retinal haemorrhages – 'scrambled egg and tomato ketchup'. There is sheathing of the vessels indicative of retinal vasculitis. Changes are usually present in both eyes.

Relevant negatives

It would be prudent to comment on the patient's general appearance and state of health.

What to tell the patient

'You have an infection affecting your eyes, which is a sign of a weak immune system. It will require intensive treatment with strong drugs to try to kill the infection and help boost your immune system. The eye is delicate and can be severely damaged by infections such as this. I will refer you to a doctor who specialises in these infections. Do you have any questions?'

What to tell the examiner – state the most likely diagnosis on the basis of the history and clinical findings

'The symptoms of this patient together with the clinical findings are suggestive of cytomegalovirus chorioretinitis.'

Offer relevant differential diagnoses

Possible causes of chorioretinitis include: HIV infection, toxoplasmosis, *Toxocara*, syphilis, *Borrelia*.

Demonstrate an understanding of the value of further investigation

Investigations would include:

- Cultures can be taken from throat and urine for cytomegalovirus
- Serological tests can be performed for HIV, toxoplasmosis, *Toxocara* and syphilis if there exists any doubt regarding the underlying diagnosis
- Vitreous sampling may be performed for microscopy, culture and polymerase chain reaction (PCR) DNA analysis but is not usually necessary

Always offer a management plan

Advice should be sought from an infectious disease physician and a medical retina specialist. Management involves treatment of any HIV infection along with systemic antiviral agents. Antiviral agents can be administered directly into the vitreous cavity by injection, or by slow-release implant.

Case 110: Optic atrophy

Instruction to the candidate

This 70-year-old woman has a history of poor vision in their right eye. Their optometrist noted an unusual appearance to their right optic disc. Please take a history and perform a focused examination. Summarise your findings to the patient and explain your investigation and management plan. A short discussion with the examiner will then follow.

Take a focused history

When and how did the visual loss happen? Does it continue to progress, or was it a sudden event?

Ask about any associated neurological symptoms.

Explore a past medical history for evidence of existing cardiovascular disease. Enquire of a family history of glaucoma.

In any patient over the age of 50 years with visual loss, ask about symptoms of temporal arteritis:

- Is there scalp tenderness (does it hurt to brush your hair?)?
- Is there jaw claudication (do you get tired chewing your food?)?
- Are there more generalised symptoms of weight loss, anorexia and general malaise?

Positive findings of a focused examination

Look for reduced visual acuity. There may be reduced visual acuity in the right eye. With the other unaffected.

There is a right relative afferent papillary defect, or possibly no direct reaction to light at all.

Colour vision in the right eye is poor. (Test with Ishihara plates, or ask about red desaturation.)

There is a reduced visual field to confrontation on the right side (large central scotoma, or possibly a reduced peripheral field), the left is normal.

Positive findings on fundoscopy include disc pallor in the affected eye. The unaffected eye may be normal.

Relevant negatives

Relevant negative findings include:

- There is a preserved consensual papillary reaction
- The optic disc cup is normal on the right
- There is no disc swelling

What to tell the patient

'The nerve at the back of the eye is pale due to the blockage in the blood vessels you had many years ago. We will check your blood pressure and cholesterol to make sure we are doing all we can to prevent the same thing happening again. Do you have any questions?'

What to tell the examiner – state the most likely diagnosis on the basis of the history and clinical findings

'The symptoms of the patient together with the examination findings are suggestive of optic atrophy.'

Offer relevant differential diagnoses

The causes of optic atrophy include:

- Previous vascular event (ischaemic optic neuropathy, central retinal artery occlusion, temporal arteritis)

- Optic nerve compression (tumour, aneurysm)
- Demyelination
- Advanced glaucoma (optic disc will be cupped)
- Previous optic nerve trauma/transection

Causes of bilateral optic atrophy include:

- Toxic and nutritional optic neuropathies
- Long-standing papilloedema, e.g. in idiopathic intracranial hypertension (the disc margins will be blurred)
- Leber's optic atrophy is an inherited cause of optic atrophy with visual loss

Demonstrate an understanding of the value of further investigation

Investigations will be guided by the likely underlying cause, e.g. neuroimaging if there is suspicion of optic nerve compression or demyelination.

In cases of cardiovascular aetiology, cardiovascular risk factors should be quantified. If there is concern regarding cardioembolic disease, holter monitoring can assess for arrhythmia.

Always offer a management plan

The cause in this case is presumed to be a previous vascular event and so no immediate intervention is required.

Ensure secondary modifiable cardiovascular risk factors are identified and treated.

Instruction to the candidate

A 20-year-old woman is referred to the emergency department with headaches. Please take a history and perform a focused examination. Summarise your findings to the patient and explain your investigation and management plan. A short discussion with the examiner will then follow.

Take a focused history

Ask specific questions about the headaches, including the site of pain, radiation of the pain, the periodicity, duration and severity. Are there any aggravating or relieving factors? Ascertain if the pain is unilateral and pulsating like migraine? Is the pain worse in the morning and associated with vomiting like a headache of raised intracranial pressure? Is it band-like and worse towards the end of the day like a tension headache?

Assess for associated features such as: nausea, vomiting (particularly in mornings), preceding aura or fortification spectra (flashing lights and jagged lines in visual field).

Take a past medical history, asking about head injury, hypertension.

Take a drug history, asking about oral contraceptive pill use, or tetracycline use.

Positive findings of a focused examination

Fundoscopy is likely to show bilateral swollen discs, with associated haemorrhages and exudates. Central venous pulsation is absent (look very carefully at the retinal veins for a rhythmic pulsation – its presence effectively rules out raised intracranial pressure, but its absence is non-specific).

Consider further examination for:

- Small central scotomata
- Other cranial nerve deficits to act as a localising sign
- Blood pressure

Relevant negatives

Visual acuity and papillary reactions are normal.

What to tell the patient

'The nerves at the back of your eyes appear swollen, which can be a sign of increased pressure inside your head. There are many causes of this. We will need to arrange some tests, including a brain scan, to find out what is the cause. Do you have any questions?'

What to tell the examiner – state the most likely diagnosis on the basis of the history and clinical findings

'This patient has papilloedema. I suspect this patient's presentation is secondary to raised intracranial pressure leading to bilateral disc swelling.' Note the term papilloedema refers specifically to disc swelling secondary to raised intracranial pressure. The key sign is the presence of normal visual acuity. Reduced visual acuity implies optic neuropathy.

Offer relevant differential diagnoses

The differential diagnosis of the causes of papilloedema includes:

- Intracranial tumour
- Idiopathic intracranial hypertension (pseudotumour cerebri)
- Intracranial abscess
- Dural sinus thrombosis
- Intracranial haematoma

The differential diagnosis of bilateral disc swelling includes:

- Malignant hypertension
- Bilateral ischaemic optic neuropathy (often seen after a major hypotensive episode)
- Bilateral central retinal vein occlusion
- Severe anaemia
- Diabetic papillitis

Demonstrate an understanding of the value of further investigation

Imaging

Urgent neuro-imaging is indicated, usually a CT of brain to rule out an intracranial mass, with CT venography to rule out dural sinus thrombosis.

Lumbar puncture

If the CT is normal, a lumbar puncture may be performed to establish the cerebrospinal fluid pressure and to allow analysis of the cerebrospinal fluid.

Automated visual field analysis, while not diagnostic, can be used to monitor chronically raised intracranial pressure such as in idiopathic intracranial hypertension.

Always offer a management plan

Management is very much dependent on the cause of the raised intracranial pressure, and may include neurosurgical management of any intracranial mass.

Dural sinus thrombosis requires systemic anticoagulation.

Idiopathic intracranial hypertension can be managed with acetazolamide treatment (a carbonic anhydrase inhibitor, which inhibits production of cerebrospinal fluid), therapeutic lumbar puncture and, if necessary, ventriculoperitoneal shunting.

Case 112: Foster Kennedy syndrome

Instruction to the candidate

A 68-year-old man is referred to your clinic with headaches associated with a gradual deterioration in vision in the right eye. His wife has noticed that he has become very forgetful. Please take a history and perform a focused examination. Summarise your findings to the patient and explain your investigation and management plan. A short discussion with the examiner will then follow.

Take a focused history

Take a brief history, focusing on both the headaches and the visual loss. Foster Kennedy syndrome is usually associated with a gradual painless loss of vision.

Explore the patient's forgetfulness. What is the degree of cognitive impairment and does the patient demonstrate insight? Is there associated incontinence (recent onset dementia with associated incontinence should be assumed to be due to an organic cause)? Are there any other neurological symptoms, specifically any disturbance of the sense of smell?

Positive findings of a focused examination

There is reduced visual acuity in the right eye. In addition, there is peripheral visual field loss in the right eye. There may be a right-sided relative afferent papillary defect, and reduced colour vision on the right. Fundoscopy shows a pale optic disc on the right, and a swollen optic disc on the left.

Consider further cranial nerve examination, particularly looking for an absent or diminished sense of smell and for further localising signs.

Relevant negatives

Visual acuity in the left (contra-lateral) eye is normal, with no visual loss (or possibly a small central scotoma).

What to tell the patient

'There is a problem with the nerve at the back of your eye preventing you from seeing so well. We will arrange for a brain scan to try to check if there is anything in particular causing it. I would like to see you straight after the scan to discuss the results and consider treatment options as these will very much depend on what is causing the nerve damage. Do you have any questions at this stage?'

What to tell the examiner – state the most likely diagnosis on the basis of the history and clinical findings

'The patient's presentation together with clinical findings point to a possible diagnosis of Foster Kennedy syndrome – optic atrophy due to a frontal tumour causing compressive optic atrophy, with contralateral papilloedema due to raised intracranial pressure.'

Offer relevant differential diagnoses

Possible causes of Foster Kennedy syndrome include a subfrontal olfactory groove meningioma (the classical presentation) or a glioma of frontal lobe or corpus callosum.

Pseudo-Foster Kennedy syndrome describes sequential (most often ischaemic in aetiology) optic neuropathy or optic neuritis. The more recently affected nerve is swollen, the nerve affected in the past is atrophic and pale.

Pseudo-pseudo-Foster Kennedy syndrome describes the history and appearance of ischaemic optic neuropathy, with co-existing meningioma.

Demonstrate an understanding of the value of further investigation

A CT scan of brain and orbits should be performed to exclude an intracranial mass.

Always offer a management plan

Neurosurgical advice on the management a causative intracranial mass should be sought.

Further reading

Kennedy F. Retrobulbar neuritis as an exact diagnostic sign of certain tumors and abscesses in the frontal lobes. Am J Med Sci 1911; 142:355–368.

Gelwan MJ, Seidman M, Kupersmith MJ. Pseudo-pseudo-Foster Kennedy syndrome. J Clin Neuroophthalmol 1988; 8:49–52.

Case 113: Thyrotoxicosis

Instruction to the candidate

Please examine this 40-year-old woman who complains of heat intolerance.

Take a focused history

Elicit the exact nature of the patient's symptoms. What does the patient or their GP mean by heat intolerance?

Are there associated symptoms of hyperthyroidism, such as:

- Sweating
- Palpitations
- Diarrhoea
- Change in mood, anxiety and insomnia
- As the patient is female, ask about menstrual symptoms such as amenorrhoea
- Questions relating to the patient's appearance
- Weight loss, reduction in dress size

Has the patient noticed a lump in their neck? Has anyone commented on the patient's eyes, specifically 'bulging' eyes? Go on to ask about pain in the eyes and any visual disturbance,

particularly dryness and double vision. Explore the past medical history and family history for autoimmune conditions.

Positive findings of a focused examination

There is a wealth of positive findings in thyrotoxicosis. Look for a thin, flushed patient wearing light clothing. Sweaty palms, noticed when shaking hands with the patient.

Examine the neck for a goitre and make a point of examining the eyes for proptosis, exophthalmos and lid lag (**Figures 5.10–5.12**).

Graves' ophthalmopathy

This is the clinical syndrome of proptosis, exophthalmos and lid lag. There is increased risk in smokers. Complications include:
- Optic neuropathy with decreased visual acuity
- Ophthalmoplegia with diplopia
- Keratitis due to failure of eye lid closure

Management options for Graves' ophthalmopathy range from simple measures such as artificial tears (to treat grittiness), to steroid use and orbital decompression.

Examine the cardiovascular system for a tachycardia and any signs of cardiac failure.

Ask the patient to stand from sitting (without using their hands) to elicit any myopathy.

Examine the shins for pre-tibial myxoedema and the toes for thyroid acropachy.

Relevant negatives

The lack of an irregular pulse suggestive of atrial fibrillation is an important relevant negative finding in the setting of thyrotoxicosis.

What to tell the patient

'From your symptoms and the clinical findings I can elicit I suspect you have a condition known as thyrotoxicosis. You may have heard of it as an over-active thyroid. I will request some investigations and refer you to the specialist endocrinology clinic for further assessment. In the meantime I will start you on a medication known as a beta-blocker which will help with some of your symptoms.'

If the patient has eye signs or symptoms, explain the complication of Graves' disease and tell them you will also refer them to the ophthalmologists.

What to tell the examiner – state the most likely diagnosis on the basis of the history and clinical findings

'This patient has symptoms and signs consistent with a diagnosis of thyrotoxicosis.'

Offer relevant differential diagnoses

The common causes of hyperthyroidism include:

- Graves' disease
- Solitary toxic nodule
- Multinodular goitre
- In the case of a tender thyroid think of thyroiditis and ask about recent viral infection

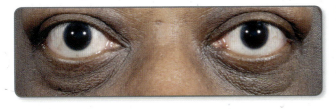

Figure 5.10 Thyroid eye disease. This patient, with hyperthyroidism, has forward protrusion of the eyeball. It is best appreciated either laterally (see Figure 5.11) or from above. Indeed, formal examination should involve standing behind the seated patient and looking down over the top of their head to see if the proptotic eyeballs can be seen in front of the forehead. Note also the peri-orbital oedema.

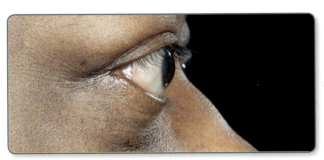

Figure 5.11 Thyroid eye disease. In this lateral view of the same patient seen in Figure 5.12, the forward protrusion of the eyeball is visible. In such patients, further eye examination would involve testing for lid lag and for any complex ophthalmoplegia, which can occur in thyroid eye disease.

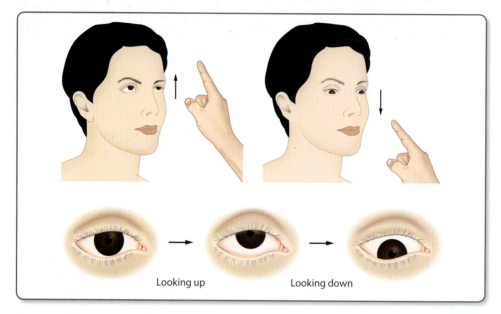

Looking up   Looking down

Figure 5.12 How to examine for lid lag. The patient is asked to focus on the examiner's finger. The finger is raised so the patient's eyes are looking toward the ceiling. The finger is then rapidly moved vertically downward. A positive finding is when the pupils move down ahead of the eye lids (there is lid 'lag') such that the superior aspect of the sclera is transiently more visible than normal.

Demonstrate an understanding of the value of further investigation

Blood testing would include:

- Thyroid profile including TSH, T4 and T3
- Thyroid autoantibody profile including
- Anti-TSH receptor antibodies
- Anti-thyroid peroxidase antibodies

Imaging options include an USS of the thyroid to identify any structural abnormality such as goitre or nodules, and an uptake scan to show the pattern of activity. Homogenous increased uptake suggests autoimmune thyrotoxicosis, a focal area of activity is consistent with a toxic nodule and absent or globally reduced uptake suggests a thyroiditis.

If there is ophthalmopathy associated with Graves' disease, the patient will need formal assessment by an ophthalmologist. Investigations may include CT or MRI of the orbits.

Always offer a management plan

Beta-blockade can help symptoms of tremor and palpitations.

Treatment options specific to hyperthyroidism include:

- Medical therapy with carbimazole or propylthyrouracil. It is important to recognise the risk of agranulocytosis on these medications, so tell the patient to present to hospital if they feel unwell or have a fever. A sore throat is a classical presenting symptoms in patients with neutropaenia
- Radioiodine therapy is an ablative treatment for thyrotoxicosis. It is contraindicated in pregnant and breastfeeding women. The use of radioiodine in autoimmune thyrotoxicosis with eye disease can worsen active ophthalmopathy. Due to the radioactive nature of radioiodine, patients receiving this treatment will be given advice on how to limit contact with other individuals depending on the dose of radioiodine they are given
- Surgical options include thyroidectomy

Case 114: Hypothyroidism

Instruction to the candidate

Please assess this 40-year-old woman who has presented with fatigue and weight gain. Discuss your findings with the patient and agree a management plan.

Take a focused history

Fatigue has a wide differential, as does weight gain. But the combination of the two, in the setting of station 5, places hypothyroidism high on the list of possible diagnoses.

Ask about the symptoms. Screen for alternative causes of fatigue such as anaemia, depression, and Addison's.

Ask about other symptoms of hypothyroidism such as:

- Intolerance to the cold. At the same time as being a history question, this is also an examination point: Is your PACES exam in the summer heat of August yet the patient is wearing a heavy jumper?
- Constipation
- Dry skin

Screen for complications of hypothyroidism such as carpal tunnel syndrome.

Explore the past medical and family history of the patient:

- Is this a patient who has previously undergone treatment for hyperthyroidism?
- Is the patient on thyroid replacement therapy? If so, when was their TSH last measured?
- Any past or family history of autoimmune conditions?
- Has the patient ever been on amiodarone?

Ensure to ask about mood as depression can occur insidiously in hypothyroidism.

Positive findings of a focused examination

On general inspection, note increased body habitus.

On closer inspection of the head and face, look for hair loss, dry skin, loss of outer third of the eyebrows.

Examine the neck for goitre. Are there any scars to suggest previous surgery such as a thyroidectomy?

Relevant negatives

Examine the cardiovascular system and comment on the absence of bradycardia, cardiomegaly and signs of cardiac failure.

What to tell the patient

'From what you tell me and from the signs I can elicit on examination, I think you may have a condition known as hypothyroidism, where the thyroid gland in the neck is underactive. I will request some blood tests to confirm this and I will refer you to the endocrinology clinic for further management.'

What to tell the examiner – state the most likely diagnosis on the basis of the history and clinical findings

'This patient has signs and symptoms consistent with a diagnosis of hypothyroidism.'

Offer relevant differential diagnoses

The differential diagnosis of hypothyroidism includes:

- Autoimmune (Hashimoto's) thyroiditis
- Iatrogenic
- Treatments for hyperthyroidism
- Amiodarone
- Hypothalamic or pituitary causes (will have decreased TSH in addition to decreased free T4)

Demonstrate an understanding of the value of further investigation

Investigations would include a thyroid profile including TSH, fT3, fT4 and autoantibodies. A full blood count should be performed to exclude anaemia as an alternative cause for symptoms. No radiology is required unless there is a goitre or palpable nodules.

Always offer a management plan

The mainstay of management is thyroid hormone replacement with levothyroxine. Monitoring is via TSH levels. Once stable, all patients should have at least once yearly TSH measurements.

Case 115: Acromegaly

Instruction to the candidate

Please examine this 53-year-old man who presents with headaches and sweating. Discuss your findings with the patient and agree a management plan with appropriate follow-up.

Take a focused history

Ask first about the symptoms mentioned in the candidate instruction. How long have they been going on for?

Go on to ask about:

- Stature, hand size and facial appearance. Have they noticed a change? In many cases, the patient will have been prompted by a relative. Ask if they have brought an old photograph to clinic and if not, ask them to bring one when they next attend. Have they gone up in shoe or glove size? Do they wear jewelry? If so, have they had to increase the size of any rings?
- Have they noticed any changes in their vision?

Screen for other associated conditions:

- Do they have diabetes?
- Ask about hypertension and symptoms of cardiac failure
- Obstructive sleep apnoea
- Does the patient complain of any lower gastrointestinal symptoms (acromegaly carries an increased risk of colonic polyps and malignancy)?

Positive findings of a focused examination

On general inspection, expect the patient to have large, puffy ('spade-like') hands and to be of tall stature.

On examining the face, you may notice:

- A prominent supra-orbital ridge (**Figure 5.13**)
- 'Coarse' facial features
- Prognathism
- Macroglossia and wide inter-dental spaces

On examination of the visual fields, seek to elicit a bi-temporal hemianopia.

Relevant negatives

If not present, comment on the absence of a displaced apex suggestive of cardiomegaly.

What to tell the patient

'It appears from what you tell me and from what clinical signs I can elicit on examination that you have a condition known as acromegaly, a condition where the body produces too much of a hormone called growth hormone. The usual cause is a benign tumour of a small gland in the head known as the pituitary gland. I think it is important that we do some tests to confirm that this is the case. These will involve some blood tests and an MRI scan of the head. We will see you again in 4 week's time with the results of those investigations. I will also write to your GP to let them know about the outcome of our consultation today. Are there any further questions or concerns that I can answer for you?'

What to tell the examiner – state the most likely diagnosis on the basis of the history and clinical findings

'This patient has symptoms and signs consistent with a diagnosis of acromegaly.'

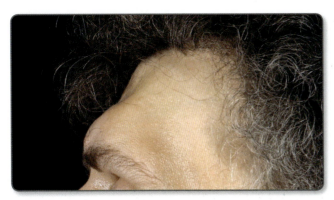

Figure 5.13 Prominent supra-orbital ridge. This patient has a clearly prominent supra-orbital ridge, as seen from the lateral view. This patient would be expected to be tall in stature and have 'coarse' facial features, with large hands. Further examination would include testing for a bitemporal hemianopia, cardiovascular examination and abdominal examination.

Offer relevant differential diagnoses

The overwhelming majority of cases of acromegaly are due to a growth hormone secreting pituitary adenoma.

Demonstrate an understanding of the value of further investigation

Blood tests would include: IGF-1, fasting glucose, HbA1c, and tests of pituitary function to screen for loss of function in other pituitary axed.

Dynamic testing is via the oral glucose tolerance test. A paradoxical rise in growth hormone level is diagnostic of acromegaly.

Due to the likelihood of a pituitary adenoma, patients with acromegaly require intracranial imaging. The modality of choice is an MRI.

Visual field testing will accurately assess any visual field defects.

If symptoms were suggestive of cardiovascular complications of acromegaly, a transthoracic echocardiogram would give evidence on cardiac structure and function.

Always offer a management plan

In cases of growth hormone secreting pituitary tumours causing acromegaly, transsphenoidal hypophysectomy is considered first line therapy. Medical therapy involves somatostatin analogues, growth hormone receptor antagonists, or dopamine agonists. Pituitary external beam radiotherapy exists as a second line for failed surgical resection.

Candidates should remember that the management of acromegaly does not solely involve addressing causative pituitary tumours. There is increased risk from cardiovascular disease, colonic polyps (complicated by malignancy), and the complications of diabetes, with these potential problems deserving of attention.

Case 116: Weight gain and easy bruising – Cushingoid appearance

Instruction to the candidate

Please assess this 43-year-old woman who has presented complaining of easy bruising and recent weight gain.

Take a focused history

How long have the symptoms been present for?

Consider causes of easy bruising. Is the patient on any medications which would put her at higher risk such as anti-platelet agents? Has the patient had any active bleeding such as epistaxis?

Screen for other symptoms of Cushing's such as amenorrhoea, increased hair growth, change in mood, or loss of libido.

Ask about important complications of Cushing's including hypertension, diabetes, and osteoporosis.

What medications is the patient on? Have they been exposed to any exogenous steroids?

Positive findings of a focused examination

On inspection, you note that the patient has centripedal obesity and a rounded plethoric facial appearance. You further inspect for:

- Interscapular fat pad (avoid using the term 'buffalo hump')
- Bruising in the context of thin skin
- Hirsutism
- Pigmented striae (**Figure 5.14**)
- Examine for proximal myopathy by asking the patient to stand from sitting with their arms crossed.
- Examine the visual fields for a bitemporal hemianopia

Relevant negatives

Make a note of the absence of signs of chronic liver disease. Chronic alcohol excess can lead to a cushingoid appearance.

What to tell the patient

'From our consultation today, I suspect you have a condition called Cushing's syndrome which is when there is too much steroid hormone in the body. This is likely what has caused your weight gain and easy bruising. I am going to request some investigations and arrange for you to be seen by one of my endocrinology specialist colleagues, who will see you promptly.'

What to tell the examiner – state the most likely diagnosis on the basis of the history and clinical findings

'This patient has a Cushingoid appearance consistent with steroid excess.'

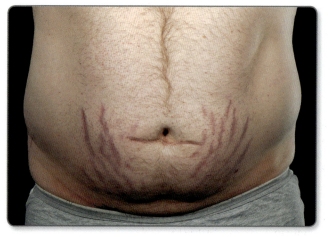

Figure 5.14 Pigmented abdominal striae. Pigmented abdominal striae are visible on the patient's abdomen. The patient has central adiposity. The infra-unblilical scar is also pigmented.

Offer relevant differential diagnoses

The differential diagnosis includes:

- ACTH-secreting pituitary adenoma (Cushing's disease)
- Excess endogenous steroid from an adrenal adenoma (Cushing's syndrome)
- Pseudo-Cushing's from conditions such as depression and alcohol excess
- Exogenous steroid use

Demonstrate an understanding of the value of further investigation

Initially, perform baseline investigations and confirm steroid excess:

- Full blood count, renal function, liver function, glucose, lipids, HbA1c, baseline cortisol and pituitary function
- 24-hour urine collections for free cortisol and overnight dexamethasone suppression test
- If urinary free cortisol elevated and failed overnight dexamethasone suppression

test, confirm the diagnosis with low dose dexamethasone suppression
- Assess whether is ACTH dependent or independent with serum ACTH value
- A high dose dexamethasone suppression tests differentiates pituitary ACTH from ectopic ACTH production

Imaging includes a pituitary MRI to identify any pituitary adenoma. If an adrenal tumour is suspected, abdominal imaging is indicated. Inferior petrosal sinus or adrenal vein sampling supplies functional anatomical information.

Always offer a management plan

The management of Cushing's depends on the underlying cause. If the cause is found to be exposure to exogenous steroid, this should be stopped.

In the final diagnosis is that of Cushing's disease, options include transsphenoidal hypophysectomy, pituitary radiotherapy, and adrenalectomy. Medical management includes drugs such as metyrapone and ketoconazole.

If a cause such as an adrenal adenoma is found, surgical removal would be warranted.

Case 117: Gynaecomastia

Instruction to the candidate

You have been asked to see this 30-year-old man, who has been referred by his general practitioner after complaining of gynaecomastia. The general practitioner notes that this young man has a high alcohol intake. Please assess the patient and inform him of your findings.

Take a focused history

The patient reports that he has noticed gynaecomastia over the past year. Consider the patient's age. There will not be a child in the exam, but the patient may be in the late 'teens, when gynaecomastia may be physiological.

Take a past medical history, seeking to identify alcohol use and a history of liver disease.

Take a drug history. Given that this is a focused history, you do not need to directly ask the patient about every drug that is known to

cause gynaecomastia. Rather, ask the patient what medications he takes and if he had started any new medications around the time he noted the gynaecomastia.

Drugs causing gynaecomastia

- Oestrogens
- Hormonal medications, including those used to treat prostate cancer
- Growth hormone
- Ketoconazole
- Spironolactone
- Many anti-cancer agents such as cisplatin, vinblastine and belomycin
- Calcium-channel blockers
- Digoxin
- Neuroleptic medications such as prochlorperazine
- Alcohol
- Marijuana

As this is a male with gynaecomastia, ask if he has noted any testicular lumps, thinking of testicular cancer. Ask about libido and erectile function.

At all stages, it is important to recognise that the patient may feel a sense of embarrassment at having gynaecomastia. Explore his concerns about his symptoms.

Positive findings of a focused examination

Examine the patient's precordium. Palpate for dense sub-areolar tissue, which should feel like a 'coiled rope' **(Figure 5.15).**

Offer to examine the testicles. Make a note of secondary sexual characteristics.

Relevant negatives

The absence of signs of chronic liver disease is an important relative negative to note.

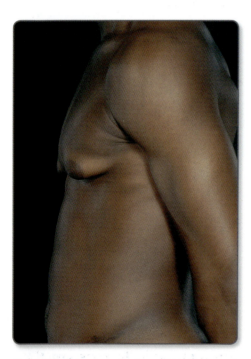

Figure 5.15 Gynaecomastia. Excess breast tissue can be seen clearly in the lateral view. Findings on palpation are discussed in the 'positive findings' section. Depending on the circumstances surrounding the patient's presentation, abdominal examination, including offering to examine the external genitalia in men, should be performed. In any drug history, common iatrogenic causes of gynaecomastia should be ruled out.

What to tell the patient

'Thank you for coming to see me today. The problem you are having, with enlargement of the male breast tissue, is known as gynaecomastia. There is a wide range of causes for this, including excess alcohol consumption. There are some serious causes of gynaecomastia, but from what you tell me and from what I can find on examination I do not think these apply to you. However, I will order some blood tests just to be sure. I will see you again in a couple of weeks with the results of these tests. I will also refer you to our community alcohol liaison team for advice on how to cut down your alcohol consumption. Do you have any other questions or concerns that I can address today?'

What to tell the examiner – state the most likely diagnosis on the basis of the history and clinical findings

'This patient has gynaecomastia.'

Offer relevant differential diagnoses

The differential diagnosis of the causes of gynaecomastia include:

- Physiological
- Due to other conditions such as liver disease, chronic kidney disease, endocrine disease
- Hormone-secreting tumours such as testicular malignancies
- Medications such as omeprazole, spironolactone and hormonal medications for prostate cancer
- Recreational drugs such as alcohol and marijuana

Demonstrate an understanding of the value of further investigation

Bloods tests including β-HCG, liver function, renal profile and prolactin level.

Further investigations such as imaging will be determined by the history and investigations. If there is concern about testicular malignancy, an ultrasound would be warranted.

Always offer a management plan

Treatment is directed to the underlying causes. Offending drugs are removed or reduced where appropriate on balance of need versus acceptable and tolerable side effects. Alcohol liaison and or drug advice should be offered where appropriate. Medical management includes use of oestrogen receptor blockers such as tamoxifen and androgens but these are used with caution. Mastectomy can be considered in severe cases.

Further reading

Tyrell CJ. Gynaecomastia: aetiology and treatment options. Prostate Cancer Prostatic Dis 1999; 2:167–171.

Mahoney CP. Adolescent gynaecomastia. Differential diagnosis and management. Paediatr Clin North Am 1990; 37:1389–1404.

Case 118: Pseudohypoparathyroidism – Albright's hereditary osteodystrophy

Instruction to the candidate

This 28-year-old woman has been referred by her general practitioner with hypocalcaemia. Please take a history and perform an appropriate examination. Following that, inform the patient of your findings.

Take a focused history

Ask about symptoms of hypocalcaemia:

- Tingling and numbness, which can be peri-oral or in the peripheries
- Carpopedal spasm and muscular cramps
- Any history of seizures, which could be due to severe hypocalcaemia

If any of the symptoms are present, assess their severity and duration.

Where general inspection suggests an inherited condition, see below, take a careful family history.

Positive findings of a focused examination

On general inspection, you note that the patient is of short stature, with obesity and a round facial appearance. On inspection of the hands, you note that the patient has a short 4th and 5th metacarpal on each hand.

Additionally, examine for clinical evidence of hypocalcaemia by assessing for the following signs:

- Chvostek's sign: hemifacial twitching due to repetitive percussion over the ipsilateral facial nerve

- Trousseau's sign: carpopedal spasm brought on by inflating a blood pressure cuff on the patient's arm

Relevant negatives

If signs of hypocalcaemia were absent they should be mentioned as relevant negatives. This would move the diagnosis from pseudohypoparathyroidism to pseudopseudohypoparathyroidism.

What to tell the patient

'From what your GP has told me and from the findings of our discussion and examination, I feel you are likely to have a condition known as pseudohypoparathyroidism. This is an inherited condition which causes low levels of calcium, one of the body salts. I will arrange for you to be referred to the endocrinology clinic. In the meantime I will request some blood tests and start you on some oral calcium supplements. Do you have any further questions or concerns I can answer for you today?'

What to tell the examiner – state the most likely diagnosis on the basis of the history and clinical findings

'The combination of the phenotypic appearance of Albright's hereditary osteodystrophy with symptoms and signs of hypocalcaemia suggest a diagnosis of pseudohypoparathyroidism.'

Offer relevant differential diagnoses

The phenotypical appearance of Albright's hereditary osteodystrophy, without evidence of hypocalcaemia, is known as pseudopseudohypoparathyroidism.

Demonstrate an understanding of the value of further investigation

- Calcium, PTH, vitamin D. Expect a low calcium with an appropriately raised PTH

- Screen for hypogonadism and hypothyroidism if clinically indicated
- The Ellsworth-Howard test involves measurement of serum and urine phosphate after intravenous PTH

Always offer a management plan

Important points in management of this condition:

- Genetic counselling
- Calcium and vitamin D replacement
- Phosphate binders if necessary

Case 119: Chronic skin conditions – plaque psoriasis

Instruction to the candidate

Examine this 42-year-old man's skin and discuss diagnosis and therapeutic options.

Take a focused history

Begin by ascertaining the age of onset of the rash and establish the areas affected. Ask specifically about scalp, genital and nail involvement as this information may not be volunteered. Explore the precipitants of plaque psoriasis, all of which may also precipitate guttate psoriasis:

- Physical or emotional stress (Koebner phenomenon)
- Infection (β-haemolytic streptococcal infection)
- Sunlight (may provoke psoriasis but also make it better)
- Drugs (beta-blockers, stopping systemic glucocorticoids, lithium, anti-malarials)
- Alcohol and smoking

Also ask about family history and any past admission to hospital with erythroderma. Ascertain smoking history and cardiovascular disease risk factors as psoriasis is associated with cardiovascular disease and diabetes. Do not forget to ask about functional impairment or disability due to the skin disease

Positive findings of a focused examination

The rash in chronic plaque psoriasis is demonstrated in **Figures 5.16–5.19**. There are well-demarcated papules or plaques of varying size, which are dull-red or salmon-pink colour. A loosely adherent silvery-white scale is noted.

Auspitz sign is demonstrated when removal of scale results in minute blood droplets (should be mentioned rather than performed).

Regarding the distribution of rash, it tends to be symmetrical, focused on extensor surfaces (of elbows, knees, knuckles), behind the ears, and the scalp hairline. The palms and soles may also be involved.

The nails may be involved (**Figures 5.20–5.21**), demonstrating pitting, onycholysis, discolouration (oil spots are pathognomonic: yellow-brown spots under nail plate) and subungual keratosis.

If the submammary, axillary and/or anogenital folds are involved, there may be glistening, sharply demarcated red plaques, with scale absent.

Relevant negatives

If appropriate, comment on the absence of arthropathy, which occurs in 10–25% of patients.

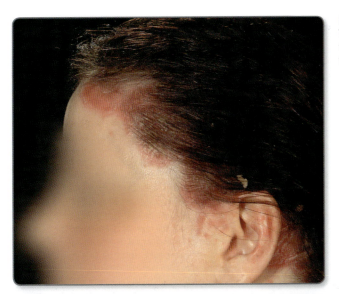

Figure 5.16 Psoriatic plaques.
The psoriatic plaques are visible on the patient's hairline and behind the ears.

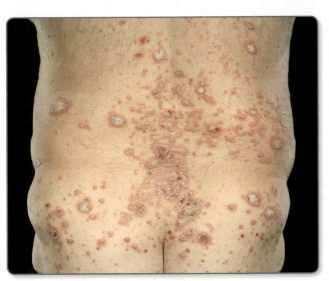

Figure 5.17 Chronic plaque psoriasis. This patient has large flat plaques covered in scale on the lower back

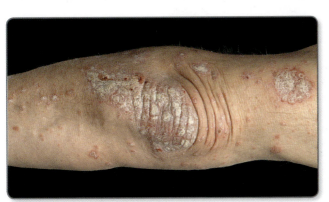

Figure 5.18 Psoriatic plaques.
The extensor surface of the elbow demonstrates the classical silver, scaly plaque of psoriasis. Note also some smaller plaques elsewhere on the upper limb.

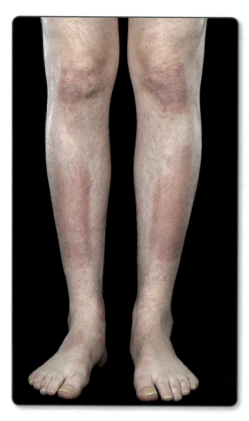

Figure 5.19 Psoriatic plaques. There are plaques on the extensor aspect of both knees, with bilateral plaques also on the shins.

What to tell the patient

'The skin changes you have suggest that you have a condition called psoriasis. It is a very common skin condition affecting 5% of the population. It is not infective or contagious. The trigger appears to be an outside event, such as a throat infection, stress or an injury to the skin. A high alcohol intake and smoking can worsen psoriasis too, as can medicines used for other conditions. Psoriasis is usually easy to recognise and no further investigations are needed at this stage. Topical treatment for psoriasis is usually effective but if the psoriasis is severe or resistant to treatment there are other options such as light therapy and systemic medication. The skin becomes less scaly and may then look completely normal. However, even if your psoriasis disappears after treatment, there is a tendency for it to return. This may not happen for many years, but can do so within a few weeks.

'I would like to bring you back to clinic in 3 months to assess your progress on the treatment I will prescribe today. I will be writing to your GP to inform him of your visit today.

'Do you have any questions or concerns that I can address today?'

What to tell the examiner – state the most likely diagnosis on the basis of the history and clinical findings

'The presence of erythematous, scaly plaques in the extensor surfaces alongside the nail findings

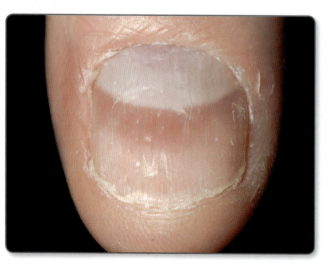

Figure 5.20 Psoriatic nails. Pitted nails in a patient with psoriasis. There is also longitudinal ridging and evidence of onycholysis at the free edge of the nail.

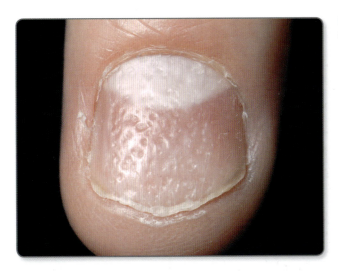

Figure 5.21 Psoriatic nails. A second example of nail pitting.

and scalp involvement is strongly suggestive of chronic plaque psoriasis.'

Key clinical features of psoriasis

History:
- Chronic
- Indolent
- Present for months and years
- Slowly changing

Examination:
- Silvery-white scale
- Well-demarcated
- Salmon pink plaques
- Extensor surfaces

Offer relevant differential diagnoses

The differential diagnosis of small scaly plaques includes: seborrhoeic dermatitis (may be indistinguishable), discoid eczema, discoid lupus, tinea corporis (usually solitary lesion; take fungal scrapes).

Apart from psoriasis, other causes of a flaky scalp include seborrhoeic dermatitis and tinea capitis.

Demonstrate an understanding of the value of further investigation

ASO titre/throat swab in suspected recent streptococcal infection.

Screening blood tests, including hepatitis serology, HIV, and TB Elispot especially if there

is widespread involvement likely to require systemic medication such as methotrexate or biologic. Liver function and lipid profile should be taken before starting acitretin, methotrexate. Renal function is monitored in patients on ciclosporin.

Always offer a management plan

Management depends on site and extent of involvement, the type of psoriasis (e.g. plaque vs guttate) and treatment tolerance. All patients, regardless of severity, require emollients and soap substitutes to control scale and protect the skin.

For localised or mild form, affecting <5% of the body surface and can be managed in the community: start with vitamin D analogues (calcipotriol/calcitriol). Not more than 100 g/week to avoid hypercalcaemia. These are often combined with potent topical corticosteroids, e.g. calcipotriol with betamethasone..

If the condition is unresponsive to first line therapy, or if the patient suffers side effects, the following can be used:

- Dithranol: inhibits DNA synthesis and oxygen free radicals. It is, however, time-consuming, irritant, and stains. Avoid on face and skin folds
- Tar preparations: act by inhibiting DNA synthesis (anti-mitotic effect). Have a strong aroma, messy, irritant
- Topical steroid ointments reduce scaling and erythema. They can cause dermal atrophy and show tachyphylaxis

For generalised or moderate-severe form refer to dermatology for consideration of phototherapy and/or systemic treatment.

Phototherapy

Narrowband UVB phototherapy is especially good for thin plaques. It is very effective when used in combination with topical vitamin D analogues.

PUVA photochemotherapy involves ingestion of 8-methoxypsoralen and exposure to UVA. Beware of long-term the side-effects, i.e. increased incidence of skin cancers.

Systemic treatment

Acitretin (may be used alone or in combination with light treatment). Combination therapy improves the efficacy of each and allows for reduced dose and duration of treatment.

Methotrexate: beware of potential liver toxicity especially in the presence of high alcohol intake, intravenous drug use, and abnormal baseline liver function.

Ciclosporin should only be used in patients without risk factors and is usually used for emergencies such as erythroderma or pustular psoriasis to induce remission. Needs monitoring of blood pressure and serum creatinine.

Fumaric acid esters and hydroxychloroquine are other alternatives.

Methotrexate and biologics, such as adalimumab, etanercept and ustekinumab and may additionally control psoriatic arthritis. Patients need to have failed conventional systemic treatment and have a DLQI and PASI >10 to qualify for treatment.

Disease monitoring

Disease monitoring can be achieved with the Psoriasis Area and Severity Index (PASI). The intensity of redness, thickness and scaling on a scale of 0–4 is assessed for a representative area for each body region. Each subtotal is then multiplied by the body surface area for that region and the results are added together to give the PASI score. The DLQI score is also helpful in assessing the impact the disease has in the patient's life.

Case 120: Atopic dermatitis or atopic eczema

Instruction to the candidate

Examine this 27-year-old woman's skin and discuss diagnosis and therapeutic options.

Take a focused history

On the basis of the clinical findings on general inspection, see below, assess for the presence of the triad of atopy – childhood eczema, asthma, and allergic rhinitis/hayfever. Screen for food allergies and/or a family history of atopy.

Ask about exacerbating factors of the patient's symptoms, such as infections, allergens (e.g. dust, grass, pollen), sweating, heat, and stress. Obtain an occupational history and potential exposure to irritants such as detergents or other chemicals. Atopic eczema is a major contributor to occupational irritant contact dermatitis. Enquire about previous treatments used and their impact. Consider asking about history of cold sores (risk of eczema herpeticum).

Assess the effect of the patient's symptoms on their daily life.

Positive findings of a focused examination

The patient may have a diffuse pattern of eczema, with widespread, dry, lichenified skin or persistent localised eczema, affecting areas like the hands and eyelids (**Figures 5.22** and **5.23** for clinical photographs of eczema) The rash is characterised by:

- Itchy erythematous dry scaly patches
- Excoriations and lichenification from chronic scratching
- Fissures (hands and feet)

Consider further examination of the hands for nail pitting or ridging.

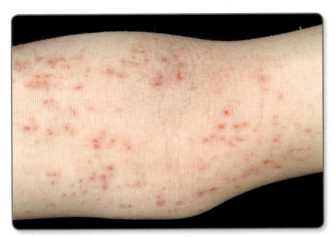

Figure 5.22 Eczematous rash. This patient, with ectopic eczema, has an itchy rash on the flexural aspect of forearm. There is thickened, dry skin (lichenified) with evidence of excoriation.

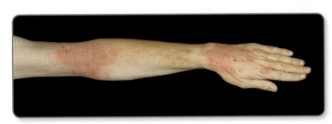

Figure 5.23 Eczematous rash. Eczematous lesions involving both the flexural aspect of the elbow and the dorsum of the hand.

Relevant negatives

The absence of signs suggestive of superimposed infection is an important negative finding.

What to tell the patient

'Atopic eczema is an inflammatory condition of the skin. In people with atopic eczema, a gene alters the skin barrier function, so irritant and allergy-inducing substances can enter the skin causing dryness and inflammation. Emollients help to protect the skin from the outside world. The inflammation is treated with topical steroids and, if severe, other treatments such as light therapy or systemic medication may be considered. I would like to see you again in 3 months time to assess your progress and discuss your results. I will also be writing to your GP about today's visit.'

What to tell the examiner – state the most likely diagnosis on the basis of the history and clinical findings

'The presence of a symmetrical, itchy, dry flexural skin rash together with a history of asthma and hayfever are strongly suggestive of a diagnosis of atopic eczema.'

> ### Diagnostic criteria for atopic eczema
>
> An itchy skin condition with three or more of:
> - Onset <2
> - Skin crease involvement
> - Dry skin
> - Personal history of atopy
> - Flexural dermatitis

Offer relevant differential diagnoses

The differential diagnosis would include allergic or irritant contact dermatitis, however in such cases the site of eruption usually confined to exposure areas.

Seborrhoeic dermatitis, another differential, is more likely in areas with sebaceous glands such as face, scalp, sternum, body folds.

Urticaria does not tend to be scaly.

Demonstrate an understanding of the value of further investigation

Investigations should seek to exclude skin infection and rule out precipitating factors. Investigations may include:

- Skin swabs and skin scrapings for suspected superimposed infection

- Laboratory blood tests, including total IgE and specific IgEs to comomn allergens, a full blood count to identify eosinophilia, and iron studies (iron deficiency can lead to pruritis)
- Patch testing is useful to exclude contact dermatitis

Always offer a management plan

All patients regardless of severity require emollients and soap substitutes.

For localised or mild disease, topical steroids are used for flare-ups, with topical immunomodulators such as tacrolimus or pimecrolimus as steroid sparing agents for maintenance or control of minor flares. For example, a patient may use topical steroids such as hydrocortisone or clobetasone butyrate ointment to the face and neck to induce clearance and introduce tacrolimus as maintenance treatment. A stronger topical steroid such as betamethasone, mometasone or even clobetasone propionate may be needed for body eczema. A soap substitute such as Dermol 500 and an emollient such as Cetraben or Epaderm should be used on a daily basis.

For generalised or moderate-severe form atopic eczema, the patient may require phototherapy or systemic treatment with immunosuppressive agents such as azathioprine, methotrexate and ciclosporine. Biologic therapies can be used for recalcitrant eczema non-responsive to conventional treatment.

Antibiotics are used for secondary bacterial infections. Antihistamines may helo reduce irritation and itching and are especially helpful at nightime.

Case 121: Pyoderma gangrenosum

Instruction to the candidate

This 37-year-old woman has been referred by her gastroenterologist for an opinion in relation to the lesion on her right lower leg. Take a short history and examine this patient's skin lesion and discuss diagnosis and therapeutic options.

Take a focused history

Establish the clinical history. Pyoderma gangrenosum is an uncommon cause of very painful skin ulceration. The lower legs are the commonest site. Establish the evolution of the lesion: Pyoderma usually starts as a small pustule, red bump or 'blood blister' which may be painful and occur either de novo or after minimal trauma. The skin then breaks down, resulting in an ulcer.

Adopt a systems-based approach to identify associated systemic disease, which is present in 50% of cases. Ask about gastrointestinal symptoms (inflammatory bowel disease), joint involvement (rheumatoid arthritis) and any history of haematological disease (myeloma).

Disease associations with pyoderma gangrenosum

- Crohn's
- Ulcerative colitis
- Diverticulosis
- Rheumatoid arthritis
- Paraproteinaemia
- Myeloma
- Leukemia
- Behçet syndrome
- Active chronic hepatitis
- PBC

Positive findings of a focused examination

Suspect pyoderma gangrenosum in the presence of a painful ulcer with characteristic purple edge and an elevated border particularly on the lower leg (**Figure 5.24**).

Pyoderma gangrenosum demonstrates pathergy (exaggerated skin injury after minor trauma). A skin prick test causes a papule/pustule/ulcer. This should not be performed in the exam.

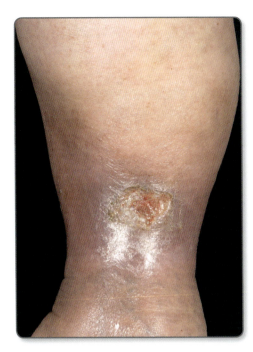

Figure 5.24 Pyoderma gangrenosum. This shallow ulcer has a classical violaceous border. The ulcer bed is granulating. If this finding is identified on clinical examination, proceed to examine for signs associated with common causes of pyoderma gangrenosum, as discussed in the text.

Perform further examination for signs of an underlying causative disease:

- Mouth ulceration e.g. Crohn's, myelodysplastic syndromes
- Conjunctival involvement
- Joint involvement e.g. rheumatoid arthritis

Relevant negatives

It is important to note the absence of lymphadenopathy, which might be present in the setting of superadded infection or in the case of an advanced squamous cell carcinoma (a differential diagnosis of pyoderma gangrenosum).

What to tell the patient

'I suspect the ulcer you have on your leg is pyoderma gangrenosum, which is a rare treatable cause of skin ulcers and is commonly associated with gastrointestinal disease, especially inflammatory bowel disease. We will have to take a small biopsy to confirm the diagnosis. The ulcer is likely to heal with treatment for your inflammatory bowel disease but if not we have other options to consider. It is likely to take some time to heal but is unlikely to require surgery or skin grafting.'

What to tell the examiner – state the most likely diagnosis on the basis of the history and clinical findings

'The history of rapid evolution of the skin ulcer in combination with a background inflammatory bowel disease is suggestive of a diagnosis of pyoderma gangrenosum.

Offer relevant differential diagnoses

The differential diagnosis of pyoderma gangrenosum includes:

- Localised gangrene
- Ecthyma
- Atypical mycobacterial infection
- Stasis ulcer
- Squamous cell carcinoma

Demonstrate an understanding of the value of further investigation

Pyoderma gangrenosum is usually diagnosed clinically. Investigations are aimed at identifying underlying disease or ruling out infection. Take a skin swab to exclude superimposed infection. If needed, a skin biopsy can be perfomed to confirm the diagnosis (taken from edge, needs to be deep).

Laboratory blood tests to exclude underlying associated disease:

- Immunology: ANA/ANCA, rheumatoid factor
- Full blood count
- Inflammatory markers raised in inflammatory bowel disease

Always offer a management plan

Treatment of the underlying disease and topical or systemic treatment for the ulcer.

Topical therapies include strong steroid ointments or intralesional steroids. Involve the tissue viability nurse for help with dressings and consideration of supplementary treatment, such as potassium permanganate. Symptom control involves simple analgesia to manage the pain of the ulcer.

Systemic options (**Table 5.2**) include oral prednisolone and immunosuppressive agents such as mycophenolate mofetil, ciclosporin and azathioprine. Biologic therapies (infliximab, etanercept, adalimumab) are also used.

Antibiotics are indicated for superimposed infection.

Table 5.2 Immunosuppressive and biologic agents for pyoderma gangrenosum and a wide range of conditions		
Immunosuppresant	**Mode of action**	**Side effects**
Mycophenolate mofetil (MMF)	Inhibits lymphocyte proliferation and antibody production	Taste disturbance, gingival hypertrophy, gastrointestinal disturbance, skin cancer, myelosuppression
Ciclosporin (CyA)	Calcineurin inhibitor	Hypertension Nephrotoxicity Hypertrichosis gingival hyperplasia/bleeding gums Ototoxicity Hyperuricaemia, tremor, paraesthesiae, skin cancer Lymphoproliferative disorders
Methotrexate (MTX)	Dihydrofolate reductase inhibitor	Myelosuppression Pulmonary and hepatic fibrosis Teratogenic Ulcerative stomatitis
Azathioprine (AZT)	Pro-drug for purine synthesis inhibitor	Bone marrow toxicity, liver, interstitial nephritis, non-Hodgkin's lymphoma, small cell carcinoma, Azoospermia
Cyclophosphamide	Nitrogen mustard alkylating agent causing cell death	Pancreatitis, cardiotoxicity, pulmonary fibrosis, SIADH, hyperpigmentation Rarely hepatotoxic/nephrotoxic
Biologics		
Infliximab	Chimeric monoclonal antibody against TNFa	Lymphoma, reactivation of hepatitis, tuberculosis, drug induced lupus, demyelinating CNS disease
Etanercept	Fusion protein, TNF inhibitor	
Adalimumab	Human monoclonal antibody against TNFa	

SIADH, syndrome of inappropriate antidiuretic hormone; TNF, tumour necrosis factor.

Case 122: Vasculitis (Henoch–Schönlein purpura)

Instruction to the candidate

This 38-year-old patient has recently been treated by his GP for suspected gastroenteritis. He presents with a rash on the legs. Please assess and suggest management.

Take a focused history

When presented with a rash and suspected systemic features always think about a diagnosis of vasculitis. The following history points should be checked for any type of suspected vasculitis:

- General symptoms: general malaise, headache, anorexia, myalgia, fever
- Eyes: episcleritis, visual loss
- Respiratory: dyspnoea, haemoptysis
- Cardiovascular: angina, heart failure
- GI: abdominal pain, diarrhoea
- Neurology: sensorimotor neuropathy, fitting, ataxia, chorea, psychosis, mood disturbance

HSP usually presents with a prodromal illness of general malaise, headache, fever and anorexia. Associated features include:

- Arthralgia: usually poly-arthralgia in ankles, knees elbows and small joints of hands
- GI upset: abdominal pain, colic, vomiting, diarrhoea
- The rash may persist after all other symptoms have settled or recurrent attacks may occur

Ask about the rash. Did it begin as a crop? Is it painful or pruritic? Commons sites include the limbs and buttocks. Is there an urticarial component? This is very common and characteristic in HSP vasculitis which may present as localised oedema or urticarial lesions.

Screen for other causes of vasculitis, such as:

- Drugs: aspirin, non-steroidal anti-inflammatories, antibiotics
- Infections such as streptococcal sore throat
- Autoimmune connective tissue disease (lupus, rheumatoid arthritis, Sjögren's)
- Blood disorders such as cryoglobulinaemia
- Renal involvement is the most serious feature of the disease, and may present as nephritic or nephrotic syndrome

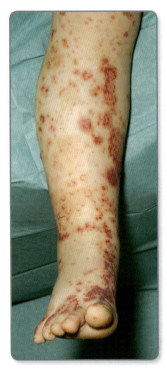

Figure 5.25 Vasculitis. There is a purpuric rash with petechiae and ecchymoses affecting the lower limb. Although in Henoch–Shönlein purpura the vasculitic rash is typically distributed over the buttocks and posterior aspect of the lower limbs, the diagnosis should be considered in the presence of any vasculitic rash. Indeed, appropriate investigations (a 'vasculitic screen') should be carried out for any patient who presents with such a rash.

Positive findings of a focused examination

Examine the legs, buttocks, and flanks. Look for palpable purpura (palpable petechiae, bright red well demarcated macules and papules with central dot-like haemorrhage). Lesions may be scattered, discrete or confluent **(Figure 5.25)**. Consider examining the abdomen.

Relevant negatives

In any patient with purpura and systemic features, it is important to note the absence of signs suggestive of meningism. Suggest a bedside urine dipstick to look for renal involvement as evidenced by proteinuria or haematuria.

What to tell the patient

'I suspect the rash on your legs and buttocks is related to your recent illness with gastroenteritis.

We will need to run some more tests to confirm. The rash should clear within 3–6 weeks but I must warn you that recurrences are common in up to half patients. This condition, called Henoch–Schönlein purpura, may occasionally affect other body organs, such as your kidneys and it is important to keep a close eye on your kidney function with weekly urine tests. Treatment is symptomatic at this stage, but I will arrange to see you again in a week's time and if the rash is spreading or your kidneys become affected, we will start you on oral steroid tablets.'

What to tell the examiner – state the most likely diagnosis on the basis of the history and clinical findings

'This man presents with a palpable purpuric eruption on his legs and buttocks and a preceding history of abdominal pain and arthralgia, which would be consistent with Henoch–Schönlein purpura.'

> **Vasculitis**
>
> Vasculitis is a group of conditions characterised by histological changes in small and medium sized blood vessels of the dermis. Vasculitis can be clinically divided into cutaneous and visceral or mixed forms.

Offer relevant differential diagnoses

The diagnosis is usually clear when all components of the syndrome are present. In young children appendicitis, mesenteric adenitis and rheumatic fever may present similarly.

Other causes of purpuric eruption can be divided into vasculitic causes, thrombocytopenic causes and non-thrombocytopenic causes. Thrombocytopenic causes include meningococcal disease, disseminated intravascular coagulation and idiopathic thrombocytopenic purpura. Non-thrombocytopenic causes include trauma, drug-induced purpura, and senile purpura.

Demonstrate an understanding of the value of further investigation

Investigations in vasculitis depend on an adequate history taking to identify triggers or altered host response. They are aimed at identifying triggers but also factors enhancing vascular injury such as coagulation as well as identification of target organ damage. Candidates should be able to identify the distinct patterns of HSP or erythema nodosum and tailor investigations appropriately as follows:

- Investigations to identify triggers and enhancing factors include:
  - Full blood count and clotting for thrombocytopenia and disseminated intravascular coagulation
  - Inflammatory markers
  - ANA (especially when very high ESR to rule out lupus)
  - Throat swab and ASO-titre to exclude streptococcal infection
  - Skin biopsy if diagnosis not clear
- Evidence of systemic involvement can be identified through the following investigations:
  - Urinalysis to look for casts and proteinuria. Red cell casts indicate glomerular injury, white cell casts acute inflammation or infection, epithelial casts severe renal tubular damage. Patients should have weekly urinalysis during the attack, at the end of the attack, and for 1–3 months after the attack has resolve.
  - Plasma creatinine
  - Blood pressure

Always offer a management plan

Therapy based on eliminating triggers and supporting host defences. Prognosis depends on systemic involvement. General measures include rest and elimination of trigger factor if identified. Underlying causes should be treated where identified. Topical steroids are given for rash. Oral steroid and immunosuppressive therapy is indicated in systemic involvement.

Case 123: Chronic venous insufficiency

Instruction to the candidate

This 65-year-old patient has been referred by his GP with difficult to manage eczema on his lower legs. Please assess her legs and suggest further management.

Take a focused history

Chronic venous insufficiency arises from failure of blood venous return (from damage to valves of deep veins or communicating veins) and raised capillary pressure. Seek to elicit the following symptoms:

- Pain: pain secondary to venous insufficiency will often present as leg heaviness or aching, worse on standing and relieved by walking (in contrast to arteriopathic pain worsening with walking and relieved by rest)
- Oedema: this will typically be worse on standing, or at the end of the day and in warm weather. Ask about shoe tightness and sleeping arrangements (often elderly people sleep in a chair with gravitational effects to legs)
- Erythrocyte extravasation: does the patient have easy bruising after minimal trauma
- Ulceration: this may be painful and worse on standing
- Itching: as a result of leaky capillaries

Regarding the past medical history, is there a history of venous thrombosis? This can lead to post-phlebitic syndrome with similar clinical appearance. Is there a history of varicose veins that an damage the valves? Screen for a history of atherosclerotic disease (important in the differential of ulceration), diabetes (may prevent healing), rheumatoid arthritis, history of anaemia or malnutrition.

Positive findings of a focused examination

In any elderly patient presenting with lower limb eczema suspect the diagnosis of chronic venous insufficiency. The cardinal features that are sought on examination are oedema, eczema, pigmentation, thickening and fibrosis with or without ulceration.

Look for stasis eczema with scaling and thickening of the skin, especially near the ankles. Acute dermatitis may also be present with exudates and inflammatory papules. Haemosiderin deposition can be found over varices and ankles.

Lipodermatosclerosis describes thickened, indurated, hyperpigmentaed skin creating classic inverted Champagne-bottle appearance of legs.

Associated features include:

- Varicose veins (superficial, enlarged, tortuous veins, best evaluated in standing position)
- Venous ulcers (**Figure 5.26**)
- Atrophie blanche: white atrophic plaques with prominent red dots within (enlarged capillary blood vessels) and surrounding pigmentation on lower legs and feet

Relevant negatives

It is important to note the presence of peripheral pulses as venous ulceration can occasionally co-exist with arterial disease.

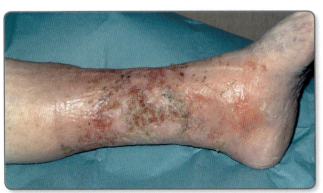

Figure 5.26 Venous ulceration.
This patient has multiple areas of shallow ulceration in the medial gaiter area of the lower limb. . Note the 'inverted champagne bottle' appearance, yellow crusting suggestive of secondary infection and shiny, woody texture of the skin around the ankles.

Take care to distinguish from other types of ulceration (**Figure 5.27, Figure 5.28** and **Table 5.3**). Look for signs of eczema elsewhere which might indicate the patient has a history of atopy and therefore predisposition to eczema or an 'autosensitisation reaction', i.e eczema that has spread to affect other areas of the body

What to tell the patient

'The changes I can see today on your lower legs are probably related to the veins in your leg being unable to efficiently pump back the blood to your heart. As a result the blood pools in your legs causing these changes we can see. We will need to run some tests to check how well both the veins and arteries in your legs function before choosing the best treatment, as it may involve compression bandaging. The most important thing you can do to help your legs is to keep them elevated. I will prescribe some emollients and topical steroid ointments until I next see you. Do you have any questions?'

What to tell the examiner – state the most likely diagnosis on the basis of the history and clinical findings

'This patient has an eczematous rash on both lower legs with signs of chronic venous insufficiency and secondary ulceration.

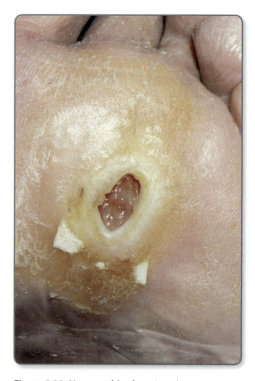

Figure 5.28 Neuropathic ulcer. Any ulcer on a pressure area, as this one is, should prompt the candidate to examine for any associate abnormal sensation and to consider conditions which can cause a peripheral sensory neuropathy e.g. diabetes.

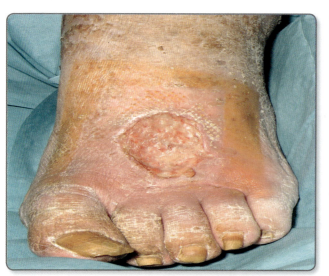

Figure 5.27 Arterial ulceration. There is a 'punched-out' ulcer on the dorsum aspect of the foot. There are associated atrophic changes. This patient would require examination of the pulses and clinical assessment for severe vascular disease.

Table 5.3 Clinical features of venous, arterial, and neuropathic ulcers*			
	Venous	**Arterial**	**Neuropathic**
History			
• Pain	Often painful Worse on standing	Painful at night	Painless
• Past medical history	Varicose veins, DVT	Arterial disease elsewhere	Diabetes or neurological disease
Sites affected	Malleolar area (medial>lateral)	Pressure and trauma sites Pre-tibial, supra-malleolar (lateral)	Pressure sites • Soles • Heels • Metatarsal heads
Ulcer characteristics			
• Size	Large	Small	Variable size
• Depth	Shallow	Deep	Variable depth
• Contour	Irregular	Sharply defined	Occasionally surrounded by hyperkeratotic area
• Base	Exudative granulating base	Necrotic base	Granulating base
Associated features			
• Surrounding skin	Warm	Cold, shiny/pale	Warm
• Peripheral pulses	Normal	Weak or absent	Normal
• Other	Leg oedema Haemosiderin deposition Lipodermatosclerosis Atrophie blance	Shiny pale skin Hair loss	Peripheral neuropathy
Investigations	ABPI Swabs Doppler ultrasound	ABPI <0.8 Doppler ultrasound Angiography	(ABPI not reliable in patients with diabetes) X-ray to exclude OM
Management	Compression bandaging	Vascular reconstruction No compression	Wound debridement Regular repositioning, footwear/nutrition

* See also Figures 5.26–5.28.
NO, nitric oxide; ABPI, ankle-brachial pressure index..

Offer relevant differential diagnoses

The differential diagnosis of a lower leg ulcer includes arterial and neuropathic ulcers, neoplasia and trauma.

The differential diagnosis of an erythematous or oedematous leg includes cellulitis/erysipelas (may be co-existent) and venous thrombosis (usually unilateral).

Demonstrate an understanding of the value of further investigation

Investigations are aimed at searching for adjuvant factors and associated disease such as anaemia and malnutrition.

Laboratory blood tests:

- Full blood count for anaemia
- Inflammatory markers

- Liver function for low albumin and serum protein
- Glucose as diabetes may discourage healing

Ulcer swabs to rule out suprimposed infection. Patch tests to identify a contact allergy if the patient has been using topical treatments and not improving
Imaging:

- Plain films to rule out rheumatoid arthritis and osteomyelitis
- Arterial and venous Doppler ultrasound to assess venous competence, thrombosis or co-existent arterial disease that may preclude compression bandaging
- Ultrasound abdomen in suspected abdominal mass causing venous obstruction

Consider ABPI measurement.

Always offer a management plan

The principles of management are aimed at reducing swelling in the leg and treating the venous dermatitis. Care is delivered through a multidisciplinary team with dermatology, vascular surgery and tissue viability nursing. Options include:

- General measures: leg elevation and exercise
- Antibiotics for secondary infection
- Compression stockings (provided no significant arterial disease) and bandaging in the presence of ulceration
- Local applications such as potassium permanganate to soak up exudates, remove slough
- Emollients
- Short-term topical steroids

Case 124: Cutaneous lupus erythematosus

Instruction to the candidate

This 34-year-old woman complains of a facial rash. Please examine the patient, ask any relevant questions and provide a management plan.

Take a focused history

In any facial rash you need to establish whether it is photosensitive or not and ask about specific precipitating factors such as sunlight and drugs. Diuretics, hydralazine, procainamide, isoniazid and anticonvulsants can all cause drug-induced lupus that remits on withdrawal of the offending drug. Sulphonamides and the combined oral contraceptive may trigger idiopathic SLE.

Screen for constitutional symptoms, such as fatigue, malaise, fever, weight loss, arthralgia and flu-like symptoms.

Proceed to a systems-based approach:

- Renal disease
- Cardio-respiratory involvement with pleuritic pain/pericarditis (serositis)
- Neurological: seizures in the absence of causative drugs, psychosis

- Thromboembolic disease and a history of miscarriage

> ### Antiphospholipid syndrome
>
> In the context of:
> - Thromboembolic disease
> - Stroke
> - Migraine
> - Miscarriages
> - Multi-infarct dementia
> - Livedo reticularis (**Figure 5.29**)
>
> Always think of antiphospholipid syndrome and test for: lupus anticoagulant and antiphospholipid antibody.

Positive findings of a focused examination

Skin

It is of paramount importance to do a full body examination after examining the presenting rash, otherwise important signs might be missed. Note that peripheral skin examination may be normal.

Face

Malar (butterfly) rash: A sharply defined erythematous, confluent, macular rash, affecting cheeks and nose and sparing the nasolabial folds (**Figure 5.30**).

Discoid lupus erythematosus (DLE) predominantly affects the cheeks, nose and ears (ocasionally the upper back and V of the neck), with red scaly patches that heal with scarring and may be associated with a scarring alopecia. It is usually not associated with systemic involvement but up to 5% of patients may progress to systemic lupus.

Discoid rash: erythematous, raised patches with scaling and follicular plugging (**Figure 5.31** and **5.32**)

Associated facial oedema may be noted. Also look at the mouth for oral ulceration and the scalp for alopecia areata or diffuse hair shedding.

Trunk/limbs

Livedo reticularis, mottled bluish discolouration of skin in a net-like pattern, may also be found when examining the limbs.

Signs in the hands may include, peri-ungual telangiectasia, digital erythema or Raynaud's phenomenon.

Further examination

Further examination should be guided by the clinical history. It may involve:

- Cardiovascular examination, looking for a pericardial rub (pericarditis) or signs of a pericardial effusion
- Respiratory examination to look for evidence of pleural effusion, pleural rub or lung fibrosis and lymphadenopathy
- Neurological examination to look for focal neurological signs, chorea or ataxia, psychosis
- Musculoskeletal examination to identify a peripheral arthropathy affecting at least two peripheral joints (present in 90% of patients). Jaccoud's arthropathy may also be noted
- An abdominal examination may reveal splenomegaly

> **Lupus erythematosus**
>
> Lupus erythematosus covers a group of related disorders, all of which can affect the skin. The spectrum ranges from the purely cutaneous type (discoid LE), intermediate type associated with internal problems (subacute cutaneous LE) to severe multi-system disease (systemic LE).

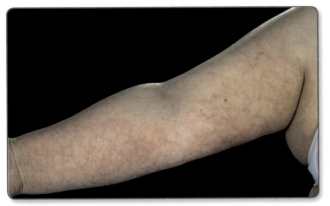

Figure 5.29 Livido reticularis. On patient's upper limb, there is a blue-purple net-like appearance of livido reticularis. May also be found in SLE.

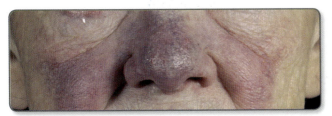

Figure 5.30 Malar rash. There is confluent erythema in a butterfly distribution. Remember to consider diagnoses other than systemic lupus erythematosus when presented with a malar rash, especially in male or in older patients, such as the malar flush of mitral valve disease.

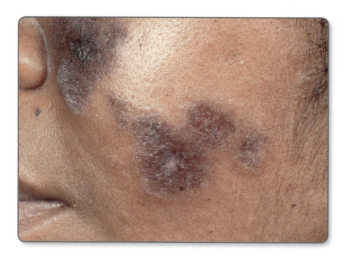

Figure 5.31 Discoid rash. This patient has a discoid, red rash on the left cheek with evidence of scarring.

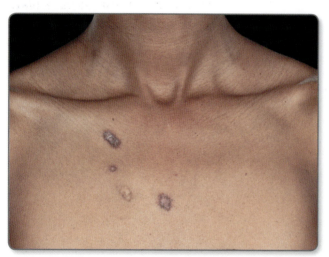

Figure 5.32 Discoid lupus. A patient with discoid lupus on the praecordium.

Relevant negatives

The absence of systemic features of SLE (as listed above) would be important relevant negatives in a patient presenting with a malar rash. Given that mitral stenosis is a differential diagnosis, the absence of auscultatory features of mitral stenosis is also important.

What to tell the patient

'I suspect you have a condition called systemic lupus erythematosus. This is an auto-immune condition that usually affects other body organs but occasionally only the skin. The most important thing you can do is to protect your skin from sunlight. There is no instant cure but many treatments are able to help it. You will require long-term follow-up. I will refer you for an opinion from the heart and nerve specialists for the symptoms you have described to me to rule out other organ involvement. I will review your progress in a few weeks' time.'

What to tell the examiner – state the most likely diagnosis on the basis of the history and clinical findings

'This patient appears to have systemic lupus erythematosus.'

Offer relevant differential diagnoses

The differential diagnosis of a malar rash includes mitral stenosis, sunburn, polymorphic light eruption, and rosacea.

Demonstrate an understanding of the value of further investigation

Investigations are aimed at confirming the diagnosis and monitoring disease activity.

A skin biopsy with immunofluorescence may be carried out. Typical biopsy features include epidermal atrophy, liquefaction degeneration of dermoepidermal junction, with fibrinoid degeneration of connective tissue and walls of blood vessels. Immunofluorescence (lupus band test) will show positive antibody deposition along the basement membrane (IgG, IgM and C3 granular or global deposits).

Haematological blood tests may show some or all of the following:

- Anaemia, which may be normocytic or due to haemolysis
- Thrombocytopaenia
- Lymphopaenia

- A raised ESR (in the context of a normal CRP)
- Renal function and urinalysis for identification of proteinuria or haematuria or red cell casts

Auto-antibody profile: The ANA is positive in 95% with anti-dsDNA antibodies being highly specific for SLE. Anti-Sm antibodies are also highly specific. Rheumatoid factor is positive in 40%. Anticardiolipin antibodies, which may give rise to false-positive tests for syphilis, are positive in antiphospholipid syndrome. Anti-Ro antibodies are characteristic in Subacute LE. If a mother with LE carries the antibody the neonate is at risk of neonatal LE with congenital heart block, hepatic and haematological involvement. Other tests include: lupus anticoagulant and complement levels (expect to be low).

Always offer a management plan

General measures involve rest and sun-avoidance or appropriate sun protection, with analgesia for arthralgia.

Hydroxychloroquine is indicated in mild disease with cutaneous or joint involvement, because of its anti-inflammatory properties. Regular renal function tests and eye checks are necessary.

In moderate/severe disease, systemic steroids and immunosuppressants are used, especially in the presence of central nervous system or renal involvement, severe illness, haemolytic crisis, and thrombocytopenia.

Other drugs may be needed to manage organ-specific complications, e.g. anticonvulsants, antihypertensives.

Think of conception and pregnancy. Fertility is not usually affected in people with SLE, but some women have a higher chance of miscarriage. Blood pressure can be affected during pregnancy in the presence of kidney involvement. Most women with mild or well-controlled SLE are likely to have an uneventful pregnancy. In the presence of maternal anti-Ro antibodies, as these cross the placenta, the baby may be born with neonatal lupus: a temporary ring-like (annular) rash and risk of congenital heart block.

Case 125: Discoid lupus erythematosus

Instruction to the candidate

This 32-year-old patient complains of a body rash. It has not responded to treatment for eczema and psoriasis. Please examine the patient and discuss diagnosis and treatment.

Take a focused history

In any facial rash you need to establish whether it is photosensitive or not and ask about specific precipitating factors such as sunlight and medication.

As with SLE screen for the presence of constitutional symptoms suggestive of systemic involvement.

Positive findings of a focused examination

The rash in discoid lupus consists of well-demarcated, red, atrophic, scaly plaques with keratin plugs in dilated follicles ('grated nutmeg'). The rash occurs in sun-exposed areas: scalp, face, ears but may also affect upper back, V-neck and dorsum of hands. This is a scarring disease therefore may leave post-inflammatory scarring and hypopigmentation.

Consider further examination for scarring alopecia or discoid lesions on the patient's scalp.

Relevant negatives

Discoid lupus usually has no systemic involvement so a wider focused examination should reveal none of the multi-system clinical signs discussed in *Cutaneous lupus erythematosus* (p. 226).

What to tell the patient

'I suspect you have a condition called discoid lupus erythematosus (DLE), which causes this kind of rash in sun-exposed areas. There is a wide range of related disorders which can damage internal organs but the type you have is usually confided to the skin and does not cause general ill health. The cause is not fully understood but it is likely to be an auto-immune condition. There is not a curative treatment, but the skin rash can improve with topical steroids and anti-malarial tablets. You should protect yourself from sunlight and always use high SpF sunscreen.

What to tell the examiner – state the most likely diagnosis on the basis of the history and clinical findings

'This patient has a scarring, discoid rash in a photosensitive distribution without systemic features, in keeping with discoid lupus erythematosus.'

Offer relevant differential diagnoses

Psoriasis is a key differential but this is usually larger, thicker scales, symmetrical, involving elbows, knees, scalp, and sacrum.

Fungal skin infection is another alternative diagnosis, but this is likely to be a solitary, annular lesion with a peripheral rim of scale.

Demonstrate an understanding of the value of further investigation

Discoid lupus has a low incidence of ANA with titres >1:16.

A skin biopsy with immunofluorescence should be performed. This will show hyperkeratosis, epidermal atrophy and follicular plugging.

The Lupus Band Test (LBT) may be positive in 90% of active lesions.

Always offer a management plan

The patient should administer topical steroids twice daily until clear (ensure you give advice regarding long-term side effects). Intralesional triamcinolone if topical steroid therapy fails. Hydroxychloroquine is an option for extensive or recurrent skin involvement (ensure pre-treatment eye tests).

Patients should wear a high SpF sunblock. Cosmetic camouflage may also be offered.

In severe cases when there is no response to anti-malarials azathioprine, mycophenolate mofetil and methotrexate may also be used.

Case 126: Skin manifestations of systemic disease – dermatomyositis

Instruction to the candidate

This 62-year-old man has been referred to the dermatology clinic with a facial rash. Please examine the patient, take any relevant history and discuss further management.

Take a focused history

In patients in whom the focused clinical examination (see below) reveals signs of dermatomyositis ensure you ask specific questions on the following:

- General malaise, fevers, weight loss
- Muscle weakness, usually symmetrical and proximal (rash often precedes myositis in 56% of patients). Such proximal weakness may be demonstrated as difficulty rising from supine position, climbing stairs, or raising arms over head
- Raynaud's phenomenon
- Lung involvement
- Arthralgia
- Dysphagia, nasal speech and regurgitation from bulbar involvement
- Gut motility problems

In patients >40 consider underlying malignancy. Lung, breast, gastrointestinal tract, and ovary are the commonest associations.

Positive findings of a focused examination

The key clinical finding is a heliotrope rash, a periorbital and malar violaceous (lilac-blue) flush with associated periorbital oedema. There may be erythema, or blue-purple patches, of other sun exposed areas such as the face, neck and upper trunk.

Go on to examine the hands for the following clinical signs:

- Gottron's papules: flat topped violaceous papules over bony prominences, especially the knuckles
- Mechanic's hands: rough, cracked skin on palms and fingertips
- Dilated capillary loops: periungual erythema with telangiectasia, thrombosis of capillary loops, infarctions

See **Figures 5.33–5.36** for clinical photographs.
Seek to elicit signs of proximal myopathy. Ask the patient to rise from a seated position. Ask them to raise their arms above their head.

Relevant negatives

A lack of obvious clinical findings pointing towards a solid organ malignancy is an important negative finding to make.

What to tell the patient

'I suspect you have a condition called dermatomyositis. It is an inflammatory condition affecting the skin and muscles and usually has a good prognosis. We will need to run some more tests to make sure no other body organs are affected and to find a possible cause. You will require treatment with oral steroids to begin with and depending on your response we will see if you require stronger agents to suppress the inflammation.'

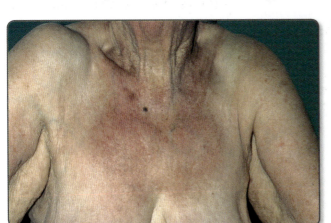

Figure 5.33 Dermatomyositis.
Photosensitive rash in a patient with dermatomyositis. Note the well-demarcated rash in a sun exposed area of the chest.

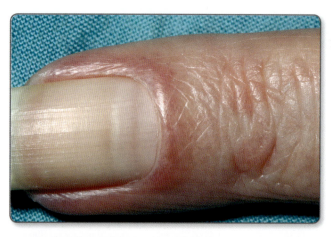

Figure 5.34 Dermatomyositis.
This patient's finger demonstrates periungual erythema and small red patches on the bony prominence of the distal interphalangeal joint. The rest of the hands should be examined to look for associated signs such as Gottron's papules. An examination of the hands is likely to be prompted by the identification of a heliotrope rash.

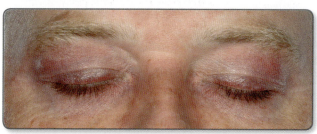

Figure 5.35 Heliotropic rash. There is a peri-orbital violaceous hue consistent with dermatomyositis. Be sure to examine other sun-exposed areas and take a close look at the hands.

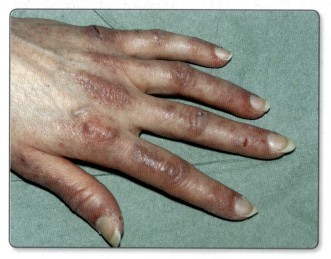

Figure 5.36 Hand signs in dermatomyositis. Gottron's papules are present on the dorsal aspect of the metacarpophalangeal and proximal interphalangeal joints. There is also rough, dry skin on the fingertips and ragged cuticles, colloquially known as 'mechanic's hands'.

What to tell the examiner – state the most likely diagnosis on the basis of the history and clinical findings

'This patient presents with a heliotrope rash and a rash in a photosensitive distribution over the chest and hands, where there are also signs of Gottron's papules and periungual erythema. There is also associated proximal muscle weakness. The most likely diagnosis is dermatomyositis.'

Offer relevant differential diagnoses

The differential diagnosis of a periorbital rash includes: seborrhoeic dermatitis, periorbital contact allergic dermatitis, ocular rosacea.

Demonstrate an understanding of the value of further investigation

Blood tests can both demonstrate autoimmune serology and give evidence of myositis. Anti-Jo1 antibodies are positive in 80% and are highly specific. ANA is positive in 40% of patients but has a low specificity. Creatine kinase may be elevated, demonstrating myositis.

- Raised CK
- ANA positive in 40% of patients but has low specificity
- Anti-Jo1 (highly specific) and anti-Mi2 (chromosomal helicase DNA binding protein)

The finding of weakness would prompt investigation with EMG, MRI, and muscle biopsy (gold standard for diagnosis).

A 12-lead electrocardiogram may demonstrate myocarditis or AV block in the appropriate clinical setting.

A skin biopsy may be performed if there is diagnostic uncertainty.

Importantly, a diagnosis of dermatomyositis would prompt an appropriate search for underlying malignancy.

Always offer a management plan

Systemic therapy options include:

- Oral steroids
- Methotrexate, cyclophosphamide, ciclosporin
- Intravenous immunoglobulin

Management is also targeted at any underlying malignancy that may have been identified. Don't forget to offer physiotherapy in the presence of muscle weakness and advise sun-protection measures.

Case 127: Alopecia areata

Instruction to the candidate

This 40-year-old woman has attended your clinic complaining of hair loss. Please assess the patient and provide a management plan.

Take a focused history

Aim to establish the type of hair loss , speed of onset (in alopecia areata the hair loss is sudden), and any potential causes. Establish if the alopecia is diffuse or localised. See **Table 5.4** for causes of hair loss according to type, which can guide the focused history according to what the patient describes and the clinical factors they describe in their past medical history. As alopecia areata often starts after a stressful even don't forget to ask and also assess the emotional impact the conditions is having on the patient.

Drug history (see **Table 5.4**), cessation of oestrogen therapy, family history of hair loss, recent surgery/pregnancy are also important to clarify when taking a hair loss history of any type.

Positive findings of a focused examination

On the scalp, look for diffuse or patchy hair loss. Alopecia areata is demonstrated by a well-circumscribed, totally bald, smooth patch(s). There are exclamation-mark hairs at the borders. The eyebrows and beard may also be affected. New hair growth may be white or gray. See **Figures 5.37–5.39** for clinical photographs.

If alopecia areata is identified. Occasionally the whole scalp is affected (Alopecia totalis) or the whole body hair is lost (Alopecia universalis). Offer to examine other hair bearing areas. Consider performing a full body examination for evidence of autoimmune disease, such as:

- Vitiligo. Well-demarcated macular de-pigmented areas in a symmetrical distribution
- Thyroid examination (autoimmune thyroid disease)

Table 5.4 Causes of hair loss according to type*		
Diffuse non-scarring	**Localised non-scarring**	**Localised/diffuse scarring**
Androgenic (male-pattern or female-pattern) • More pronounced after menopause (see Figure 5.40)	Alopecia areata • Auto-immune disorders especially pernicious anaemia, vitiligo, autoimmune thyroid disease	Burns/irradiation • Chemical or thermal • X-rays
Endocrine • Hypothyroidism • Hypoadrenalism • Hypopituitarism	Infections • Ringworm • Secondary syphilis	Infection • Shingles • kerion
Nutrition • Iron deficiency • Zinc • Protein	Trauma/traction	Lichen planus
Telogen effluvium Stressors • High fever • Childbirth • Surgery • Other stress		Discoid lupus erythematosus
Drugs • Allopurinol • Beta-blockers • Carbimazole • Warfarin		
* See also Figures 5.37–5.40.		

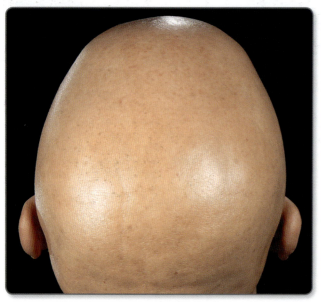

Figure 5.37 Alopecia totalis. This patient has complete hair loss.

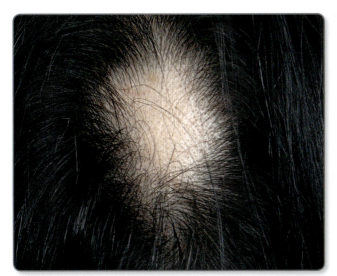

Figure 5.38 Localised alopecia areata. This patient has a well circumscribed, bald, smooth patch with small broken hairs in the periphery ('exclamation mark' hairs).

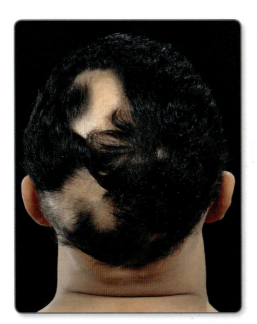

Figure 5.39 Multi-site localised alopecia areata. This patient has multiple areas of hair loss.

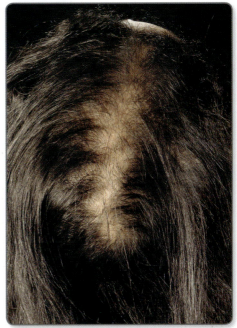

Figure 5.40 Female pattern hair loss - androgenic alopecia. This patient has thinning over the vertex with parting of the hairline. In contrast male pattern baldness results in a receding frontal hairline that progresses to a bald patch on the top of the head.

- Addison's disease may be suggested by the finding of diffuse hyperpigmentation, accentuated on exposed body parts and maximal on face, areolae, genitalia, knees, knuckles, palmar creases, lips, gums, tongue. There may also be buccal hyperpigmentation

Relevant negatives

If no signs suggestive of an underlying autoimmune disease were found, this would be an important negative finding to report to the examiner.

What to tell the patient

'It appears that you have developed a type of hair loss called alopecia areata, which consists of small, round patches of baldness on the scalp. This type of hair loss is associated with an inflammatory response but the exact cause is unknown. It is thought that the immune system attacks the growing hairs. The chances of hair growing back are generally good when the patch is small. Re-growth occurs from the centre of the patch and is often white at first but usually regains colour. There is a chance there will be complete re-growth within one year but further episodes may occur in the future. Topical steroids may help induce hair growth. People who suffer with alopecia areata are more likely to develop other auto-immune conditions such as thyroid disease or diabetes and as such it will be important that we screen for these.'

What to tell the examiner – state the most likely diagnosis on the basis of the history and clinical findings

'This patient has a solitary patch of hair loss with exclamation-mark hairs on the edge without peripheral signs of auto-immune disease. This is in keeping with alopecia areata.'

Offer relevant differential diagnoses

Hair loss has a wide differential, the different subtypes of which are discussed in **Table 5.4**.

Demonstrate an understanding of the value of further investigation

Investigations are aimed at identifying the cause of hair loss and at identifying any underlying autoimmune disease.

To investigate for hair loss:

- Iron studies and ferritin
- ANA
- Serum zinc
- Thyroid function tests
- Prolactin, LH, FSH, testosterone, SHBG

In suspected cases of Addison's, perform a 9 am cortisol, check serum electrolytes and perform stimulation tests as appropriate.

In suspected thyroid disease check thyroid function tests and test for the presence of thyroid auto-antibodies.

Always offer a management plan

In addition to treating any identifiable underlying cause, management of alopecia areata involves the use of short courses of potent topical steroids followed by topical immunomodulators such as tacrolimus. Intralesional steroids are another option for small patches. More widespread disease may require oral courses of steroids. The patient should be warned that when the treatment stops alopecia may recur. Patients can also obtain wigs on prescription while they are waiting for re-growth to occur.

Any co-existing vitiligo is managed with topical steroid alternating with topical protopic, phototherapy, and cosmetic camouflage.

Case 128: Sarcoidosis

Instruction to the candidate

This 47-year-old man has come back to clinic for the results of his lung function tests, which show some reduced lung capacity. He also complains of a rash on his lower legs. Take a brief history, perform a focused examination and explain your findings to the patient.

Take a focused history

Look for clues in the instruction and think of skin problems in association with lung disease, focusing the history accordingly. Ask about the onset and duration of the rash and whether it is painful. Erythema nodosum usually presents with erythematous, painful lumps on the lower legs but other sites such as the arms may also be affected.

Ask about other causes of erythema nodosum:

- Sore throat (streptococcal infection)
- TB
- Pregnancy
- Oral contraceptive pill
- NSAIDs

Respiratory involvement with reduced lung capacity is suggestive of sarcoidosis.

Enquire about constitutional symptoms such as fatigue, weight loss, arrhythmia, or night sweats.

Assess for systemic involvement:

- Pulmonary: ask about cough, shortness of breath, chest pain
- Eyes: red or watery eyes
- Cardiac: chest pain, palpitations
- Central nervous system: headaches, confusion, malaise
- Musculoskeletal: arthralgia, arthritis
- Kidney stones: hypercalcaemia may lead to nephrocalcinosis. Make sure you ask about loin pain, haematuria

Positive findings of a focused examination

Skin lesions are present in up to 35% of patients with sarcoidosis **(Figures 5.41, 5.42)**. Note that 1/3 of patients with cutaneous sarcoidosis may not have other organ involvement. Skin manifestations of sarcoid include:

- Erythema nodosum: tender bumps on the shins
- Lupus pernio: large dusky blue or violaceous, soft infiltrates (nodules and plaques) cheeks and nose
- Papules and plaques: purple-red, thick, circular lesions
- Calcinosis cutis

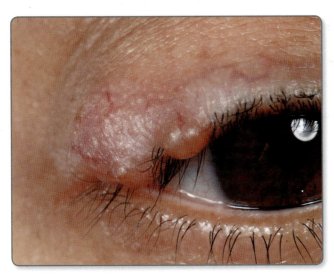

Figure 5.41 Cutaneous sarcoid lesion on the upper eyelid. Small cutaneous lesions on the left upper eyelid in a patient with sarcoidosis. Cutaneous manifestations of sarcoidosis occur in approximately 30% of cases.

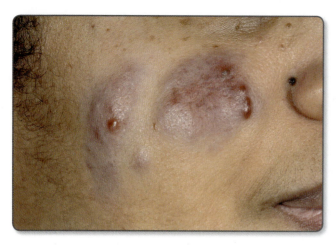

Figure 5.42 Cutaneous sarcoid lesions on the right cheek.
Multiple, dusky-purple plaque-like lesions on the patient's right cheek, consistent with lupus pernio. Similar large bluish-red and dusky purple infiltrated nodules and plaque-like lesions can be found on nose, cheeks, ears, fingers and toes.

Examine the hands for individual swelling of digits and popular violaceous/brown lesions on the dorsum.

Perform a systemic examination to look for other features of sarcoidosis:

- Lung involvement (90% of cases): apical fibrosis
- Eyes (30%): uveitis, conjunctivitis
- Liver (40%): look for hepatomegaly that may be accompanied by splenomegaly
- Heart (5–25%): cardiomyopathy or arrhythmias
- CNS (1–5%): Bell's palsy, neuropathy
- Musculoskeletal (2–38%): ankle, elbows, wrists, hands arthritis or arthralgia
- Examine all patients for lymphadenopathy and presence of enlarged parotids

Relevant negatives

In a patient with suspected sarcoidosis, the absence of systemic features is an important negative finding. In other cases of erythema nodosum, it would be important to exclude the afore-mentioned causes.

What to tell the patient

'I suspect you have a condition called sarcoidosis, a disease that can cause inflammation on many body parts. It is not cancerous or infectious. It most commonly presents with a rash on the legs and joint pains, but it may often affect other body organs, such as the lungs. The lung tests you had show there is mild involvement of the lung tissue. I will organise a CT scan of your chest, with high resolution to look closer at the lungs. In general

in most patients, sarcoidosis resolves without relapse, but small proportion of patients are left with some permanent lung damage.

'In most mild-to-moderate cases, no treatment is required apart from observation. Sometimes oral steroids are needed to reduce the inflammation. I will see you in 3 months' time with the results of all the other tests. I would like you to see an ophthalmologist to look at your eyes.'

What to tell the examiner – state the most likely diagnosis on the basis of the history and clinical findings

'This patient presents with painful, tender, erythematous lumps on the lower legs, in keeping with erythema nodosum. The most likely cause given the lung function is sarcoidosis.'

Offer relevant differential diagnoses

In cases where the main finding is erythema nodosum, offer a range of possible alternative causes, such as:

- Medications, such as the oral contraceptive pill, sulphonamides, salicylates and NSAIDs.
- Inflammatory bowel disease
- Tuberculosis
- Infections, such as streptococcus, mycoplasma
- Pregnancy

Demonstrate an understanding of the value of further investigation

Laboratory blood tests which would support a diagnosis of sarcoidosis would include:

- Lymphopaenia on full blood count
- Raised serum angiotensin converting enzyme
- Hypercalcaemia: if this is high, a 24-hour urinary calcium excretion can be performed
- Abnormal liver function tests
- Raised ESR

A skin biopsy of the cutaneous lesion may show non-caseating granulomata.

Further investigations may include:

- A plain chest radiograph to look for bilateral hilar lymphadenopathy. A high-resolution CT can confirm lung involvement

- A 12-lead electrocardiogram will identify any bundle branch block or arrhythmia
- Slit lamp examination

Always offer a management plan

Erythema nodosum usually requires no treatment but may take 3-6 weeks to settle. Recommend bed rest and NSAIDs to reduce discomfort.

With regards to sarcoidosis, in most cases no treatment is required and the disease may resolve spontaneously after a few months. Initial treatment is with systemic corticosteroids, especially in the presence of lung disease, uveitis, hypercalcaemia, neurologic or cardiac complications. Other options may include hydroxychloroquine, methotrexate, axathioprine or anti-TNFa agents.

Cutaneous lesions may be treated with topical or intralesional steroids. Laser surgery can be used for severe, disfiguring plaques.

Case 129: Tuberous sclerosis

Instruction to the candidate

Please examine this 35-year-old woman's skin. She is also being investigated for blackouts. Tell the patient what you think the most likely diagnosis is.

Take a focused history

Tuberous sclerosis is an uncommon autosomal dominant disorder with variable expression. 50% of patients will have new mutations. The key features may not appear until after puberty. Establish the onset of the features identified on clinical examination and positive family history.

Enquire about associated conditions such as epilepsy, learning difficulties, autism spectrum of disorders, and renal problems.

Positive findings of a focused examination

Key findings in tuberous sclerosis include (**Figures 5.43–5.45**):

- Ash leaf macules (hypomelanotic macules): These are off-white, polygonal or thumbprint

or confetti macules. If you see any ash leaf macules you need to inspect the whole body to identify more. Three or more white spots at birth are suggestive of tuberous sclerosis. Ash leaf macules fluoresce under Wood's light. In terms of distribution, the most common place to find Ash leaf macules is the trunk, followed by the lower extremities

- Adenoma sebaceum/angiofibromas: These are 0.1–0.5 cm diameter dome-shaped, confluent, small erythematous glistening papules. They can be skin-coloured or red and are commonly found on the centre of the face and in the perinasal region
- Shagreen patches are skin-coloured connective tissue naevi, found on the buttock and back
- Periungual fibromas (Koenen tumours) are smooth, firm, flesh-coloured nodules that emerge from the nailfolds

Relevant negatives

If having identified any of the key clinical features of tuberous sclerosis any of the other key features were absent, these would be

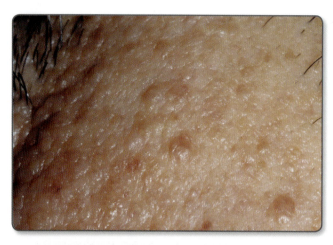

Figure 5.43 Multiple angiofibromas. These papules are small and coalescent. As with any finding consistent with a diagnosis of tuberous sclerosis, it should prompt examination for the other known clinical findings. If they are present they should be reported as positive findings. If not present, they should be included as relevant negative findings.

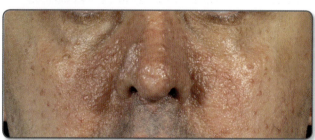

Figure 5.44 Adenoma sebaceum as a clinical finding in tuberous sclerosis. Multiple small, pink spots across the cheeks and nose.

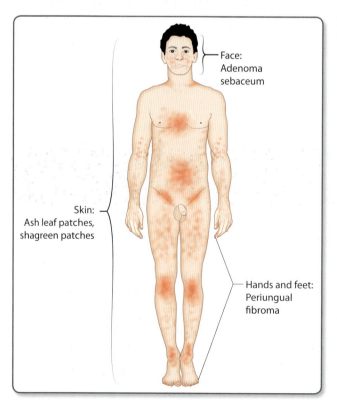

Figure 5.45 Tuberous sclerosis. Clinical signs in tuberous sclerosis.

Face:
Adenoma
sebaceum

Skin:
Ash leaf patches,
shagreen patches

Hands and feet:
Periungual
fibroma

mentioned as relevant negatives. Other relevant negatives would include a lack of cognitive deficit and the absence of abdominal masses (tuberous sclerosis is associated with renal, hepatic and GI hamartomas).

What to tell the patient

'The marks I have seen on your skin today suggest you have tuberous sclerosis. It is a complex genetic condition caused by an alteration in a gene. We will arrange for you to have multi-professional care and I would therefore like you to see an ophthalmologist to check your eyes, a neurologist as well as your GP at regular intervals to keep an eye on your blood pressure. If you are planning to have a family you ought to be seen by a specialist for genetic counselling as tuberous sclerosis is a condition that you can pass on to your children. Most people with tuberous sclerosis will live a normal lifespan and any problems related to the condition will be monitored and managed. I will be writing to your GP to inform him of your visit today.'

What to tell the examiner – state the most likely diagnosis on the basis of the history and clinical findings

'This patient's skin examination has revealed multiple hypomelanotic macules and a facial rash around the cheeks and nose consistent with adenoma sebaceum and thus a diagnosis of tuberous sclerosis. The blackouts are suggestive of epileptic fits which as commonly associated with tuberous sclerosis.'

Offer relevant differential diagnoses

A differential diagnosis of Ash leaf macules includes other white spots such as: vitiligo, tinea versicolor, post-inflammatory hypomelanosis.

Demonstrate an understanding of the value of further investigation

Important investigations to mention to the examiner include:

- CT or MRI head for tuberous masses
- Echo to exclude cardiac hamartomas
- Ultrasound of the renal tract for cysts and hamartomas

Always offer a management plan

Principles of management would include genetic counselling and appropriate specialist referral for system specific complications (in this case and in the absence of further information, the patient's blackouts could be due to either cardiac or neurological complications).

Laser surgery can be performed on angiofibromas.

Case 130: Neurofibromatosis

Instruction to the candidate

This is a 23-year-old woman who is concerned about her skin appearance. Please examine her skin and discuss the diagnosis with her.

Take a focused history

As the examination section below demonstrates, this patient has signs consistent with neurofibromatosis. In such cases, seek to elicit the following clinical features:

- Duration: all children with NF-1 have café au lait macules by 15-years of age
- Precocious puberty (especially seen in association with optic tumours)
- Learning difficulties and epilepsy
- Enquire about central nervous and eye involvement (optic nerve tumours can cause visual loss)
- Hearing defects (more common in NF2)
- Hypertension secondary to renal artery stenosis or phaeochromocytoma

Positive findings of a focused examination

See **Figures 5.46–5.51** for clinical photographs for the following clinical signs of neurofibromatosis:

- Café au lait macules are flat, coffee-coloured patches of skin. They usually appear in the 1st year of life and increase in number with age. If you find more than 6 café au lait macules proceed to look for other manifestations of neurofibromatosis

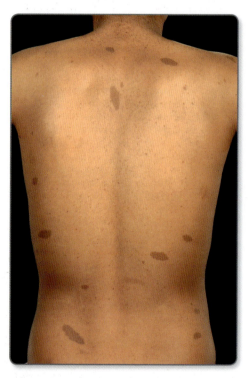

Figure 5.47 Multiple café au lait macules. This patient's back demonstrates multiple café au lait macules. There is freckling on the whole area of the back (non-specific) and freckling at the base of the neck.

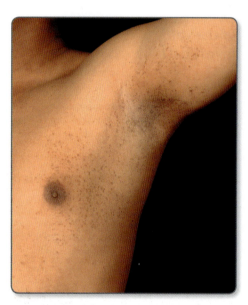

Figure 5.46 Axillary freckling as a clinical finding in neurofibromatosis. Example of freckling in the left axilla and surrounding area. In neurofibromatosis, freckling can also occur in the groin, the base of the neck and the submammary areas. It is usually present by the age of 10.

Figure 5.48 Single neurofibromas. An isolated, flesh-coloured papule consistent with a neurofibroma.

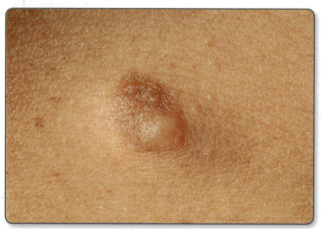

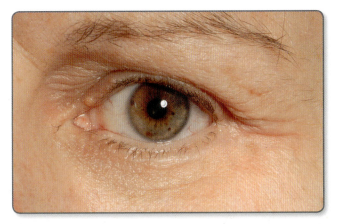

Figure 5.49 Lisch nodules in neurofibromatosis. This patient has brown-coloured pigmented lesions on the iris. On further examination with a slit-lamp and with clinical examination, associated signs of neurofibromatosis would be indicated.

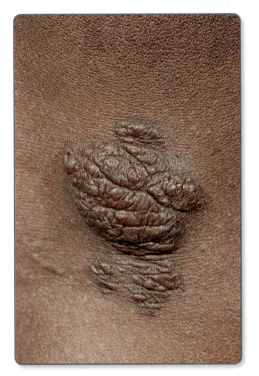

Figure 5.50 Neurofibroma. Superficial, soft tumour of the skin on the lower back.

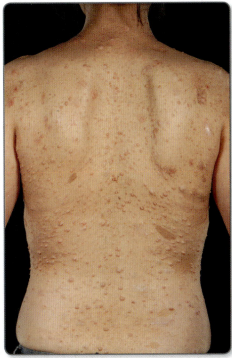

Figure 5.51 Multiple cutaneous neurofibromata. In this patient there are also café au lait macules present.

- Freckling is apparent in the axillae, groin, neck base and sub-mammary areas. They usually appear by 10-year of age
- Neurofibromas can take on a number of forms. Most commonly they appear as flesh-coloured papules, soft, button holed, easily pushed into the skin. Their number increases with age. They can also be nodular or plexiform

- Lisch nodules – tiny tumours on the iris of the eye

Relevant negatives

Important relevant negative findings include the absence of signs suggestive of tuberous sclerosis, which as discussed below is in the differential diagnosis for causes of café au lait spots.

What to tell the patient

'Examination of your skin suggests a condition called neurofibromatosis. This is a genetic condition which causes abnormalities of the skin but also in the nervous system and other organs. As you are concerned about your skin appearance I will arrange for you to see a dermatologist to discuss the treatment options. Furthermore, we will arrange for specialist review to discuss the genetic nature of this condition. Do you have any further questions or concerns I can address for you today?'

What to tell the examiner – state the most likely diagnosis on the basis of the history and clinical findings

'The clinical examination has revealed multiple cafe au lait spots, axillary freckling and multiple neurofibromas. These findings would be in keeping with a diagnosis of neurofibromatosis type I.'

> ### Diagnostic criteria for neurofibromatosis type 1
>
> For a diagnosis to be made, two out of the following seven features need to be identifies:
> - > 6 café au lait macules
> - > 2 neurofibromas
> - Axillary or groin freckling
> - >2 Lisch nodules
> - Optic glioma
> - Bone deformity, e.g. sphenoid
> - First degree relative with two criteria

Offer relevant differential diagnoses

The differential diagnosis of disease associations of café au lait spots includes tuberous sclerosis, McCune–Albright syndrome and urticaria pigmentosa. Remember also that café au lait spots can be a normal finding in healthy individuals (especially if they number <6).

Skin lesions which may appear to be similar to neurofibromas include leiomyomas (red-brown smooth, firm papules or nodules, often painful) and common nevi (although they are softer than neurofibromas and compressible).

Demonstrate an understanding of the value of further investigation

Slit-lamp investigation will confirm the presence of Lisch nodules, which are pigmented iris hamartomas and are part of the diagnostic criteria for neurofibromatosis type 1. X-rays for bone deformities. Annual blood pressure measurement. Regular skin survey for sarcomatous change of neurofibromas.

Where appropriate, MRI can be used to exclude optic pathway and central nervous system involvement. Genetic testing for confirmation (NF1 chromosome 17, NF2 chromosome 22).

Always offer a management plan

Management is multi-disciplinary involving primary care, geneticist, neurologist, and ophthalmologist. Genetic counselling and appropriate investigation of family members is appropriate.

Carbon dioxide (CO_2) laser, dermabrasion or surgical excision can be used for disfiguring facial neurofibromas. Consider the psychological impact the condition may have, the risk of isolation and loneliness.

> ### Neurofibromatosis type 2–key facts
>
> - Autosomal dominant
> - Much rarer than NF1
> - Café au lait spots
> - Bilateral vestibular schwannomas (acoustic neuromas)
> - Juvenile posterior subscapular lenticular opacity
> - Schwannomas of other cranial nerves
> - Meningiomas

Case 131: Osler–Weber–Rendu syndrome (hereditary haemorrhagic telangiectasia)

The hallmark of this condition is the presence of muco-cutaneous telangiectasia and arteriovenous malformations (pulmonary, hepatic, cerebral, and spinal). Red nodules and starry telangiectasia are found on mucous membranes and skin (**Figures 5.52** and **5.53**).

The patient may present with a history of epistaxis and GI bleeds. They may also have neurological symptoms due to TIA or stroke. Cardiac symptoms or signs may be present due to high-output cardiac failure secondary to arteriovenous malformations. There may be liver dysfunction.

Management is of complications. Genetic counselling is important due to the autosomal dominant inheritance of this condition.

Case 132: Port-wine stains (capillary vascular malformation)

Port-wine stains are well-defined, large, flat patches, purple or dark red in colour, which are found usually on face but can present anywhere in the body (**Figures 5.54** and **5.55**). If present in a trigeminal nerve supplied dermatome, think of Sturge–Weber syndrome (this is associated with microcephaly, brain calcification, seizures). Laser treatment can be performed for cosmesis.

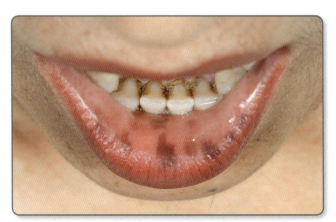

Figure 5.52 Hereditary haemorrhagic telangiectasia. Mucosal telangiectasia in a patient with the rare, autosomal dominant condition of hereditary haemorrhagic telangiectasia.

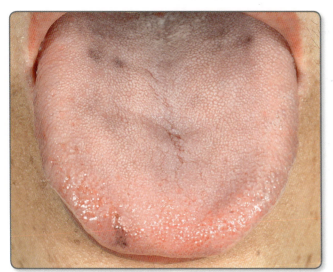

Figure 5.53 Tongue lesions in hereditary haemorrhagic telangiectasia. The same patient as in Figure 5.58, with a further mucocutaneous lesion, this time demonstrated on the tongue. In such patients the skin should be examined carefully for cutaneous telangiectasia. Enquire about symptoms of anaemia. Has the patient been given a diagnosis of hereditary haemorrhagic telangiectasia? Have they had to have any interventions in the past?

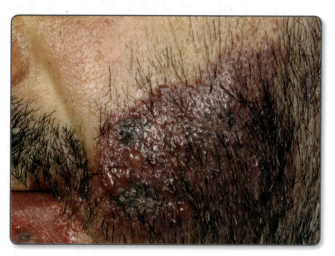

Figure 5.54 Port-wine stain.
The large, purple red patch on the patient's left cheek is consistent with a port-wine stain.

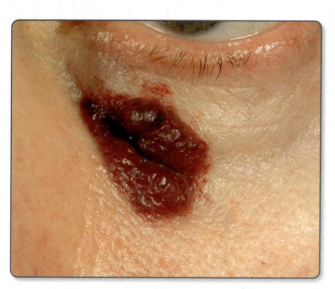

Figure 5.55 Port-wine stain. This example of a port-wine stain is situated under the eye.

Case 133: Ankylosing spondylitis

Instruction to the candidate

This 30-year-old man has been experiencing back pain. Please take a brief history, perform an appropriate examination and present your findings to the examiner.

Take a focused history

Use the history to elicit whether this back pain in a young male is mechanical, or whether it is associated with stiffness and decreased mobility. Ankylosing spondylitis will be high in your mind given the presenting symptom and the patient demographic (age <45), so take the time to ask about rheumatological symptoms as well.

Remember to ask about function (what can the patient not do because of the symptoms) and explore the patient's concerns and questions.

What is their occupation? While the PACES candidate may be focusing on detecting iritis to demonstrate their knowledge to the examiner, the young, previously healthy man working in a manual job may be more concerned about potential loss of income.

Positive findings of a focused examination

Inspect the spine for deformity (**Figures 5.56** and **5.57**) and make a functional assessment by asking the patient to look up towards the ceiling, noting limitation.

Assess for reduced flexion of the lumbar spine by performing Schober's test. Get the patient to stand in front of you, facing away from you. Find L5 level. With a pen, make two marks in the midline, one 5 cm below L5 and one 10 cm above. Ask the patient to touch their toes. Measure the distance between the two marks on the patient's back. If the distance between the two marks is now less than 20 cm (that is to say it has increased by less than 5 cm), this is indicative of reduced lumbar spine flexion.

Examine for associated findings:

- Examine the lungs for apical lung fibrosis
- Examine the cardiovascular system for the early-diastolic murmur of aortic regurgitation, with or without a collapsing pulse and other peripheral signs of aortic regurgitation
- Dry eyes

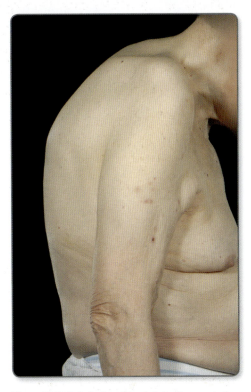

Figure 5.56 Ankylosing spondylosis. Exaggerated thoracic kyphosis, as part of a 'question mark spine' in a patient with ankylosing spondylosis.

Relevant negatives

It is important to note the absences of psoriatic plaques and abdominal scars, either of which may suggest an alternative diagnosis of back pain (see differential diagnosis below).

What to tell the patient

'The symptoms you describe and the clinical signs I have found on examination suggest you may have a condition known as ankylosing spondylitis. The main manifestation of this condition is reduced mobility of the spine,

'We will have to order some investigations to look more closely at the spine. These will involve plain X-rays in the first instance and then likely some more advanced imaging such as MRI scans. We will also take some blood tests that will tell us about the levels of inflammation in the body,

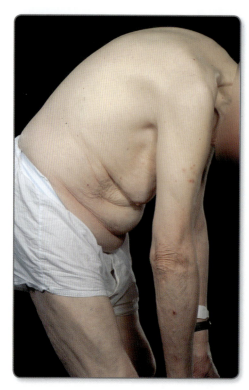

Figure 5.57 Reduced flexion of the lumbar spine in ankylosing spondylitis. This can be confirmed clinically by performing Schober's test.

'I will arrange for you to be seen in the rheumatology clinic with the results of these investigations. Until then I will prescribe you some anti-inflammatory medications and arrange for you to be seen by the physiotherapy team,

'Are there any other questions or concerns that I can address for you today?'

What to tell the examiner – state the most likely diagnosis on the basis of the history and clinical findings

'This patient has signs and symptoms consistent with a diagnosis of ankylosing spondylitis.'

The British Society of Rheumatology advises the use of modified New York diagnostic criteria for ankylosing spondylitis. The modified New York criteria divides cases into 'definite' and 'probable' ankylosing spondylitis based on clinical (pain, stiffness, loss of lumbar spinal mobility, loss of chest expansion) and radiological criteria (the presence and grade of sacroiliitis).

Offer relevant differential diagnoses

The differential diagnosis for back pain in a young male includes:

- Mechanical
- Traumatic
- Ankylosing spondylitis
- Other spondyloarthropathy: reactive arthritis, psoriatic arthritis, enteropathic arthritis

Demonstrate an understanding of the value of further investigation

Initial investigations will include appropriate imaging modalities and blood tests.

Imaging would include:

- Plain spinal radiograph: the main radiological evidence to tell the examiner about is that of sacroiliitis, which in the majority of cases will be bilateral. Other features include cervical spine involvement and syndesmophyte formation, which can lead to spinal fusion
- MRI spine can detect inflammatory changes and is now included in the ASAS classification for diagnosis of spondyloarthritis
- Blood tests would include inflammatory markers and rheumatoid factors.

Additionally, an electrocardiogram will demonstrate any atrioventricular conduction abnormality, of which there is a higher risk in ankylosing spondylitis. In addition, the presence of a collapsing pulse, diastolic murmur, or any other clinical evidence of aortic regurgitation would demand a transthoracic echocardiogram to assess the aortic valve and root (aortic regurgitation).

Always offer a management plan

Management is multi-disciplinary in nature, with physiotherapy and occupational therapy teams involved to help maintain function.

Medical therapies involve:

- Analgesia (WHO pain ladder), specifically NSAIDs
- Biologicals (anti-TNFα drugs). The British Society of Rheumatology guidelines (2004) recommend anti-TNF therapy for those with Disease which meets modified New York Criteria. Note that DMARDs are not effective for spinal symptoms

Monitoring for depression – remember that these are young patients who may have been extremely active previously so are at risk of depression.

Use the Bath Ankylosing Spondylitis Activity Index (BASAI) for disease monitoring. It incorporates current medications, gender, age and questions about pain and swelling over the previous week to assess disease activity. Whilst in a station 5 case where you make a de novo diagnosis of ankylosing spondylitis it is likely not necessary to actually use BASAI, if the patient tells you they have a known diagnosis of ankylosing spondylitis, it will impress the examiner if you use it as part of your focused assessment (assuming time allows).

Further reading

Jang JH, Ward MM, Rucker AN, et al. Ankylosing spondylitis: patterns of radiographic involvement—a re-examination of accepted principles in a cohort of 769 patients. Radiology 2011; 258:192–198.

Rudwaleit M, van der Heijde D, Landewé R, et al. The development of Assessment of Spondylo Arthritis international Society classification criteria for axial spondyloarthritis (part II): validation and final selection. Ann Rheum Dis 2009; 68:777–783.

The British Society for Rheumatology (BSR). BSR guidelines for prescribing TNF-alpha blockers in adults with ankylosing spondylitis. London; BSR, 2004.

van der Linden S, Valkenburg HA, Cats A. Evaluation of diagnostic criteria for ankylosing spondylitis. A proposal for modification of the New York criteria. Arthritis Rheum 1984; 27:361–368.

Garrett S, Jenkinson T, Kennedy LG, et al. A new approach to defining disease status in ankylosing spondylitis: the Bath Ankylosing Spondylitis Disease Activity Index. J Rheumatol 1994; 21:2286–2291.

Case 134: Marfan syndrome

Instruction to the candidate

Please examine this 22-year-old woman who has been complaining of shortness of breath. Following an examination and history, discuss your findings with the patient. A discussion with the examiner will then follow.

Take a focused history

After having made the spot diagnosis of Marfan syndrome in a patient who is tall and thin, with long arms and arachnodactyly (see positive findings of focussed examination below), ask the patient about:

- Her shortness of breath (see cardiac history). Does she have any known cardiac valvular abnormalities? Has she ever had a pneumothorax?
- Is there a confirmed diagnosis of Marfan's?
- Family history: it would be a mistake to only explore the family history of the patient's ancestors. Remember to include questions about descendants. A proportion of cases are new mutations so there may be no family history
- Visual defects: is the patient myopic (the most common symptom)?
- Is there any arthritis due to joint laxity? The candidate may miss this aspect of the disease if they focus too much on the cardiovascular manifestations

Positive findings of a focused examination

A sensible focused examination would include:

- Get the patient to stand: ask for a measuring tape and measure both their height and their arm span. Compare the length of their trunk to the length of their legs. Look at the fingers: are they long and thin demonstrating arachnodactyly?

- Assess for joint hyper-extensibility
- Inspect the praecordium for pectus deformity (**Figure 5.58**)
- Auscultation the heart, listening specifically for the ejection diastolic murmur of aortic regurgitation. Examine for a collapsing pulse. If a murmur or collapsing pulse is present, go on to examine for other signs of aortic regurgitation. Also, listen carefully for any mitral valve prolapse/regurgitation that might be present
- Assess the eyes, is there heterochromia?
- Do they have a high-arched palate? (**Figure 5.59**)

Relevant negatives

It would be important to note the absence of a midline sternotomy, which would indicate previous aortic and/or cardiac complications.

What to tell the patient

'You have features consistent with a diagnosis of a defect in one of the heart valves. This is known as aortic regurgitation. This may be a complication of a congenital syndrome known as Marfan syndrome. We will need to order some investigations to assess the heart valve lesion and I will be arranging for you to see a cardiologist in the near future. Do you have any further questions or concerns I can address today?'

What to tell the examiner – state the most likely diagnosis on the basis of the history and clinical findings

'This patient has symptoms and signs consistent with a diagnosis of aortic regurgitation as a complication of Marfan syndrome. Marfan syndrome is an autosomal dominant condition (with variable penetrance) affecting connective tissue, due to a mutation in the FBN-1 gene on chromosome 15, which codes for the protein fibrillin-1.'

Whilst it is easy for a candidate in MRCP PACES to comment that a patient is 'likely' to have Marfan syndrome, the Ghent criteria for making a formal diagnosis are extensive. They cover the following systems: Skeletal, Ocular, Cardiovascular, Pulmonary, Skin, Dura, family/Genetic history. While most candidates would consider it an inefficient use of time to

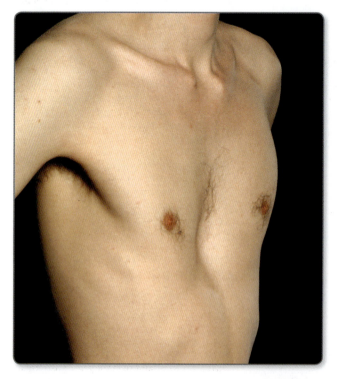

Figure 5.58 Pectus deformity in Marfan syndrome. This patient, with an underlying diagnosis of Marfan syndrome. Note the defect in the centre of the chest.

Offer relevant differential diagnoses

You can choose to give the examiner any of a range of differential diagnoses. For example, you could give a differential diagnosis of shortness of breath in a patient with Marfan syndrome:

- Aortic regurgitation
- Mitral valve disease
- Spontaneous pneumothorax
- Respiratory failure due to pectus deformity

Demonstrate an understanding of the value of further investigation

This patient will require a full cardiac work-up, firstly to confirm aortic regurgitation and secondly to assess its severity. See Chapter 1 for details but this will include a 12-lead electrocardiogram, a plain chest radiograph, and a transthoracic echocardiogram. The plain chest radiograph will also serve to rule out any pneumothorax.

Always offer a management plan

An important aspect of management of patients with Marfan's (and particularly important in this case) is the prevention and management of cardiovascular complications.

Key factors in the management of this condition include:

- Beta-blockade
- Regular (and often) clinical and echocardiographic assessment to monitor for progressive aortic root dilatation
- Consideration of prophylactic aortic root surgery when diameter >45 mm
- Regular ophthalmological assessment is also an important aspect to impress upon the examiner. This is a young woman so counselling must be given regarding pregnancy. When one considers the issues surrounding Marfan's in pregnancy, it is natural to concern oneself with the increased risk that a pregnancy confers on the mother. She has an increased risk of aortic dissection, an event that occurs in 4.5% of pregnancies involving patients with Marfan's. Any discussion with the examiner should include mention of the multi-disciplinary approach to managing a pregnant patient with Marfan's, with a team of obstetricians and cardiologists with expertise in the field. Genetic counselling will also need to be given to the patient regarding the autosomal

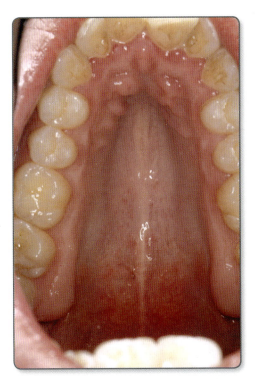

Figure 5.59 High-arched palate in Marfan syndrome.
Use a pen torch to look inside the patient's mouth.

memorise the whole list of criteria, the body system titles can be used as an aide memoir during the history and examination to ensure you are covering all the relevant points.

The criteria go on to state the requirements for a diagnosis of Marfan's. Note that these requirements are different for the index case, and for relatives of the index case.

Key clinical features of Marfan syndrome

- Tall stature
- Arm span > height
- Trunk length > leg length
- Arachnodactyly
- Pectus deformities
- Aortic regurgitation due to cystic medial necrosis
- Mitral valve prolapse or regurgitation
- Upward lens dislocation (the fact that in homocystinuria the lens dislocation is downwards is a dichotomy loved by examiners but almost entirely useless in the daily clinical practice of a general physician)
- Aortic dissection
- Spontaneous pneumothorax

dominant nature of inheritance and the implications for children in the event of a successful pregnancy

Further reading

Yuan SM, Jing H. Marfan syndrome: an overview. Sao Paulo Med J 2010; 128:360–366. De Paepe A, Devereux RB, Dietz HC, Hennekam RC, Pyeritz RE. Revised Diagnostic Criteria For The Marfan Syndrome. Am J Med Genet 1996; 62:417–426.

Dean JC. Marfan Syndrome: Clinical Diagnosis and Management. Eur J Hum Genet 2007; 15:724–733.

Lind J, Wallenburg HC. The Marfan syndrome and pregnancy: a retrospective study in a Dutch population. Eur J Obstet Gynaecol Reprod Biol 2001; 98: 28–35.

Case 135: Turner syndrome

Instruction to the candidate

Please examine this 19-year-old woman who has been complaining of recurrent urinary tract infections. Following your assessment, inform the patient of your findings. A short discussion with the examiner will follow.

Take a focused history

Ask about the recurrent urinary tract infections. How often does she get them? What antibiotics has she taken in the past? Ask about sexual intercourse, is there a correlation? Has she been investigated for this already with an ultrasound of the urinary tract?

Ask about her past medical history. Given findings of general inspection with evidence of small stature, webbed neck (may be hidden by hair) and, a 'shield' chest deformity, ask specifically about Turner syndrome.

Ask about other features of Turner syndrome:

- The key cardiovascular manifestations are the presence of a bicuspid aortic valve, aortic coarctation, and mitral regurgitation. Bicuspid aortic valve occurs in up to 30% of patients with Turner syndrome when assessed by transthoracic echocardiography in conjunction with MRI. Coarctation of the aorta occurs in 6.6% of patients and mitral regurgitation occurs in 7.4%
- Gynaecological complications such as ovarian failure

- Failure of growth. At what age was it noticed that her growth was lagging behind that of her peers? Was it this that led to her diagnosis? Has she had any treatment for small stature such as growth hormone therapy or oxandrelone?
- Are there any neurological or behavioural complications?

Positive findings of a focused examination

The examination should seek to elicit findings both to confirm your diagnosis of Turner syndrome and to elicit any abnormality that can help in your assessment of the patient's recurrent urinary tract infections.

A brief auscultation of the heart would identify any concurrent aortic stenosis or coarctation.

The clinical features of Turner syndrome include:

- General inspection: short stature
- Hands and arms: nail dysplasia, cubitus valgus, short fourth metacarpal, single palmar crease
- Head and face: low-set ears, retrognathia (posterior positioning of the mandible), Low posterior hairline, webbed neck, epicanthal folds, ptosis, strabismus
- Praecordium: pectus deformity, widely-spaced nipples, coarctation of the aorta, aortic stenosis (secondary to bicuspid valve)

Relevant negatives

Important relevant negative features would include the absence of signs of active infection such as fever, tachycardia and any abdominal tenderness (suprapubic and/or renal angle).

What to tell the patient

'The recurrent urine infections are most likely due to kidney problems associated with a condition called Turner syndrome. It will be necessary to obtain an ultrasound of your kidneys and bladder to investigate the cause further and discuss potential management options with the results in clinic. It may be possible to place you on a preventative daily antibiotic in the interim to reduce the symptoms and prevent further complications.'

What to tell the examiner – state the most likely diagnosis on the basis of the history and clinical findings

'This patient has signs and symptoms consistent with recurrent urinary tract infection, likely as a renal complication of Turner syndrome.'

Offer relevant differential diagnoses

As with most obvious spot diagnoses you can choose your differential, in this case the differential diagnosis for recurrent urinary tract infection.

The differential diagnoses for renal manifestations in Turner syndrome include:

- Double collecting systems
- Hydronephrosis
- Horseshoe kidney

Demonstrate an understanding of the value of further investigation

To investigate this patient's recurrent infections, the following tests would be requested:

- Urine dipstick and mid-stream urine for microscopy, culture and sensitivity
- Blood tests including white cell count and inflammatory markers to look for active infection
- Renal tract ultrasound scan is a key investigation as it identifies any structural abnormality of the renal tract such as those listed in the box on renal complications
- While not necessarily directly applicable to the presenting complaint, mention to the examiner that the patient would require (at some stage)
- Karyotyping: likely done at a very young age
- Transthoracic echocardiography to identify valvular or aortic abnormality
- Blood pressure monitoring

Always offer a management plan

Principles of management can be divided into managing the recurrent urinary tract infection (antibiotics where appropriate, hygiene advice, urology and renal referral if needed) and that of the underlying Turner syndrome. This would include regular cardiovascular assessment, genetic counselling, and endocrine referral for ovarian failure or growth failure.

Further reading

Davenport ML. Approach to the patient with Turner syndrome. J Clin Endocrinol Metab 2010; 95: 1487–1495.

Sachdev V, Matura LA, Sidenko S, et al. Aortic valve disease in Turner syndrome. J Am Coll Cardiol 2008; 51:1904–1909.

Carvalho AB, Guerra Júnior G, Baptista MT, et al. Cardiovascular and renal anomalies in Turner syndrome. Rev Assoc Med Bras 2010; 56:655–659.

Case 136: Tremor

Instruction to the candidate

You are the SHO in the neurology clinic. A 48-year-old man has been referred by his GP complaining of tremor. Please assess him and inform him of your management plan.

Take a focused history

Identify the characteristics of the tremor:

- Onset and severity
- Resting versus intention or postural
- Unilateral or bilateral

Ask the patient is the tremor is something that they have noticed, or if it has been mentioned by a relative/carer? A patient with an essential tremor or cerebellar dysfunction may be more likely to notice their tremor than a Parkinsonian patient.

Consider the differential diagnosis of tremor (see below). Does the patient have any associated symptoms that would identify an underlying diagnosis?

Be sure to ask about alcohol intake. In benign essential tremor, symptoms are often alleviated by alcohol, with a propensity for alcohol dependence. Alternatively, alcohol may be the underlying cause of any cerebellar disease, with resultant tremor. Additionally, with regard to essential tremor, be sure to take a family history to screen for an inherited or genetic component.

Assess the impact of the tremor on the patient's quality of life. Even in benign essential tremor, there is considerable associated morbidity, with potential for significant impairment and disability as a consequence. It is therefore important that you assess, and are seen to assess, the functional and psychosocial effects of the tremor.

Positive findings of a focused examination

Inspect the patient to assess for the presence of a resting tremor, looking specifically for a pill-rolling Parkinsonian tremor. It may be necessary to utilise distraction to elicit a resting tremor. Screen for postural or action tremor, often by performing a hand or cerebellar examination. A re-emergent tremor can often be useful in distinguishing between a subtle essential tremor and the resting tremor of Parkinson's.

Perform a neurological examination to assess for:

- Parkinsonian signs – pill-rolling resting tremor, expressionless face, clasp-knife rigidity with cog-wheeling
- Cerebellar signs: ataxia, dysdiadochokinesia, nystagmus, past-pointing, intention tremor, slurred speech, hypotonia

Relevant negatives

Relevant negative findings would include any of the above clinical signs, which are absent (see positive findings).

What to tell the patient

'From what you tell me and from examination findings, I believe you are suffering from what is known as benign essential tremor, where a tremor exists that can be exacerbated by social situations. I can reassure you that I can find no evidence of Parkinson's disease, cerebellar dysfunction or any other sinister cause of tremor. The initial management in benign essential tremor is lifestyle modification, with avoidance of caffeinated drinks and ensuring you get good quality and duration of sleep.

'If you feel strongly about the severity of the impact of the tremor we can consider using a medication called propranolol to attempt to control it. This medication is from a family of drugs called beta-blockers. Side effects of this drug include feeling fatigued but are tolerated well.

'I think we should discharge you from the clinic today, and continue care through your GP to whom I will write a letter. However, if you feel things are getting worse I am more than happy for the GP to refer you back to see me again. Do you have any further questions or concerns I can address for you today?'

What to tell the examiner – state the most likely diagnosis on the basis of the history and clinical findings

'The patient history and clinical examination are consistent with a diagnosis of benign essential tremor.'

Offer relevant differential diagnoses

Important causes of tremor include:

- Benign essential tremor
- Parkinsonism
- Cerebellar dysfunciton

Remember that in a young person, in addition to considering benign essential tremor, you should consider Wilson's disease if any cerebellar disorder is present.

Demonstrate an understanding of the value of further investigation

If the history and examination are suggestive of benign essential tremor then no investigations are necessary. Should there be present features that are consistent with either Parkinsonism or cerebellar dysfunction then the appropriate investigations should be requested (See *Intention tremor and problems with co-ordination – cerebellar syndrome*, p. 92 and *Central cord syndrome – syringomyelia*, p. 93).

Always offer a management plan

It is important to counsel the patient on lifestyle adaptations, which can help with the symptom burden. For example, limiting the intake of caffeinated drinks, ensuring adequate sleep levels and avoiding stress where possible are all important.

The first-line pharmacological management of benign essential tremor is beta-blockade with propranolol. If that is ineffective, the anticonvulsant primidone can be used.

NICE has recently released a consultation document relating to deep brain stimulation for essential tremor, but most candidates would correctly wish to avoid such discussions in the PACES examination.

If the patient has reported a significant alcohol intake, you should seek to counsel them about the dangers of using alcohol to control their tremor and, if appropriate, refer them to community alcohol liaison services.

You can also inform the patient that there is a National Tremor Foundation to provide help and support to those with tremor.

Further reading

Louis ED. Treatment of essential tremor: are there Issues we are overlooking? Front Neurol 2012; 2:91
National Tremor Foundation. www.tremor.org.uk.

Case 137: Seizures

Instruction to the candidate

You are asked to review a 48-year-old man on the acute medical ward who was admitted overnight with new-onset seizures. Please assess him and inform him of your management plan.

Take a focused history

On introducing yourself to the patient, you notice that he has multiple cutaneous neurofibromas.

Ask about the seizures: Are they generalised, partial, or complex-partial (complex-partial are more common on NF1 however all seizure types can occur). Has the patient had any investigations for the seizures? Have they been started on any anti-epileptic medications? Ask about the patient's occupation – does it involve driving (an important point in the patient with seizures)?

Confirm that the patient has already been given a diagnosis of NF1 (this is likely). Ask him about any complications that have occurred in the past.

Ask (tactfully) about academic progression, as learning difficulties can be a feature. Explore the effect on the patient's life, their questions and their concerns.

Positive findings of a focused examination

Confirm on examination the presence of neurofibromata, being mindful of alternative diagnoses such as multiple lipomata or Dercum's disease.

- Ask to see the patient's axillae and note the presence of axillary freckling
- Look for and comment on the number of café au lait macules
- Inspect the eyes for evidence of Lisch nodules affecting the iris

Relevant negatives

Perform a full neurological examination to assess for any focal neurological deficit.

What to tell the patient

'From what you have told me and the findings of my examination it appears that the seizures you have experienced are most likely a complication of your neurofibromatosis. I will be requesting some investigations to rule out other causes of seizures and I will refer you to a neurologist for specialist management. They may choose to start you on anti-epileptic medications. In the meantime, I must inform you that the licensing authorities stipulate that you should not drive following a seizure. As this is likely epilepsy secondary to neurofibromatosis, this period of time would be of one year's duration, however the neurologist will advise you further. I can give you some written information if you would like. Do you have any further questions or concerns that I can address at the current time?'

What to tell the examiner – state the most likely diagnosis on the basis of the history and clinical findings

'This patient describes seizures on a background of symptoms and signs consistent with a diagnosis of neurofibromatosis type 1, an autosomal dominant condition due to a mutation on chromosome 17.'

Offer relevant differential diagnoses

The differential diagnosis for café au lait macules includes:

- Tuberous sclerosis
- Normal finding in healthy individuals (especially if <6)
- McCune-Albright syndrome (café au lait macules, bony deformities and fractures, endocrine abnormalities)
- Urticaria pigmentosa

Demonstrate an understanding of the value of further investigation

For the patient's seizures, they will require:

- Electroencephalogram
- Intracerebral imaging: MRI is the imaging modality of choice

Always offer a management plan

The patient would warrant specialist neurological referral for initiation of anti-epileptic medications. The patient also needs to be counselled on rules regarding driving after seizures.

Further reading

Ferner RE. The neurofibromatoses (review article). Pract Neurol 2010; 10:82–93.

Brems H, Chmara M, Sahbatou M, et al. Germline loss-of-function mutations in SPRED1 cause a neurofibromatosis 1-like phenotype. 2007; 39:1120–1126.

Gutmann DH, Aylsworth A, Carey JC, et al. The diagnostic evaluation and multidisciplinary management of neurofibromatosis 1 and neurofibromatosis 2. J Am Med Assoc 1997; 278:51–57.

Chapter 6

History taking (station 2)

Candidate information

Scenario

You are the registrar in the Rapid Access Chest Pain Clinic. You are asked to see a 58-year-old woman who has been referred by her GP due to chest pain of recent onset. Her 12-lead electrocardiogram has been commented on by the referring GP as being unremarkable. Please take a full history from the patient. An examination is not required. Explain your working diagnosis to the patient and formulate a plan of action including any further investigations or management options. Thereafter be prepared to discuss the case with the examiner.

Actor information

You have attended today because you are worried about the exertional chest discomfort you have been having recently. You are particularly worried about your risk of a heart attack.

Prior to entering the room

The differential for chest pain is broad. It is useful to consider the common causes by system: cardiac, pulmonary, gastrointestinal, vascular and musculoskeletal. As ever, open questioning will allow you to best evaluate the value of further questioning on any given topic. However, there are often clues in the written instructions that will guide your thought process. Where chest discomfort is described as exertional, immediately one should be alert to the possibility of ischaemic heart disease. In taking a cardiac history, be mindful that a strong candidate will establish a working diagnosis, risk stratify the patient, and construct a management plan that will involve clear explanations to the patient avoiding jargon. Additionally, one should explore thoroughly the patient's underlying ideas and preconceptions as to the cause of their symptoms.

On entering the room begin with open questioning

In the first instance open questioning should be used to subsequently guide a more focused exploration of the symptoms, in particular asking about:

- Site
- Nature of the pain
- Onset – insidious/acute
- Context
- Duration
- Frequency of symptoms
- Alleviating/exacerbating factors

Allow the patient to describe the nature of the pain using her own language. Try to avoid giving exemplars of types of pain, to avoid misinterpretation and maximise the diagnostic value of the history.

The differential diagnosis can then be narrowed by the characteristics of the pain revealed in the history:

Cardiac

- Myocardial ischaemia – pressure or crushing sensation, exertional, relieved by rest, radiating to the arm or jaw, associated diaphoresis and autonomic features
- Pericarditis – constant, aggravated by breathing or swallowing, relieved on sitting forward
- Myocarditis – similar to pericarditis, systemically unwell, fever or recent viral illness, often with features of heart failure
- Dissection – acute tearing pain, often radiating to the back

Respiratory

- Pulmonary embolism – pleuritic with dyspnoea, cough and haemoptysis possible
- Pleurisy – painful, difficult breathing, often post pneumonia or viral infection
- Pneumothorax – acute onset shortness of breath and pain

Gastrointestinal

- Ulcer – recurrent, epigastric, improved with food or antacids in a smoker or in the context of excessive alcohol
- Gastro-oesophageal reflux – burning, radiating from epigastrium to centre of chest, worse on lying flat and post meals in patient with risk factors
- Oesophageal dysmotility – insidious onset, related to swallowing

Musculoskeletal

- Strain – reproducible long-standing pain with history of heavy lifting or recent infection with chronic cough
- Costochondritis – focal reproducible tenderness aggravated with movement
- Fractures – history of trauma, pain with movement

Infective

- Herpes zoster – unilateral, band-like, burning.

> **Open questioning suggests a diagnosis of angina**

With this diagnosis, closed questioning should focus on the following

A typical history of angina will involve all of:
- Constricting or pressure-like discomfort in the anterior chest, neck, shoulder, or arm
- Pain precipitated by a clear trigger, most commonly physical exertion or stress
- Relief after a period of rest or use of sublingual nitrate within minutes

Where a patient describes any of the above it is important that you are seen to clarify each of the three points. Consider using the Canadian Cardiovascular Classification – grading severity related to triggers:

Class I – strenuous or prolonged physical activity
Class II – vigorous physical activity: walking rapidly, climbing multiple flights of stairs
Class III – symptoms with everyday living activities: walking, stairs, emotional stress
Class IV – angina at rest

Focus on precipitating and relieving factors – most commonly physical exertion resulting in increased myocardial oxygen demand limited by atherosclerotic disease, but be mindful of the alternatives including decubitus and variant (also known as Prinzmetal's) angina. Decubitus angina where there is a clear history of heart failure, occurring on lying flat due to increased return to the heart and resultant strain. Variant angina, particularly in younger women with no atherosclerotic risk factors, occurring at rest and in cycles, thought to be secondary to vasospasm.

Despite being prepared for a history of

stable chest pain, always ensure that there are no crescendo or rest symptoms consistent with unstable angina or acute coronary syndromes.

Establish exercise tolerance as accurately as possible, usually the distance on the flat that the patient can tolerate before onset of symptoms. Commonly, where it proves difficult to quantify distance, patients relate better to the number of flights of stairs. Sometimes it is more useful to establish whether the distance has decreased recently, limited by pain or shortness of breath, thus relative as opposed to absolute distance is key. Exercise tolerance will give both an indication as to the severity of disease but also prove useful in monitoring disease progression, particularly after initiation of management and future clinic review.

Identify associated symptoms. Enquire as to the presence of autonomic features including sweating, dry mouth and nausea. In some patients shortness of breath represents the predominant feature of their angina and proves more troublesome than chest discomfort.

Succinctly combine past medical and social history to achieve a review of the patient's cardiac risk factors. It can be useful to ask a general question such as 'Other than the episodes of chest discomfort that are clearly troubling you, how is the rest of your health?' This demonstrates empathy and moves the conversation on without seeming like you are running through a prescribed list. If the patient replies that she is otherwise well, it is useful to proceed with 'there are a few questions that I ask everyone at this stage, would that be alright' followed by each of the modifiable and non modifiable risk factors. If she informs you that she has diabetes, clarify when it was diagnosed, whether it is diet, tablet, or insulin controlled, what her blood sugar control is like and whether she is experiencing any recognised complications. With regard to modifiable risk factors enquire as to control, compliance with medication and most recent review. Be prepared to swiftly cover hypertension, hypercholesterolaemia and smoking cessation in a similar fashion. A history of recreational drug use, in particular cocaine, is also important, and needs to be sensitively addressed.

A final review of symptoms and risk factors offers you the ability to take stock of the history thus far and allows you to summarise the information that you have gleaned.

'To summarise, you have been experiencing

central chest discomfort that sometimes moves into your neck after physical exertion for the last 6 months. These symptoms seem to be starting after two flights of stairs and force you to stop. The discomfort passes after a couple of minutes. It has been happening three times a week but you are concerned that it is occurring more frequently lately. You never experienced these symptoms at rest. Is there anything else that we haven't discussed that you think is important and that I should know about?'

Explore concerns, ideas, and expectations

Question – 'Have you had any thoughts or concerns about what may be causing these symptoms?'
Answer – 'Is this a heart attack?' or 'Does this mean I am going to have a heart attack?'
Question – 'How have these symptoms been affecting your life?'
Answer – 'I worry that this will affect my ability to work and my husband was recently made redundant.' or 'Does this mean I cannot drive?'

What to tell the patient

By exploring their ideas, concerns and expectations, often the working diagnosis will be offered by the patient and you will be in a position to confirm and clarify.
   'The symptoms that you describe sound very much like angina. Have you heard of angina/what do you understand by the term?'
   Offer a working diagnosis, explore understanding, ensure clear explanations, and formulate a plan of action.
   'The discomfort that you experience when you are walking up stairs I think is coming from your heart. This is a common condition and is due to a narrowing of the blood vessels that supply your heart with blood. The heart pumps blood to the rest of the body, supplying oxygen to allow your body to work. But the heart itself needs blood and oxygen which are supplied by the coronary arteries. Over the years, the coronary arteries can become narrowed. The narrowing is made worse by smoking, a fatty diet, and other conditions like diabetes. When you are sitting at rest, the amount of blood that your heart needs to do its job can be supplied by your narrowed arteries. But when you ask your heart to pump faster or harder, when you are climbing stairs for instance, the narrowed arteries prevent sufficient blood from flowing to your heart muscle and it responds with pain.

That is why, when you rest and your heart rate slows down, with time the pain goes away.'
   Check the patient understands. 'Angina is chronic but can be treated. There are medications that you can take to improve your symptoms and the amount of exercise that you can do. It is important that we treat your symptoms and try to stop the narrowing from getting worse to prevent you from having problems in the future. Importantly we want to avoid problems like a heart attack.'

What to tell the examiner

Summarise the clinical case

'This patient described symptoms consistent with a diagnosis of angina. This is most commonly caused by atherosclerotic disease for which she does (or does not) have risk factors. The requirement for functional or anatomical tests is dependent on the likelihood of coronary artery disease. That likelihood is dependent on how typical the history of angina is, the patient's age and gender and the presence of risk factors.'

Investigations

'I would review a 12-lead electrocardiogram, and check fasting lipids and blood glucose in order to risk stratify their cardiac profile. Resting echocardiography should also be considered for LV function assessment. ECGs in angina may show evidence of previous infarction, hypertrophy, or nonspecific ST-segment and T-wave abnormalities. A resting ECG alone does not establish or refute the diagnosis.'
   'In this case, I would assess their calculated likelihood of coronary artery disease (as per NICE guidelines) and use this to decide on the most appropriate investigation to perform. Options include coronary CT scanning (calcium score with or without CT coronary angiography), functional testing, or invasive coronary angiography. If the patient's likelihood of coronary artery disease is calculated as being greater than 90%, then no further tests are necessary to reach a diagnosis of angina (however, further investigations may be used, depending on the patient's clinical presentation to aid decisions on revascularisation).'

Management

Initiation of management and choice of medication should always be discussed with the patient. Give a brief overview, and then discuss details with the examiner.
   Management should be considered as

optimisation of modifiable and non-modifiable risk factors (involving both lifestyle changes and medical therapies), pharmacological secondary prevention, and PRN and regular symptom relief medication.

- In addition to dietary advice, smoking cessation, and moderation of alcohol consumption, it is often necessary to aid a patient in pacing their daily activities, managing stress and anxiety, and offering advice with regard physical exertion and sexual activity. Conservative management in this regard can be complex and require significant input from primary care.
- Secondary prevention measures: Aspirin (or clopidogrel if aspirin intolerant) and statin therapy should be prescribed for all stable coronary artery disease patients, with ACE inhibitors (or angiotensin receptor blockers if intolerant) if there is coexisting hypertension, diabetes mellitus or heart failure.
- Anti-anginal drug treatment.
  In the first instance a short-acting sublingual nitrate should be used. In providing GTN spray for symptom relief, one should explain to the patient how to administer the short-acting nitrate. Furthermore, instruct her to use it immediately before any planned exercise or exertion. Also, warn the patient that side effects such as flushing, headache and light-headedness may occur and to sit down or find something to hold on to if feeling light-headed after use.
  Beta-blockers or a calcium channel blocker are first-line treatment for stable angina, using synergistically (a non-rate limiting calcium channel blocker when added to a beta-blocker) where symptoms are not controlled on mono-therapy. Anti-anginal drugs prevent attacks of angina by decreasing myocardial oxygen consumption (by lowering heart rate, blood pressure, myocardial loading, or myocardial contractility) or by increasing myocardial oxygen supply (by increasing coronary blood flow). Where patients are intolerant of beta-blockers or calcium channel blockers, or both are contraindicated, second line treatment with one of the following is considered (depending upon heart rate, blood pressure and tolerance):

- Isosorbide mono-nitrate (ISMN)
- Ivabradine
- Nicorandil
- Ranolazine

In cases of chest pain of recent onset, where investigations suggest significant coronary artery disease or evidence of inducible ischaemia, invasive angiography with a view to coronary intervention should be considered.

Further reading

National Institute for Health and Care Excellence (NICE). CG95, Chest pain of recent onset: assessment and diagnosis of recent onset chest pain or discomfort of suspected cardiac origin. London, NICE, 2010. National Institute for Health and Care Excellence (NICE). CG126, The management of stable angina. London; NICE, 2011.

Case 139: Irregular pulse

Candidate information

Scenario

As the registrar on the acute medical take you are asked to see the following GP referral: I would be grateful if you would review this 76-year-old man who has been experiencing palpitations over the last year. I reviewed him in the surgery today after he presented having suffered a dizzy spell associated with his palpitations for the first time, resulting in a fall and minor head injury, although he denies losing consciousness. This man is a stoical type and this is the first time he has brought these symptoms to my attention, which I am concerned may be related to atrial fibrillation in view of an irregularly irregular pulse of 100 beats per minute. His blood pressure today was 162/90 mmHg. Many thanks.

Please take a history from the patient, offer an explanation for his symptoms and discuss your findings with the examiner.

Actor information

You have recently been experiencing palpitations and dizziness. On one occasion you have actually fallen over with these symptoms. Your GP has told you today that you have an irregular pulse. You are concerned that you have also been told that irregular pulses cause strokes, and you wish to know how likely or unlikely this is.

Prior to entering the room

Despite the suggestion of atrial fibrillation, be wary of a presumptuous diagnosis. Allow a description of the episodes or symptoms before attempting to narrow the differential. The age of the patient might bias towards a potential diagnosis of atrial fibrillation, but all arrhythmias should be considered especially if there is a history of preexisting cardiac disease.

Be mindful that this consultation will focus on the underlying causes of atrial fibrillation, symptoms from atrial fibrillation, and consideration of embolic cerebrovascular event risk with the need for anticoagulation and/or warfarin counselling.

On entering the room, begin with open questioning

Encourage the patient to best describe the palpitations in his or her own words. Often patients will describe fluttering, racing, or simply pounding and an awareness of their heartbeat, others will describe missed beats. Diagnostic yield from description alone is poor and the need to capture episodes on a 12-lead electrocardiogram paramount, however one can narrow the differential based on the nature, onset, rate, duration and termination of palpitations. In this case, focus upon the rhythm and rate. Establishing the irregularly irregular nature and the rate will be best achieved by asking the patient to tap out the beat with his finger.

In such cases, the history can serve to establish some fundamental features of the diagnosis. Firstly, is this new onset atrial fibrillation and further, is it possible to classify between paroxysmal, persistent and permanent?

Atrial fibrillation can be classified as:

- Acute – onset within 48 hours
- Paroxysmal – episodes that terminate spontaneously within 7 days, most often

episodes last less than 24 hours. Diagnosed after 2 or more discrete episodes

- Persistent – episodes lasting more than 7 days, requiring pharmacological or electrical cardioversion to terminate. Labelling someone as having persistent atrial fibrillation implies that there is still an intention to attempt rhythm control to achieve sinus rhythm
- Permanent – persisting for more than 1 year. Labelling a patient as having permanent AF implies pursuance of a rate-control strategy

The duration and frequency of palpitations will be key in attempting to classify atrial fibrillation from the history alone. Useful lines of enquiry will relate to the number of palpitations experienced in the average, day, week, or month and whether the patient feels that their pulse ever returns to 'normal'.

Open questioning suggests a diagnosis of atrial fibrillation

With this diagnosis closed questioning should focus on the following

In considering the patient's past medical history, medication and social history, it is possible to swiftly cover the common causes and triggers of atrial fibrillation:

Past medical history

Atrial fibrillation is common secondary to cardiac disease that affects the atria including congestive heart failure, coronary artery disease, hypertensive heart disease, and rheumatic heart disease. Such aetiologies are more common in the elderly population and generally result in persistent or permanent atrial fibrillation.

Cardiac causes

- Ischaemic heart disease
- Valvular pathology, most commonly mitral valve disease resulting in raised left atrial pressures
- Hypertension
- Heart failure, whereby AF is commonly an accompanying pathology

Non-cardiac causes

Thyroid disease, infection, pulmonary embolism and hypothermia can all precipitate atrial fibrillation, as can electrolyte abnormalities.

Ensure to enquire about the patient's caffeine, smoking, and alcohol intake, and also a history of stress and anxiety.

Where a potentially symptomatic episode has been eluded (as in this case) it is vital to understand the exact circumstances surrounding the event. Clearly define the features and relationship of the symptoms to the palpitations then screen for any other symptoms, such as breathlessness, palpitations, and syncope. Symptoms in atrial fibrillation can be classified using the EHRA classification:

I. No symptoms
II. Mild symptoms – those that do not affect normal daily activities
III. Severe symptoms – those that affect normal daily activities
IV. Disabling symptoms – those that cause the patient to stop normal daily activities

Stratify risk

a. *Embolic risk*: Ask about a history of heart failure, hypertension, diabetes mellitus, previous stroke or TIA, or previous vascular disease
b. *Bleeding risk*: In addition to previous questions, specifically ask about previous bleeding episodes or use of anticoagulation, renal disease, liver disease, and other medications such as NSAIDs

Explore concerns, ideas, and expectations

Be prepared for varying themes, introduced by the patient, which may change the direction of the consultation. With common conditions such as atrial fibrillation, often there will be a twist for which you should be prepared. As always ideas, concerns and expectations can be used to lead into diagnosis, investigation and management. The patient may offer statements such as:

- 'I think this is happening because I have been drinking too much since the death of my wife'
- 'I was very frightened by the fall, will it happen again?'
- 'My GP told me I would have a stroke, I am very upset. What did he mean?'
- 'My GP told me I would need to take medication for the rest of my life, I don't like pills. Do I have any choice in the matter?'

What to tell the patient

'I think you have a condition called atrial fibrillation which is causing an erratic heart rate which you are experiencing as palpitations and may have been responsible for your recent dizzy episode. Have you ever heard of atrial fibrillation, or know anything about it?'

Where you are reviewing a patient referred by a GP or colleague it is likely that some form of discussion has already occurred in rationalising the need for a specialist clinic appointment. As such, gauging the patients understanding is a good way to start and often makes the process of explaining the need for further investigation with ECG, blood tests and echocardiogram, easier.

Tell the patient that you will arrange some investigations, starting with a 12-lead electrocardiogram.

Treatment options should be explained succinctly, explaining:

- The potential to treat an underlying cause revealed by the results of investigations, or avoid triggers elucidated in the history
- The potential need to slow the heart to prevent further dizzy episodes
- The choice of medications to slow the heart or the potential to stop further palpitations and restore normal sinus rhythm may be influenced by the results of the investigation, including the echocardiogram. It would be sensible to arrange a further clinic appointment with the results, or admit to hospital for investigation if sufficient concern about symptoms
- Explain the risk of complications from atrial fibrillation, specifically that of an embolic cerebrovascular event and the need for anticoagulation. This will involve use of the CHA2DS2 VASC score (see below) which is more likely to come up in discussion with the examiner, but a brief explanation of risk and choice of anticoagulation with the patient is prudent

What to tell the examiner
Summarise the clinical case

Reaffirm the working diagnosis and classification of atrial fibrillation. Succinctly reiterate the need to investigate as outlined with the patient to confirm the diagnosis and screen for underlying causes. Where ECG demonstrates sinus rhythm and paroxysmal AF is suspected, discuss the need for ambulatory investigation. The emphasis of your discussion should then be placed upon the principles of management, rhythm versus rate control, and rationale for anticoagulation.

Investigations

The necessary investigations in a case of atrial fibrillation may include:

- A 12-lead electrocardiogram which may demonstrate atrial fibrillation at that time. There may also be evidence of ischaemia and/or structural heart disease
- Holter monitoring may be required if the 12-lead ECG demonstrates sinus rhythm (i.e. to achieve the diagnosis). Furthermore, ambulatory monitoring helps to assess for the adequacy of rate control in patients with known AF and also to help identify any other concomitant arrhythmias
- Transthoracic echocardiography can give aetiological information such as confirming the presence of valvular disease or the presence of LV dysfunction. Furthermore it can aid in the assessment of risk stratification for cardioembolic disease

Management

Patients with AF should be offered an individualised, tailored package of care. The main principles of management in atrial fibrillation can be summarised as:

- Rate control vs rhythm control
- Risk stratification for anticoagulation
- If possible, identify and treat the underlying cause

Rate versus rhythm control

Rhythm control is offered to patients:

- in whom it would be more suitable based upon clinical judgement (such as young individuals, for example)
- who develop heart failure secondary to the AF
- with new-onset AF
- in whom AF has a reversible cause

Rhythm control strategies include drugs, electrical cardioversion, and ablation procedures (pulmonary vein isolation). Drug therapy is individualised to the patient. Flecainide, for example, can be used in the absence of underlying ischaemic or structural heart disease, whereas amiodarone may be used in the presence of structural heart disease or heart failure. The relative benefits and risks, particularly side-effect profiles, of these common drugs need to be considered on an individual patient basis.

Otherwise, rate control is offered. Emphasize that rate versus rhythm control has no difference on long-term outcome, with patients offered rhythm control more likely to experience side-effects of therapy or intervention (hence this is reserved for those in whom the benefit outweighs the risk). Rate control is achieved initially with a beta-blocker or a rate-limiting calcium-channel blocker, with digoxin as adjunctive therapy if first line monotherapy has failed. Long-term digoxin monotherapy is only considered for sedentary individuals. Amiodarone is not recommended for long-term rate control. Difficult cases of poorly controlled ventricular rate despite medical therapy may require a pacemaker with AV node ablation strategy.

Anticoagulation

The need for anticoagulation relates to the inherent risk of embolic stroke related to atrial fibrillation, which is increased in the presence of other risk factors. The CHA2DS2-VASc score is a scoring system which aims to risk stratify patients suffering from atrial fibrillation with the intention of identifying those who would benefit most from anticoagulation. It uses the following factors to assess stroke risk: heart failure, hypertension, age, diabetes, cerebrovascular disease, vascular disease, patient sex. Aside from patients undergoing cardioversion or intervention, long-term anticoagulation is not offered to patients under 65 years with AF and no risk factors other than their sex (i.e. a CHA2DS2-VASc score of 0 for men or 1 for women). Otherwise, men with a score of 1 can be considered for anticoagulation, and anticoagulation is offered to all patients with a score of 2 or more.

In at risk patients with suitable safety profiles, formal anticoagulation with warfarin or the novel oral anticoagulants (NOACs, such as apixaban, dabigatran, and rivaroxaban) is recommended for reducing the risk of stroke. Aspirin has no role as monotherapy in the contemporary management of stroke prevention in AF.

Bleeding risk must always be taken into account. An important additional scoring system is the HAS-BLED score, which attempts to quantify the risk of bleeding. This is an important tool in considering anticoagulation therapy particularly in older patients where there is a history of previous bleeding such as peptic ulcers or cerebral haemorrhage, excess alcohol intake, chronic liver or kidney disease, poorly controlled hypertension or on a background of poly-pharmacy. Combining CHA2DS2-VASc and HAS-BLED scores allows you to consider the risk versus benefit of anticoagulation in atrial fibrillation.

In complex patients, or those with poor symptom control, consider referral to an electrophysiology specialist service where interventional options such as ablation can be considered.

Further reading

Fuster V, Rydén LE, Asinger RW, et al. ACC/AHA/ESC guidelines for the management of patients with atrial fibrillation: executive summary a report of the American College of Cardiology/American Heart Association task force on practice guidelines and the European Society of Cardiology committee for practice guidelines and policy conferences (committee to develop guidelines for the management of patients with atrial fibrillation) developed in collaboration with the North American Society of Pacing and Electrophysiology. Circulation 2001; 104:2118–2150.

Camm JA, Kirchhof P, Lip GYH, et al. Guidelines for the management of atrial fibrillation. Eur Heart J 2010; 31:2369-2429.

Camm AJ, Kirchhof P, Lip GY, et al. Guidelines for the management of atrial fibrillation: the Task Force for the Management of Atrial Fibrillation of the European Society of Cardiology (ESC). Eur Heart J 2010:2369–2429.

National Institute for Health and Care Excellence (NICE). CG180, The management of atrial fibrillation. London; NICE, June 2014.

Lip GY, Nieuwlaat R, Pisters R, Lane DA, Crijns HJ, et al. Refining clinical risk stratification for predicting stroke and thromboembolism in atrial fibrillation using a novel risk factor-based approach: the euro heart survey on atrial fibrillation. Chest 2010; 137:263–272.

Lip GY, Frison L, Halperin JL, Lane DA. Comparative validation of a novel risk score for predicting bleeding risk in anticoagulated patients with atrial fibrillation: the HAS-BLED (Hypertension, Abnormal Renal/Liver Function, Stroke, Bleeding History or Predisposition, Labile INR, Elderly, Drugs/Alcohol Concomitantly) score. J Am Coll Cadriol 2011; 57:173–180.

Case 140: Palpitations

Candidate information

Scenario

As the medical registrar on-call, you are asked to review a patient in Accident and Emergency. A 22-year-old male student has been experiencing palpitations recently. It is a stressful time of year with end of year examinations looming. His observations are unremarkable, HR 68, BP 122/81. Resting 12-lead electrocardiogram is normal. Please take a history from the patient, tell them what you think is wrong and discuss your findings with the examiner.

Actor information

You have recently noticed an unnerving sensation of feeling your heart beat at rest. You are very concerned about this, which is an added stress on top of your upcoming exams. You do not feel dizzy or collapse with your palpitations. You do not take any regular medications or drugs.

Prior to entering the room

In general when considering palpitations the importance is placed upon distinguishing between those that are harmless requiring reassurance only versus those that carry more serious adverse outcomes necessitating intervention. 'Palpitation' is a non-specific term relating to an increased and subjective awareness of the heart beating. Palpitations commonly reflect a change in cardiac rate, rhythm or contractility. Accurate diagnosis requires capture of an electrocardiogram during an episode of palpitations. Thus, the history should serve in the first instance to risk stratify patients to decide on appropriate reassurance versus referral or admission for observation, monitoring or treatment.

On entering the room begin with open questioning

Encourage the patient to describe the palpitations in his own words. Often patients will describe fluttering, racing, or simply pounding and an awareness of their heartbeat, others will describe missed beats. Diagnostic yield from description alone is poor and the need to capture electrocardiographic evidence during symptoms is paramount, however one can narrow the differential based on the nature, onset, rate, duration and termination of palpitations. It is often more useful to ask the patient to tap out the beat to better assess rate and rhythm.

For all palpitations, to narrow the differential, consider the following:

- Nature, rate and rhythm – speed of onset and offset, estimated rate, regular or irregular?
- Duration and frequency
- Termination – use of valsalva, knowingly or unknowingly by holding their breath or 'popping' their ears
- Precipitants – stress, anxiety, sleep deprivation, caffeine, drug use (prescription or recreational), pregnancy

Consider associated features – red flags prompting possible admission or expedient referral as certain associated symptoms raise suspicion of a more serious underlying pathology:

- Light-headedness, severe dizziness or syncope (particularly if injury occurs from syncope)
- Tunnel vision
- Chest pain
- Breathlessness

Patients sometimes complain of missed or skipped beats. On further questioning it may transpire that the sensation is one of an isolated pounding, or of a weak or strong extra beat. This would raise the suspicion of ectopic beats. Commonly they occur at rest, rarely with compromise and require firm reassurance from the outset particularly on a background of no previous cardiac disease (which is an imperative piece of past medical history to establish, see below). Ectopics tend to disappear with exercise.

A fast irregularly irregular heartbeat, often with sudden onset and offset will require investigation, treatment and referral with the presumption of paroxysmal atrial fibrillation.

Symptoms of sudden onset and offset associated with a heartbeat which is often too rapid to count, likely regular but occasionally difficult to ascertain due to the rate, and associated with symptoms of breathlessness, chest tightness or dizziness raise the suspicion of supraventricular or ventricular tachycardias.

Consider a summary of differential diagnosis based on the history

- Extra or missed beats, isolated, thumping sensation:
  - Premature atrial or ventricular beats – benign normal variant
  - Intermittent atrioventricular block
- Irregular:
  - Atrial fibrillation or flutter
- Sudden onset and termination, regular, recurrent lasting for seconds or minutes to hours:
  - Supraventricular arrhythmias
    - Atrial tachycardia
    - Atrioventricular re-entry tachycardia (AVRT), including Wolff–Parkinson–White
    - Atrioventricular nodal re-entry tachycardia (AVNRT)
  - Ventricular arrhythmias
    - Sustained or non-sustained ventricular tachycardia (VT)
    - Polymorphic VT
- Palpitations during exercise or stress:
  - Sinus tachycardia
  - Exercise can induce supraventricular or ventricular tachycardia, particularly polymorphic VT in patients with pre-existing long QT
  - Ischaemia induced arrhythmia, often ventricular
- Medication or recreational drug use:
  - Drug-induced palpitations. Think of illicit drugs and also of drugs that prolong the QT interval on the ECG
  - Palpitations associated with emotional distress or general anxiety may not have an underlying arrhythmia, but should be considered as a diagnosis of exclusion after organic arrhythmia has been ruled out

Where the history does not conform to a classical pattern, be sure to establish the key features with prompting where appropriate and aim to review with the results of further investigation.

> ## Open questioning suggests a diagnosis of fast palpitations

With this diagnosis closed questioning should focus on the following

A review of symptoms should cover those of potentially causative disorders. Where anxiety and stress form a predominant feature of the history relating to palpitations be sure to consider hyperthyroidism and rarer diagnoses such as phaeochromocytoma:

- Hyperthyroidism – palpitations in the context of heat intolerance, weight loss, and tremor would be useful screening questions
- Phaeochromocytoma – palpitations in the context of headaches, sweating and diaphoresis on a background of hypertension would be strongly suggestive

Where the review of symptoms are vague and centre around tiredness, lethargy and breathlessness think of anaemia. Screen for predispositions such as haematological disorders or for symptoms such as menorrhagia and rectal bleeding.

Consider the past medical history. Ask specifically about any previous history of cardiac disease (including ischaemic, congential, or valvular heart disease or heart failure) thyroid disorders, and previously diagnosed hypertension if not suggested by the review of symptoms. Structural heart disease, especially mitral valve disease, with which palpitations are a common finding. Also congenital abnormalities and cardiac surgery. In the family history screen for arrhythmias and sudden cardiac death.

Be alert to the use of medication with adrenergic effects, predisposing to palpitations, such as β-agonists or theophyllines in the treatment of asthma, levothyroxine in the treatment of hypothyroidism, or commonly over the counter remedies for flu and cold that contain pseudoephedrine. Be aware that certain medication can inadvertently induce palpitations and prolong the QT interval predisposing to ventricular tachycardia. These include:

- Anti-arrhythmia medication – amiodarone, quinidine, sotalol
- Macrolide antibiotics – erythromycin, clarithromycin
- Antihistamines – terfenadine
- Anti-depressants

In the social history, attempt to quantify the intake of caffeine and alcohol, and where possible establish any potential link with onset of symptoms to intake or increase in consumption. Smoking habits may be a useful indicator of stress levels and serve as a sensitive way in which to broach the subject – 'Is there any particular reason that you have been smoking more recently?', 'Do you smoke more when you are stressed? Do you feel more stressed recently?'

You must ask about illicit drug use, especially in the younger patient. Explain to the patient that it is a standard, confidential question with no judgement or suspicion attached. Directly ask about common recreations drugs including cocaine, ecstasy and amphetamines.

Explore concerns, ideas, and expectations

What do they think is causing the palpitations?

Is it affecting his ability to study? Has his sporting performance decreased, is he reluctant to push harder or perform to his best for fear of symptoms?

Awareness of palpitations can be heightened in depression or anxiety thus screening is prudent.

What to tell the patient

Without electrocardiographic evidence of the causative cardiac rhythm disturbance (if any) it is impossible to give the patient a definitive diagnosis. It is possible, however, to inform the patient of a range of likely differential diagnoses, and to reassure them (if possible) regarding risk stratification based on the absence of red flag symptoms. Inform the patient of the necessary investigations that will be organised with the aim to reach a diagnosis. Further advise the patient on any lifestyle modifications which can be implemented with the aim of symptom reduction, e.g. managing stress. Inform the patient of any follow-up which is necessary.

What to tell the examiner

Summarise the clinical case

'The patient has intermittent palpitations without suggestion of red flag symptoms. Apart from stress due to examinations, there are no obvious precipitating features.'

Investigations

Standard screening of all palpitations will involve a resting 12-lead electrocardiogram (to assess the resting cardiac rhythm and to identify signs of structural heart disease or arrhythmia potential such as long QT interval), together with echocardiography particularly in cases of suspected underlying structural heart disease. Routine blood testing with full blood count to rule out anaemia, quantification of electrolytes, and importantly thyroid function testing. Where appropriate, urinary catecholamines dependent upon clinical context.

Ambulatory electrocardiogram monitoring is used to identify the cardiac rhythm at the time of symptoms. The duration of monitoring is variable, usually between 24 hours to 1 week.

Implantable loop recorders are typically used in situations where a diagnosis has not been reached despite extensive ambulatory monitoring and/or where the time period between symptoms is sufficiently long such that a 24-hour or 1 week long period of monitoring is thought to have a low diagnostic yield.

Electrophysiological studies are also an option, typically utilised following review at an arrhythmia clinic.

Management

The specific management of palpitations varies widely depending on the underlying diagnosis. For the patient in this specific case, no drug treatments are necessary based on the evidence provided to the candidate. The patient should be reassured and advised regarding stress management. Any specific treatments would depend on reaching a specific diagnosis following the results of investigations.

Case 141: Ankle swelling

Candidate information

Scenario

You are the cardiology SHO. A 68-year-old woman, with an established diagnosis of heart failure, attends for her 6-monthly review in the outpatient clinic complaining of increasing ankle swelling. Please make an assessment and formulate a management plan.

Actor information

You were diagnosed with heart failure approximately 2 years ago. Your symptoms have deteriorated slightly in the past few months. You can only manage to walk about half a mile on the flat and you would like to be able to do more.

Prior to entering the room

In considering a patient review, it will be important to attempt to gather a past history of the condition and use this in gauging the severity and importance of any new symptoms. Although this type of station appears simpler

given the diagnosis, the pitfalls of a greater depth of patient understanding and complex management issues typically makes these encounters harder. That said, PACES does not assume in-depth specialist knowledge, and the approach to the station should cover common themes, in a generalist fashion, adopting a holistic approach. Be mindful that you have been specifically asked to formulate a management plan and thus taking even the most thorough history alone will not be sufficient. Indeed, regardless of whether it is specifically stated in the instruction, the strong candidate will always strive to offer a management plan and suitable time frame for further review or specialist opinion.

On entering the room begin with open questioning

Greet the patient and open the dialogue in such a way that allows them to direct you to areas of concern whilst potentially offering you useful information. If, in starting the conversation you ask specifically about their ankle swelling, it prohibits the patient from giving you general insight into the potential aetiology of their heart failure, and time since last review or diagnosis. For example, a question such as 'How have you been and how can help you today' may be met with a response such as – 'Well doctor, life since my heart attack 6 months ago has been terrible, and now my ankles have started to swell up too, I just cannot cope', or 'Things have been going wonderfully since I last saw you in December doctor, I am back playing bowls again and have even become involved with the Cardiomyopathy Society like you suggested. I went to a fundraiser last week but fear I over did it and now I have noticed my ankles are swelling somewhat'.

Where possible aim to establish:

- The nature of the heart failure – relating to ischaemic heart disease; hypertension; valvular pathology; arrhythmias; infiltrative disease or cardiomyopathy
- The time since diagnosis or last review
- The patient's general state of health and whether symptoms improving, staying the same or worsening

After that, probe with regard to the ankle swelling. Enquire as to the onset of symptoms, insidious or acute, and duration, intermittent or persisting over a long-period of time. Be sure to gain a clear picture of the symptoms including the extent of the swelling: Is it limited to the ankles or does it extend to the knee above? Is the swelling pitting? Are there associated signs? Establish whether this is a recurrent problem and seek to identify associated symptoms of heart failure including:

- Shortness of breath
- Chest pain
- Palpitations
- Paroxysmal nocturnal dyspnoea
- Orthopnea

Be seen to relate the symptoms to exercise tolerance and gauge her disease severity in terms of the New York Heart Association (NYHA) classification.

NYHA defining severity in relation to exercise limitation by symptoms:

- I – no symptoms and no limitation in ordinary physical activity
- II – mild symptoms of shortness of breath or stable angina with slight limitation on ordinary activity
- III – marked limitation in activity
- IV – severe limitation, symptoms at rest

The question worth considering in this case will be whether the symptoms reflect a worsening or progression of disease requiring optimisation or whether this is non-compliance with medication resulting in symptoms but no worsening of disease.

Establish current management and look to consider common side effects to explain non-compliance. Tactfully approach this subject. Many patients will resent the position in which they have been placed, with chronic illness, limitation on lifestyle and the burden of polypharmacy. Fairly innocuous side effects may have a significant bearing on quality of life in this context. Be mindful to screen for depression and end-of-life decisions. It is not uncommon for this scenario to end up in a 'my life's not worth living any more' discussion.

Alternatively consider recent changes in medication, withdrawal or altered dosing, or addition of new medication in relation to onset of symptoms.

> ## Open questioning suggests a diagnosis of heart failure

With this diagnosis closed questioning should focus on the following

Of medication side effects

- ACE inhibitors – cough, hypotension
- Diuretics – urgency, night time waking, and incontinence. Dizziness and leg cramps
- Beta-blockers – lethargy, wheeze (contraindicated in asthma)
- Nitrates – headache and dizziness
- Aldosterone antagonists – fatigue and headaches

Of alternative causes of ankle swelling

Be mindful, despite the known diagnosis of heart failure, that where there is doubt you should consider the alternative causes of lower limb swelling. Does the swelling appear to be unilateral or bilateral? Where the former is prominent and acute in onset, rule out deep vein thrombosis. Venous insufficiency may be suggested by dependent oedema and by a history of symptoms worsening throughout the day. Screen for causes of hypoalbuminaemia, hepatic disease, or renal insufficiency. Consider on the basis of pitting versus non-pitting, in the latter thinking about lymphoedema. Finally screen for inflammatory processes with resultant oedema including infection or arthritis.

Explore concerns, ideas, and expectations

Where you are reviewing a chronic condition the emphasis will be placed on identifying potential reasons for exacerbations and the patient's ideas will be key in offering insight to this. Medication compliance will be central to this as outlined above. It will be important to address the patient's concerns of a worsening of their condition, outline the potential for investigation and understand their expectations for management. Establishing whether the patient expects more medication, is prepared to try a change in regime or titration of dosing, or whether they have heard about the potential for implantable devices will guide the conversation about further management.

What to tell the patient

Inform the patient of the working diagnosis. Explain to them the need for investigations to both confirm the diagnosis and to influence management decisions. Tell the patient you would like to perform some blood tests, repeat the ECG to assess for any new arrhythmias, and review the function of her heart with an echocardiogram.

Inform the patient that they will need to start some medications to treat the heart failure.

Summarise the case, and reaffirm the need for review with the results of the investigations outlined. Titration of a loop diuretic dose may be prudent as an initial management option where renal function is not of concern. Alternatively, management change may centre on compliance, and areas such as increasing morning, and reducing evening, doses of diuretics to reduce nighttime waking or deal with incontinence issues.

What to tell the examiner

Summarise the clinical case

Succinct summary of patient history including:

- Understanding from patient of the aetiology of their heart failure
- Current symptoms and NYHA grading
- Current management
- Working diagnosis re: exacerbating factors

Investigations

Initial investigations in cases of suspected heart failure will include:

- Serum BNP, which should be raised
- A 12-lead electrocardiogram: In symptomatically and echocardiographically-severe heart failure it is important to note the QRS duration as this has management implications (cardiac resynchronisation therapy)
- A plain chest radiograph will demonstrate the cardio-thoracic ratio and also demonstrate any active pulmonary oedema
- A transthoracic echocardiogram is diagnostic
- In severe systolic dysfunction, with or without a dilated left ventricle, a period of ambulatory ECG monitoring will help to exclude the presence of ventricular arrhythmia
- Cardiac MRI for tissue characterisation in the evaluation of cardiomyopathy or infiltrative diseases

Management

In addition to addressing aetiological and exacerbating factors, the management of heart failure due to left ventricular systolic dysfunction should involve:

- Institution of prognostic therapy where possible with beta-blockade and ACE inhibition
- Symptomatic therapy with diuretics
- In patients with severe systolic dysfunction, mineralocorticoid receptor antagonists such as spironolactone (or eplerenone in ischaemic cardiomyopathy) are indicated

Biventricular pacing with cardiac resynchronisation may relieve symptoms and reduce heart failure hospitalisations for patients who have severe, symptomatic heart failure and a widened QRS on ECG.

Further reading

McMurray JJ, Adamopoulos S, Anker SD, et al. ESC Guidelines for the diagnosis and treatment of acute and chronic heart failure 2012: The Task Force for the Diagnosis and Treatment of Acute and Chronic Heart Failure 2012 of the European Society of Cardiology. Developed in collaboration with the Heart Failure Association (HFA) of the ESC. Eur Heart J 2012; 33:1787–1847.

Case 142: Raised lipids

Candidate information

Scenario

You are the registrar in the cardiology clinic reviewing a 56-year-old man, referred to the outpatient clinic due to raised lipids on blood testing. His serum lipid profile is:

Total cholesterol	6.7 mmol/L
Triglycerides	3.4 mmol/L
HDL cholesterol	0.8 mmol/L
LDL cholesterol	4.4 mmol/L

Please take a history from this man and discuss the significance of the blood test results with him.

Actor information

On recent review at your local GP practice, you were told that your blood tests for cholesterol were abnormal. You are surprised, given that you consider yourself to have a healthy lifestyle. You are otherwise well.

Prior to entering the room

Conscious of the fact that hyperlipidaemia in itself does not cause symptoms, the strong candidate will consider the propensity for associated conditions such as peripheral vascular and coronary artery disease.

On entering the room begin with open questioning

Whenever the explanation of results is required it is important to establish the reasoning behind ordering them, what prompted the investigation and how they relate to a patient's ongoing health issues and management. The results require context. It is useful to open the dialogue with a review of the patient's understanding and expectations from the consultation. The nature of the results should guide you in this respect.

'I understand you have attended to receive the results of your blood tests. Before we discuss them, can you tell me what you understand about lipids and what you were expecting these tests to show?'

The nervous, anxious or demanding patient may not allow such an approach, insisting on delivery of the results before entering into a dialogue. In such circumstances, it will be necessary to package or frame the results.

Rather than merely informing the patient that your lipids seem to be raised and require further attention, consider the following approaches:

'We have performed a screen of your lipid levels. Commonly we do this as part of a general health check or when we are concerned about a patient's risk for heart disease or vascular disease. In your case, I would like to know more about the reason for performing your tests as it would appear that some of the levels are raised. Were you expecting this?' followed by 'What do you understand to be the implications of raised lipid levels?'

It may then be necessary to field questions from the patient, which will influence the direction of the rest of the history. The strong candidate will try to obtain a clear background for the test results. In narrowing your diagnosis in a structured manner, attempt to distinguish between primary and secondary causes of dyslipidaemia. Thereafter, while dyslipidemia itself usually causes no symptoms, probe for resultant symptomatic vascular disease, principally coronary artery disease and peripheral arterial disease.

Patients with primary disorders may present with:

- Eyelid xanthelasmas
- Prominent corneal arcus at a young age
- Tendon (commonly achilles, knee and elbow) or cutaneous xanthomas
- Pancreatitis – acute episodes may occur in patients with significantly elevated triglyceride levels

Common primary (familial) causes, most usefully categorised based on whether cholesterol, triglyceride or both are prinicipally raised:

- Familial hypercholesterolaemia
- Familial hypertriglyceraemia
- Familial combined hyperlipidaemia (raised cholesterol and triglycerides)

Importantly, a low HDL confers susceptibility to premature atherosclerosis and should also be considered.

Secondary, acquired, causes include:

- Sedentary lifestyle with poor diet – excessive intake of saturated and trans fats. (Most common cause of dylipidaemia)
- Diabetes mellitus
- Alcohol excess

- Chronic kidney disease
- Hypothyroidism
- Cholestatic liver disease such as primary biliary cirrhosis
- Medication including: thiazides diuretics, beta-blockers, retinoids, highly active antiretroviral treatment, and glucocorticoids.

The patient may be asymptomatic, or complain of symptoms related to the complications of hyperlipidaemia, such as angina or intermittent claudication.

Thus, dyslipidemia is suspected in patients with characteristic physical findings or complications resulting from atherosclerotic disease, and primary lipid disorders are suspected when patients have physical signs of dyslipidemia, suffer the onset of premature atherosclerotic disease, or have a strong family history of hyperlipidaemia or atherosclerotic disease.

> ## Open questioning suggests a diagnosis of raised lipids

With this diagnosis questioning should focus on the following

Where raised lipids are of concern, focus closed questioning on risk stratification using the QRISK2 risk assessment tool to assess cardiovascular disease risk for the primary prevention. Using the results of the lipid screen (total cholesterol and HDL) combined with knowledge of other cardiovascular risk factors (smoking history, blood pressure, diabetes, family history of cardiovascular disease) and past medical history (including AF, chronic kidney disease, blood pressure treatment and rheumatoid arthritis), it is possible to estimate a 10-year risk of having a heart attack or stroke. This can also be presented to the patient as their 'heart age' relative to their actual age, and their relative risk of having a cardiovascular event compared to an average individual of the same age, gender and ethnicity.

Do not use a risk assessment tool to assess cardiovascular disease risk in patients with type 1 diabetes, known cardiovascular or significant chronic kidney disease, or inherited lipid disorders. These people are already at increased cardiovascular risk.

Explore concerns, ideas, and expectations

Upon being afforded the opportunity, the patient may offer concerns such as the following:

- 'I think this has happened because I have eaten too much fast food, can the damage be reversed?'
- 'I don't understand, I don't smoke and eat healthily, how can this be the case?'
- 'My friend takes a pill for his cholesterol and eats whatever he wants, can I just do that?'
- 'Does this mean I will have a heart attack?'

What to tell the patient

The patient should be informed of: the working diagnosis; the current management plan; and the implications on the patient's cardiovascular health.

What to tell the examiner

Summarise the clinical case

The discussion with the examiner should include investigations, management and statements to the examiner that the candidate understands the role of lipid therapies in modifying cardiovascular risk.

Investigations

Establish the potential for treating the other modifiable risk factors and the secondary causes of hyperlipidaemia as discussed above:

- Routine blood tests including full blood count, renal function, electrolytes and liver function
- Ensure the lipid profile was a fasting sample, explain and repeat if necessary
- Check fasting glucose and an HbA1c
- Check thyroid function
- Calculate body mass index

Management

Initial management will involve dietary and exercise advice to achieve weight loss and improvement in lipid profile together with alcohol moderation and smoking cessation. The challenge will be to encourage the patient to understand their risk status and work together to improve their profile. If these measures are ineffective, lipid-lowering drugs should be considered.

Encourage a diet low in fat:

- Total fat intake less than 30% total energy intake
- Saturated fat less than 7% total energy intake
- Less than 300 mg/day cholesterol
- Replace saturated fats, where possible, with mono-unsaturated and polyunsaturated fats

- Combined with 5 portions of fruit and vegetables per day and 2 portions of fish per week. It will be worth referring to a dietician to achieve an optimal 'cardioprotective' diet

Physical activity is recommended as 30 minutes of physical activity a day (or cumulative 10 minute sessions throughout the day), of at least moderate intensity (brisk walk, using stairs, cycling), at least 5 days a week.

If the patient does not currently suffer from ischaemic heart disease, peripheral vascular disease and has no history of stroke then primary prevention treatment with a statin is only recommended where the risk of developing such disease is high, (QRISK2 10-year risk of greater than or equal to 10% of developing cardiovascular disease) or if lifestyle modification has been ineffective. If however, the patient has a history of any form of atherosclerotic disease, they are inherently deemed high risk and the stratification process is not necessary when deciding on whether to commence lipid lowering treatment (they are classed as requiring secondary prevention treatment, with first line recommendation being atorvastatin 80 mg).

Treatment for the primary prevention of cardiovascular disease should be initiated in people who have a 10% or greater 10-year risk of developing cardiovascular disease, and in all adults with type 1 diabetes who fit one of the following criteria: are older than 40 years, have had diabetes for more than 10 years, have established nephropathy, or have other cardiovascular risk factors. First line therapy in such individuals is atorvastatin 20 mg. If there are potential drug interactions or contraindications, a lower dose or lower intensity preparation such as pravastatin may be chosen. Fibrates and nicotinic acid should not routinely be considered for primary or secondary prevention, and specialist opinions should be sought in those with especially high cardiovascular risk (such as inherited dyslipidaemia), and in secondary prevention patients with intolerances to multiple statins.

Advise patients to read the drug information leaflet carefully, paying particular attention to possible interactions (such as grapefruit juice, for example). If there is any history of previous generalised myalgia, irrespective of previous statin use, check creatine kinase levels. Patients should seek medical attention if they develop muscle pains on statins, and creatine kinase levels measured (with statin use stopped and future management re-evaluated). Asymptomatic patients should not have creatine kinase levels routinely measured.

Liver transaminases should be measured at baseline, 3 months and 12 months. Statin therapy should be continued unless these are over 3 times the upper limit of normal.

Lipid levels should be monitored 3 months after starting or changing therapies, aiming for at least 40% reduction in non-HDL cholesterol, and at least annually thereafter.

Further reading

National Institute for Health and Care Excellence (NICE). Lipid modification: cardiovascular risk assessment and the modification of blood lipids for the primary and secondary prevention of cardiovascular disease. Clinical guideline 181. London; NICE, July 2014.

Case 143: Hypertension

Candidate information

Scenario

You are the registrar in the general medical clinic. You are asked to review an anxious 30-year-old man in the general medical clinic, referred by his GP in view of two previous BP measurements of 158/90 and 165/88 mmHg. The GP has been unsure as to whether to start treatment in a patient this age, he is currently on no medication, and has thus far advised the patient to stop smoking and improve his diet. Please take a history from this man and discuss with him your management plan.

Actor information

You have been seeing your GP recently because of high blood pressure, which was initially noted at a well-man clinic. You are keen to know whether you need to take any tablets for your blood pressure. You also wish to know the reason why you have high blood pressure.

Prior to entering the room

Hypertension is usually asymptomatic, with symptoms heralding either a severe, uncontrolled manifestation, or as the result of long standing disease – the symptoms of end-organ damage. Essential hypertension is common and offers little in the way of history; however, secondary hypertension may involve complex constellations of symptoms relating to renal or endocrine disorders. While hypertension is a common finding with age, in the young it should alert suspicion and prompt thorough investigation. The strong candidate will be prepared to think laterally in this regard, and make use of a review of symptoms to guide further lines of enquiry when thinking about the secondary causes of hypertension.

On entering the room begin with open questioning

It is sensible to start with a general statement in this case, perhaps reiterating the GP's concerns, to get a feeling for the patients understanding and appreciation of the reason for his attendance.

'I understand you have been referred to the clinic by your GP because he is concerned about your blood pressure. Can you tell me more about that?'

Alternatively, adopt the 'How can I help you today?' approach and lead in to the GP's concerns having established the patients understanding of why he has attended.

In such a station it can be difficult to avoid the inevitable rush towards closed questioning, but taking clues from the scenario eluding to an anxious patient it is important to encourage a dialogue and avoid dominating the situation. It is possible that the emphasis of the station will centre around sensitive subjects such as a family history of similar symptoms with death of a relative, worrying features like headaches that the patient has previously omitted to mention to the GP, or areas such as drug use. Alternatively, the nervous disposition may be intended as a reference to white coat hypertension and a barrage of questions may serve to merely exacerbate the patient's nerves at the outset.

Where it hasn't been detailed in the information or GP referral, elicit the circumstances in which the blood pressure readings were taken and first noted to be high. Ensure the patient was calm, rested with no recent exertion or caffeine or drug ingestion. And establish the timing between readings. Does the patient ever remember being told he had a normal blood pressure?

Begin prompting when necessary, and enquire as to the general features of uncontrolled hypertension or end organ damage. In so doing, attempt to gauge the severity of the problem. Ask specifically about headaches, visual disturbance, epistaxis, palpitations and any urinary abnormalities (haematuria or frothy urine).

It will be useful to explain to the patient why you are asking these questions – I need to understand how your blood pressure is affecting you. Sometimes it can cause headaches or problems with your sight, other times it can increase the work of your heart possibly causing pain, breathlessness or palpitations, and sometimes it can cause problems with your kidneys and affect your urine. Have you experienced anything along those lines?'

Narrow the differential – it may be necessary to screen the patients past medical and family history at an early stage in the consultation; however, this can be useful to the structure of the consultation – 'How is the rest of your health' and 'How is your family's health? Are you aware of any conditions that run in the family?' can form relatively open questioning in themselves. Furthermore, the answers to such questioning may better direct the closed questioning that follows.

Be alert for a family history of atherosclerosis, dyslipidaemia and vascular disease. Enquire about renal disorders such as polycystic kidneys and also consider diagnoses such as phaeochromocytoma.

> ## Open questioning suggests a diagnosis of hypertension

With this diagnosis, closed questioning should focus on the following

A review of symptoms may be more effective than asking questions about each of the known causes of secondary hypertension, but it is important to screen for symptoms related to the following conditions:

Cardiovascular

- In older patients, and those with risk factors, consider ischaemic heart disease. Chest pain, palpitations, reduced exercise tolerance with breathlessness, ankle swelling and lethargy.

Orthopnoea and paroxysmal nocturnal dyspnoea
- Intermittent claudication, rest pain, and poor circulation with cold extremities
- Coarctation of the aorta may be worth considering, and while this will have a paucity of symptoms, early claudication may be a feature or suggested by surgery for congenital heart defects

Renal

Lethargy, oedema, pruritis and nausea, while indiscriminate, may suggest renal disease and uraemia. Changes in urine and urination, as mentioned above, may suggest renal parenchymal disease such as glomerulonephritis, infiltrative disease, previous recurrent pyelonephritis with scarring, or obstructive uropathy. Renovascular disease is common and may be idiopathic or relate to the cardiovascular aetiologies discussed above.

Endocrine

- Phaeochromocytoma – labile blood pressure with intermittent episodes of headache, palpitations, flushing, sweating and nausea
- Hyperthyroidism – anxiety, palpitations, sweating, tremor, diarrhoea, weight loss, and potentially eye signs dependent upon the cause
- Cushing's disease or syndrome (hypertension secondary to sodium retention) – Cushingoid facies may be evident on general inspection, enquire as to steroid use, weight gain, striae, easy bruising and proximal myopathy
- Conn's syndrome – lethargy, generalised weakness and muscle cramps secondary to hypokalaemia
- Acromegaly – headaches, visual disturbance, changes in appearance and notable changes in shoe size

'White-coat' hypertension

Relates to raised measurements in a health care setting compared to normal levels during ambulatory measurement. This is a diagnosis of exclusion however, and abnormal, erratic, readings should always prompt consideration of the possibility of phaeochromocytoma or unacknowledged drug use.

Despite being told that the patient is on no medication, enquire as to over-the-counter items such as cold remedies containing pseudoephedrine, which may inadvertently raise measurements. Where the history pertains to a woman, remember that the oral contraceptive can cause hypertension and will be an important feature of subsequent management. Similarly, hypertension in pregnancy is a topic in its own right, but would prompt consideration of pre-eclampsia. If the scenario involves failure of initial management, be sure to investigate compliance, particularly related to side effects, in addition to considering medication that may interact with common anti-hypertensives.

A comprehensive social history will clarify and quantify caffeine (including carbonated energy drinks), alcohol intake and smoking pack years. Get a feel for how his diet has changed as mentioned in the information, particularly in relation to salt intake. Attempt to estimate the amount of exercise he is undertaking as a guide to the value of lifestyle intervention in considering further management options. Ask specifically about illicit drug use, particularly ecstasy, cocaine and amphetamines. Screen for source and levels of stress and anxiety.

Explore concerns, ideas, and expectations

Ask the patient if there is anything he thinks may be causing his high blood pressure? Are there underlying concerns with a family history of related conditions such as aneurysms or stroke?

What to tell the patient

'Raised blood pressure can be a problem even if you don't have any obvious symptoms, so managing it is all targeted at lowering your long term risk of complications. In particular, the effects of raised blood pressure on the cardiovascular system, to reduce the risk of heart attack or stroke, and the effects on small blood vessels in the eyes and kidneys. However, firstly we should confirm the diagnosis. I would like to repeat the measurement today and depending upon the result consider monitoring your blood pressure over a 24-hour period using a portable machine to confirm whether it is truly raised and warrants treatment.'

Depending on the scenario, it may be necessary to discuss, in depth, the underlying causes and the need for further investigation. While hypertension is a common finding with age, in the young it should alert suspicion and prompt thorough investigation. Explain the difference between essential, secondary and white-coat hypertension.

'I would also like to arrange some simple investigations which will include looking at the back of your eyes, tracing your heart with a 12-lead electrocardiogram, and testing a sample of your urine to look for the unwanted effects of chronically raised blood pressure.'

'I would like you to persevere with your achievements thus far in changing your diet and stopping smoking. These are important general health considerations from which you will benefit greatly. The most common reversible causes of raised blood pressure are smoking and alcohol, and with regard to the latter I would like you to moderate your intake before our next review if possible. Your GP has asked me to consider whether we need to start medication, and certainly I agree that this may be necessary to avoid serious complications in the future such as heart disease and stroke. But first it is important that we confirm the diagnosis, and rule out any other treatable causes. I suggest we organise the various tests we have discussed and review the situation in a couple of weeks' time. Does that sound agreeable?'

What to tell the examiner

Summarise the clinical case

Report to the examiner the main findings of the patient's history.

Investigations

A diagnosis of hypertension is made using three raised blood pressure measurements, taken in a suitable setting with the arm at rest at the level of the heart. Avoidance of preceding exertion and stimulation with substances such as nicotine or caffeine is important. Use an appropriately sized cuff and, for accuracy, ensure manual blood pressure measurements in cases of an irregular pulse.

Certain clinic readings should prompt immediate action, including:

- 220/120 mmHg or higher, or 180/110 mmHg with signs of papilloedema and/or retinal haemorrhage – treat as malignant hypertension with same day admission to hospital
- 180/110 mmHg – start anti-hypertensive treatment immediately and monitor response closely thereafter

There is a trend towards the use of 24 hour ambulatory blood pressure monitoring (ABPM) or home blood pressure monitoring (HBPM) to improve the accuracy of diagnosis where clinic readings have been persistently above 140/90 mmHg. When using clinic or home ambulatory blood pressure monitoring devices, ensure that they are validated by the British Hypertension Society (list of validated devices available on their website).

Formal diagnosis is considered as stage 1 or stage 2 hypertension based on the interpretation of blood pressure results:

- Stage 1 hypertension – clinic readings greater than 140/90 mmHg and average (ABPM or HBPM) greater than or equal to 135/85 mmHg
- Stage 2 hypertension - clinic readings greater than 160/100 mmHg and average ABPM or HBPM greater than or equal to 150/95 mmHg.

Management options will depend upon the classification of hypertension as above and further risk stratification. All patients with stage 2 hypertension should be started on medication. Offer antihypertensive treatment to those patients with stage 1 disease if aged less than 80 years and one or more of the following:

- end-organ disease
- established cardiovascular disease or 10 year cardiovascular risk of > 20%
- renal disease
- diabetes

Secondary hypertension may be more likely:
- younger patients (< 40 years)
- hypokalaemia and hypernatraemia suggestive of adrenal disease
- elevated serum creatinine and reduce eGFR suggestive of renovascular disease
- sudden onset, labile, or worsening blood pressure

Specific tests to consider (in appropriate selected cases):

- Blood tests – urea, creatinine and electrolytes, plasma glucose and serum lipids. Thyroid function tests. 9 am cortisol, dexamethasone suppression testing, and plasma aldosterone:renin activity ratio where appropriate
- ECG
- Imaging with renal USS including Doppler assessment of renal artery prompting magnetic resonance angiography if stenosis suspected.
- Echocardiogram particularly if ECG suggests hypertrophy
- 24-hour urine collection for catecholamines

Management

Lifestyle advice should be discussed – diet, smoking, alcohol and exercise changes should be outlined to the patient. For patients without indications for immediate drug therapy this will include 6 months of implementation of lifestyle changes to observe their effect, before considering the need for pharmacological intervention if blood pressure remains raised and no secondary cause is identified.

Choice of medication is dependent upon age, as defined by NICE guidelines on use of ACE inhibitor, diuretics, calcium channel blockers and beta-blockers. The aim is to achieve systolic pressure < 140 mmHg and diastolic < 90 mmHg. In diabetes, tighter control is desirable. In those aged over 80 years with treated hypertension, a target of < 150/90 has been proposed.

Specialist referral should be made (to renal or endocrinology) where investigations suggest secondary cause requiring further assessment and/or management.

Further reading

National Institute for Health and Care Excellence (NICE). CG127, Hypertension: clinical management of primary hypertension in adults. London; NICE, 2011.

Case 144: Breathlessness and wheeze – new diagnosis of asthma

Candidate information

Scenario

You are the SHO in the respiratory clinic. A 22-year-old man has presented several times to Accident and Emergency over the last year with acute episodes of breathlessness associated with cough and wheeze. He is in generally good health but has complained to his GP of aches and pains in his hands, linked to his job in construction, for which he takes over the counter painkillers. Please assess the patient and offer a management plan.

Actor information

You have been having intermittent breathing problems over the past year. Your doctor mentioned this might be partially related to the medications you have been taking for the pains in your hands.

Prior to entering the room

In any scenario dealing with shortness of breath, cough, or wheeze, be alert to the context of the symptoms. These symptoms are common to a wide range of conditions. Where there is doubt, proceed by considering the speed of onset to effectively narrow the differential and prompt further targeted lines of questioning. Attempt to classify according to sudden, acute, or chronic onset:

Causes of sudden onset breathlessness include:

- Pneumothorax: this typically presents with sudden onset dyspnoea or pleuritic pain. In asthma or COPD patients it may present as sudden deterioration in the patient's clinical condition
- Pulmonary oedema: symptoms and signs include wheeze, anxiety, pink, frothy sputum, sweating, tachycardia, and peripheral shutdown. It may be preceded by myocardial infarction, positive cardiac history or risk factors for cardiac disease
- Pulmonary embolism: typical features include pleuritic chest pain, haemoptysis, and respiratory distress. Risk factors include a family history or previous thrombosis, immobility including long haul travel/prolonged bed rest, surgery, stroke, malignancy, thrombophilia, pregnancy or postpartum, and the oral contraceptive pill
- Aspiration: aspiration of vomit, state of decreased consciousness, e.g. during epileptic attack, recent stroke
- Anxiety: hyperventilation caused by stress or emotion
- Anaphylaxis: upper airway swelling threatening patency, rash, haemodynamic instability possible in the atopic patient

Causes of acute onset breathlessness include:

- Asthma: episodic breathlessness, triggered by allergens or exercise, associated wheeze, diurnal variation, demonstrating reversibility with improvement on inhalation of β-agonist

- Infection: productive cough, pleurisy, mucupurulent or green sputum, associated fever, rigors, general malaise
- Lung tumours: associated cough, haemoptysis, weight loss, general malaise and anorexia, smoking history
- Pleural effusion: pleuritic chest pain
- Cor pulmonale: fatigue, syncope. Usually history of chronic lung disease, pulmonary vasculature disorders and neuromuscular disease
- As a compensatory mechanism for metabolic acidosis

With regard to chronic breathlessness, consider cardiac versus respiratory. Also, be mindful as to other chronic conditions that may result in breathlessness secondary to generalised fatigue or anaemia.

Respiratory causes of breathlessness

Pulmonary vasculature:

- Pulmonary hypertension: chest pain, fatigue, syncope

Interstitium:

- COPD: usually older patients, history of smoking, productive sputum, dyspnoea, wheeze, recurrent chest infections, chronic bronchitis or bronchiectasis. Acute exacerbations may present with infective symptoms or pulmonary oedema due to resultant diastolic dysfunction
- Fibrosing alveolitis: dry cough, exertional dyspnoea, malaise, weight loss, arthralgia
- Bronchiectasis: persistent productive cough, purulent sputum
- Cystic fibrosis: recurrent infections on a background of poor growth

Chest wall:

- Neuromuscular – myasthenia gravis/motor neuron disease

On entering the room begin with open questioning

Wheeze can be difficult to establish from history alone and often the term is used by patients in a non-specific manner. Cough may in fact be the only presenting feature in asthma. Consider the diagnosis in younger patients who appear otherwise well. When considering a new diagnosis, the key is to elicit the main features of asthma, and identify triggers. The cardinal features to expect are: shortness of breath or difficulty breathing,

cough that is often nocturnal, and chest tightness with or without wheeze. Symptoms are usually episodic with diurnal variation, or consistent with exposure to an environmental or occupational trigger. Bearing these features in mind, start by open questioning looking to identify common themes between recurring episodes.

Gauge the severity of the symptoms and resultant impairment:

- Frequency of symptoms
- Timing of symptoms
- Impact upon normal activity

Open questioning suggests a diagnosis of asthma

With this diagnosis closed questioning should focus on the following

Continue closed questioning and seek to establish a clear profile of potential triggers: infections, pets, dust, cold weather, damp air, stress/emotion, and drugs. Clarify working conditions and any resolution of symptoms when away from the work place. Establish the impact of exercise on symptoms and quantify exercise tolerance. Evaluate evidence of sleep disturbance with nocturnal symptoms. Specific features that would be in favour of a clinical diagnosis of asthma include:

- History of atopy: commonly eczema or hayfever
- Family history of atopy commonly found in close family members
- History of childhood asthma predisposes to, or represents recurrence of, disease in adulthood
- Drug history: symptoms worse after aspirin, NSAIDs or beta-blockers

With regard to occupational asthma, ask:

- Does the patient have symptoms during the week but not weekends or periods of holiday?
- Does the patient experience irritation of the eyes or nose in the work place?
- Do colleagues complain of similar symptoms?

Look to exclude other known causes of dyspnoea from the past medical history and elicit risk factors for other aetiologies. Importantly, exclude a cardiac history, as evidenced by concomitant chest pain, palpitations or dizziness. Be seen to consider the importance of an infective component and the contribution of smoking. A significant pack year smoking history should prompt consideration of a chronic obstructive pulmonary disease, although co-existing disease is possible.

Thereafter, employ a review of symptoms as a means of evaluating recognised conditions associated with asthma including acid reflux, polyarteritis nodosa (PAN), Churg–Strauss, and allergic bronchopulmonary aspergillosis (ABPA). It will not necessarily be important in this scenario to pursue such themes but the strong candidate will at the very least demonstrate an awareness of these conditions.

- Acid reflux: retrosternal burning pain, worse after meal and on lying flat, metallic taste in the mouth
- PAN: fevers, abdominal pain, general malaise and weight loss, arthralgia. Suspect in multisystem symptoms including renal, vascular, cardiac, CNS, GI and skin
- Churg–Strauss: asthma, eosinophilia and systemic vasculitis
- ABPA: wheeze, cough, sputum, dyspnoea, recurrent pneumonia

Explore concerns, ideas, and expectations

Themes to prepare for include:

- Patients that raise concerns are their ability to continue to work in current employment in the face of occupational asthma – balancing the need to earn an income and support a family against personal health for instance
- Consider difficulties with smoking cessation – I've tried to quit smoking before, I just can't do it
- Preconceptions surrounding the implications of the diagnosis, both relating to severity and limitations of daily life
- Stigma associated with carrying or using an inhaler in younger patients, particularly of school age

What to tell the patient

Communicate a working diagnosis of asthma. Explain the main features in lay terms, focusing on the concept of triggers causing hypersensitive airways to constrict or tighten with resultant wheeze and difficulty in breathing. Achieving a shared understanding will be beneficial in implementing management centred upon:

- PEFR chart to attempt to confirm the diagnosis
- Identifying triggers and attempting to minimise contact/exposure

- Timely clinic review
- Trial of inhalers – 'reliever' to counteract symptoms caused by constriction. Consider discussing the principals of inhaler technique
- Ensuring patient safety in the interim period – paramount to educate as to red flags symptoms that would necessitate urgent medical review

Specific to this case, the patient will have told you that he has been taking NSAIDs for joint pains in the hands. Tell the patient you will change him onto a different class of painkillers, aiming to eliminate the respiratory side effects while maintaining effective analgesia. Tell him that, if his hand symptoms become particularly troublesome you will arrange for him to be seen by a rheumatologist.

What to tell the examiner
Summarise the clinical case

'This patient describes symptoms consistent with occupational asthma. It is possible that the use of analgaesia has contributed to the episodes he describes, and it would be important to distinguish the relative importance of this and the likely environmental allergen in the work place.'

Investigations

The likelihood or certainty of a formal diagnosis should influence the initial course of action – gauged on the symptoms described and/ or available test results such as PEFR when symptomatic or formal spirometry.

If high probability: Proceed to treatment trial and continue to maintenance treatment if response satisfactory. If response is poor, check inhaler technique and compliance. Consider a course of steroids if the patient is symptomatic at the time of clinic review.

If low probability: Explore symptoms further and consider investigations required to establish alternative diagnosis. Always be prepared to re-consider the diagnosis.

Intermediate probability: Further investigations and treatment trial before confirmation of diagnosis. Objective evidence provided by spirometry: if $FEV1/FVC < 0.7$ consistent with an obstructive picture consider trial of treatment, particularly where reversibility can be demonstrated. If $FEV1/FVC > 0.7$ investigate further.

Low FEV1 or PEFR: A normal spirometry reading in asymptomatic patients is not exclusive of the diagnosis.

Management

Management considerations likely to be discussed will include the avoidance of known triggers, identifying others, encouraging smoking cessation and weight reduction in obese patients with evidence of GORD. Thereafter, medical treatment will be as outlined by the British Thoracic Society guidelines:

Step 1   Inhaled short-acting β_2-agonist
Step 2   Add inhaled steroid 200–800 µg/day
Step 3   Inhaled long-acting β-agonist. If inadequate response increase inhaled steroid to 800 µg/day. Budesonide/ formoterol in a single inhaler as rescue medication instead of a short-acting β-agonist is an option
Step 4   Increase inhaled steroid up to 2000 µg/day or add leukotriene receptor antagonist, SR theophylline, β_2-agonist tablet
Step 5   Daily steroid tablet: Maintain high dose inhaled steroid up to 2000 µg/day. Specialist input

Arrange regular review especially as treatment is stepped down. Consider severity, side effects, duration on current dose, patient preferences in changing treatment. Maintain on lowest possible dose of inhaled steroid. Complete control as assessed by:

- No daytime or nocturnal symptoms
- No rescue medication
- No exacerbations
- No limitations on activity or exercise
- Normal lung function (FEV1/PEF > 80% of predicted)

Further reading

British Thoracic Society (BTS) and Scottish Intercollegiate Guidelines Network (SIGN). British guideline on the management of asthma. London and Edinburgh; BTS and SIGN, 2012.

Case 145: Shortness of breath and wheeze – established diagnosis of asthma

Candidate information

Scenario

As the respiratory SHO in clinic you are asked to see a new referral. A 19-year-old referred by his GP due to poor asthma control in the community. Please take a history from the patient, offer an explanation and propose a management plan, before discussing the case with the examiner.

Actor information

You have had asthma since childhood. You have found you are increasingly dependent upon your inhaler with minimal relief and significant impact upon your daily living. More recently you have required treatment via Accident and Emergency for severe attacks.

Prior to entering the room

Be clear as to the accepted incremental and stepwise increase in management according to BTS guidelines. It may be worth scribbling these down to avoid confusion. Poor inhaler technique should be considered before assuming the need for a change in medication. Also be seen to consider and rule out poor compliance.

On entering the room begin with open questioning

Use open questions to find out how long they have had asthma for, who made the diagnosis, their exact symptoms. Was their asthma ever under complete control? Has anything changed recently? Does the patient have any idea why their asthma may not be under good control now?

Aim to establish the following:

- Degree of control by asking about daytime or nocturnal symptoms
- Use and frequency of rescue medication
- Number of exacerbations (including hospital admissions and use of antibiotics)
- Limitations on exercise or other activity and context of exacerbations

Are there symptoms that make an alternative diagnosis more likely? Sudden exacerbation of symptoms may indicate underlying pneumothorax, while the presence of constitutional symptoms may signify underlying Churg–Strauss especially in the context of eosonophilia.

Review peak flow diary (if the patient keeps one). Completely controlled asthma should have FEV1/PEF ratio > 80% of predicted or best effort.

Establish compliance and inhaler technique as well as exact current asthma regime and whether they have been on a stronger regime.

> ## Open questioning suggests a diagnosis of poorly controlled asthma

With this diagnosis closed questioning should focus on the following

Review the patient's past medical history, medications, allergies and social setup, especially smoking and occupation. Take a careful drug history to ensure they are not taking any medication that worsens asthma, such as NSAIDs, beta-blockers or aspirin. Check for side effects of medications such as tachycardia, tremor or anxiety from β-agonists.

Occupational history:

- Establish if symptoms are worse while at work and improve when not working such as during the weekend
- Establish a job description and contact with materials
- Concomitant rhinoconjunctivitis is often seen
- High-risk occupations include food processing or baking, sprays, animal work/farming, healthcare, metal or wood work, fumes

Explore concerns, ideas, and expectations

How is the condition affecting the patient's daily life?

What to tell the patient

'From what you are telling me today I don't think your asthma is under best possible control. If you could make one thing better for your asthma what would that be?'

Where there is suspected concomitant pathology, or an alternative diagnosis, propose to organise further tests to ensure there is nothing underlying the exacerbation of symptoms.

'I think it is important we revisit the smoking situation as I really think stopping will significantly help your symptoms and improve the quality of your life. There are ways in which we can help out achieve this if you have decided to try.'

'In the first instance, I suggest you keep a peak flow diary. You would be writing down your peak flow scores regularly; this will help you see when your asthma is improving or not. This way you can tell yourself what is happening in your lungs, record how well you have been and how effective are the medicines you are taking. It can be a major tool for helping you controlling your asthma yourself and prevent major exacerbations. Finally if you would like to, I can arrange for you to see the asthma specialist nurse to review your inhaler technique and give you some helpful tips.'

Offer a personalised self-management plan with simple verbal and written instructions and advice on what to do in an emergency. Provide asthma medicine card. Finish by saying: 'I suggest we also implement some changes in your medication today and review your symptoms in 3 months' time.'

What to tell the examiner

Summarise the clinical case

'This young man with a long history of asthma since childhood is no longer well controlled on a combination of inhaled steroids and long-acting $β_2$-agonist. I suspect his deterioration might be a combination of poor adherence to treatment and poor inhaler technique. There are no symptoms suggestive of other underlying disease.'

Investigations

If an alternative diagnosis is possible, investigate accordingly.

- Peak expiratory flow measurement or spirometry
- Prick testing may identify potential exacerbating allergens if the history is suggestive

Management

Patient education regarding asthma and control, importance of keeping a PEF diary and how to alter their medication in response to changes in symptoms or PEF. General lifestyle advice including smoking cessation, weight loss, and avoidance of known allergens. Check inhaler technique and consider alternative delivery device if necessary.

Medication changes:

- Use the step-approach (under new asthma diagnosis)

For exercise-exacerbated asthma, if patient is otherwise controlled on inhaled steroids the following can be added:

- Leukotriene receptor antagonist
- Long-acting β-agonist
- Oral β-agonist
- Theophylline
- Inhaled short-acting β-agonist immediately before exercise

Arrange regular review to step down treatment when and if appropriate. Consider severity of asthma, side effects of treatment, time on current dose and if beneficial effect is achieved. Aim to maintain on lower possible dose of inhaled steroid. Aim to review every 3 months with an aim to decrease the doses of steroids by 25–50% each time. If response is not as expected consider alternative diagnosis.

Additional themes worth considering:

- Asthma in pregnancy. Educate about importance of good asthma control during pregnancy. Long acting β_2-agonist, inhaled steroids and oral theophylline are safe in pregnancy. Leukotriene antagonists may be continued in women who have significantly benefited prior to pregnancy. Oral steroids should be reserved for severe asthma. Treatment of acute asthma should be the same as for the non-pregnant women

Further reading

British Thoracic Society (BTS) and Scottish Intercollegiate Guidelines Network (SIGN). British guideline on the management of asthma. London and Edinburgh; BTS and SIGN, 2012.

Case 146: Wheeze – established chronic obstructive pulmonary disease

Candidate information

Scenario

A 72-year-old man, who was diagnosed with COPD 4 years ago by his GP, has been having frequent exacerbations. As the respiratory SHO in the outpatient clinic, please take a history from the patient, offer him your impression of the case, and discuss your findings with the examiner.

Actor information

You saw your GP recently because you are concerned that your breathing problems are getting worse. You seem to be getting more frequent chest infections. Additionally, you have noticed you cannot walk as far as you used to be able to before getting breathless.

Prior to entering the room

Given that this man has a known diagnosis of COPD, it will be important to quantify his exercise tolerance and frequency of exacerbations. The candidate will need to establish disease severity and consider adjusting the management plan accordingly.

On entering the room begin with open questioning

Begin with open questions, which will give a chance to the patient to address their main symptoms and concerns regarding their COPD.

Enquire about the disease course and duration. Is it predominantly chronic bronchitis or emphysema? Chronic bronchitis is defined clinically as productive cough on most days for

3 months of 2 successive years. Emphysema is a histological diagnosis with enlarged air spaces distal to terminal bronchioles and destruction of alveolar walls.

Find about their current symptoms including cough, regular sputum production, wheeze and limitations on activity and daily living.

Ask about symptoms of weight loss, effort tolerance, waking at night, ankle swelling, fatigue, chest pain and haemoptysis.

Assess the degree of breathlessness using the Medical Research Council dyspnoea scale as follows:

Grade 1   Troubled only on strenuous exercise
Grade 2   Dyspnoea on exertion or walking uphill
Grade 3   Walks slowly on level ground or has to stop when walking at own pace
Grade 4   Stops for breath after 100 m or after a few minutes on level ground
Grade 5   Too breathless to leave house or when dressing/undressing

Open questioning suggests a diagnosis of COPD

With this diagnosis closed questioning should focus on the following

Deterioration of symptoms in COPD can be due to acute and/or chronic causes.

Acute causes include:

- Non-infective exacerbation: rapid and sustained worsening of symptoms beyond day-to-day variations without infective symptoms or signs
- Infective exacerbation: the commonest presentation, fever, rigors, green sputum
- Pneumothorax: from ruptures bullae, will present as sudden deterioration, cough, sudden onset dyspnoea or pleuritic chest pain. More common in patients with bullous disease
- Cor pulmonale: dyspnoea, fatigue and syncope usually in patients with long-standing COPD

Chronic causes include:

- Cor pulmonale
- Non-compliance with treatment
- Natural disease course

Also consider:

- Bronchiectasis: frequent infections, persistent cough and copious purulent sputum with occasional haemoptysis

- Alpha-1 antitrypsin deficiency: suspect in patients young patients < 40 with emphysema. Consider in patients with chronic liver disease, gallstones and dyspnoea

Continue closed questioning find out if there is past medical history of cardiac disease, establish current COPD regime, check on vaccination history especially flu jab and pneumococcus.

Explore concerns, ideas, and expectations

Take a careful social history focusing on smoking and current psychosocial issues as these can be prevalent in COPD patients.

Discuss functional aspects including strength and exercise tolerance. Screen for commonly encountered situations such as social isolation and increased periods of sedentary activity, often stemming from a fear of breathlessness resulting in avoidance of any strenuous activity. Disease progression can be correlated to muscle wasting, particularly of the proximal lower limbs and this is reflected in decreased strength or inability to stand from a seated position unaided.

What to tell the patient

'It seems you are experiencing regular exacerbations which means your COPD is not very well controlled at the moment. What do you think might be causing this?

'I would propose we run some tests to check your lung function and change your inhaler treatment accordingly.

'We also need to teach you how to manage exacerbations early to avoid having a severe exacerbation. I can give you a course of antibiotic and steroid tablets to keep at home. I would like you to start the oral steroids if you experience increasing breathlessness and it is interfering with your daily activities, and starting the antibiotic when your sputum becomes purulent. However, you should contact your doctor if your symptoms fail to improve.'

Take into account patient's needs and preferences in achieving an informed decision about treatment. Smoking cessation is important but not always possible. Often, involving pulmonary rehabilitation is the most effective way of achieving patient education, improving compliance and encouraging smoking cessation in a motivated environment with like-minded individuals. Pulmonary rehabilitation also enables targeted strength training to improve outcomes and developing the ability to cope with symptoms including breathlessness.

What to tell the examiner

Summarise the clinical case

'This patient with long-standing COPD who is still a heavy smoker is still breathless with frequent exacerbations despite taking a long-acting β-agonist. This has resulted in frequent hospitalisations. There are no symptoms in the history suggestive of progression to cor pulmonale or a lung malignancy but I would like to examine the patient in full before proceeding to stepping up his treatment and offering some other management advice.'

For suspected cor pulmonale: Examine patient for tachycardia, raised JVP, right ventricular heave, loud P2, pansystolic murmur, hepatomegaly and oedema.

Investigations

Assess the severity of COPD with post-bronchodilator spirometry in line with NICE clinical guidelines

Mild   : FEV1 > 80% of predicted
Moderate   : FEV1 50–79%
Severe   : FEV1 30–49% predicted
Very severe : FEV1 < 30%

Management

General measures include:

- Smoking cessation advice: offer nicotine replacement therapy together with a behavioural support programme. Medications include varenicline for patients who have expressed a desire to quit smoking
- Dietary advice and weight loss
- Mucolytics
- Offer vaccination to flu and pneumococcus
- Offer pulmonary rehabilitation +/- theophylline: pulmonary rehabilitation is suitable in patients including recent hospitalisation, functionally disabled (MRC grade 3 and above) but contraindicated in unstable cardiac disease
- Multidisciplinary team involvement including physiotherapy for chest exercise, dietetic advice to reduce BMI, occupational therapy for help with activities of daily living, social services, palliative care team for end-stage COPD

With regard drug treatments, if the patient is breathless and/or has exercise limitation,

consider a long-acting β-agonist (LABA) on a regular basis or a long-acting muscarinic antagonist (LAMA) on a PRN basis.

For patients with stable COPD who remain breathless or have frequent exacerbations and persistent breathlessness:

If FEV1 is < 50% of predicted
- LABA and inhaled corticosteroid in combination inhaler or LABA and LAMA if corticosteroid contraindicated or not tolerated or
- LAMA QDS (but stop LABA)

If FEV1 is > 50% of predicted
- LAMA QDS without LABA

Persistent exacerbation and/or breathlessness in patients taking LABA and inhaled steroid irrespective of FEV1:
- LAMA, LABA and inhaled corticosteroid

Teach inhaler technique and/or provide spacer. Nebulisers are an option for patient's breathlessness despite maximal therapy with inhalers.

Oral corticosteroids are not routine for chronic management. They are usually effective for exacerbations as short courses of treatment. Some patients with advanced COPD may need maintenance with oral steroids if they cannot be successfully weaned off after an exacerbation.

Theophylline can be used in combination with β-agonists and muscarinic antagonists after trials of short acting and long acting treatment has failed. Note that it interacts with macrolides and fluoroquinilones and you need to warn the patient if they develop an infective exacerbation and require treatment with antibiotics.

The aim of treatment is to minimise the impact of exacerbations by giving self management advice on responding to symptoms of exacerbation, starting appropriate treatment, using NIV, hospital at home, etc.

On review check for improvement in: symptoms, daily living, capacity, speed of symptom relief

Other management considerations

Long-term oxygen therapy should be considered in patients with severe COPD (FEV1 30–49% predicted). They need to fulfill the following criteria with measurement of arterial blood gas on 2 occasions 3 weeks apart when well:

- Pao_2 < 7.3 kPa for stable disease
- Pao_2 > 7.3 < 8 kPa when stable and

- Secondary polycythaemia
- Peripheral oedema
- Nocturnal hypoxaemia
- Pulmonary hypertension

Ambulatory oxygen therapy is a suitable option for patients on LTOT who want to use oxygen outside the home and have exercise desaturation and $Pao_2 < 7.3$ and improve on oxygen.

Patients with hypercapnia or acidosis on LTOT may require long term NIV.

Surgical options do exist for appropriately selected patients such as lung volume reduction surgery or rarely lung transplantation. Candidates should however, ensure they have a firm grasp on the medical management of COPD before beginning discussions on the much less commonly used surgical options.

Case 147: Haemoptysis in the returning traveller

Candidate information

Scenario

You are the medical registrar on call. You have been asked to see a 30-year-old man, who has recently returned from a prolonged stay in rural sub-Saharan Africa, has presented with frank haemoptysis. Please take a history from the patient, offer a management plan based on a working diagnosis, and discuss your findings with the examiner.

Actor information

You have recently returned from a year-long trip to Zambia, where you were working for a healthcare NGO. You have been troubled with a persistent cough for some time now. Recently, you have noticed that you have started to cough up what looks to you like blood.

Prior to entering the room

A travel history with relevant destinations can be useful if considering a differential and tailoring the approach to history taking. A sensible approach would be to consider diseases endemic to the area visited, however, avoid jumping to too many assumptions and risk overlooking basic information in your quest for an exotic diagnosis.

On entering the room begin with open questioning

- Let the patient talk to you about their symptoms

- Take a careful travel history including all areas visited and any stop-overs
- Find out if they were travelling alone and what accommodation was used
- The use (or otherwise) of preventative measures such as pre-travel immunisations and malaria prophylaxis should help you narrow your differential
- Symptoms of fever, lassitude, night sweats, weight loss, anorexia, cough, sputum, haemoptysis are highly suggestive of TB

Open questioning suggests a diagnosis of tuberculosis

With this diagnosis closed questioning should focus on the following

Explore other important causes of haemoptysis, such as:

- Pneumonia: fever, purulent sputum, productive cough, headaches, myalgia
- Bronchial cancer: more chronic presentation, weight loss, cough, sputum with flecks of blood, general malaise, anorexia, smoking history
- Pulmonary oedema: dyspnoea, fatigue, orthopnoea, PND, chest pain, nocturnal cough, pink frothy sputum, previous cardiac history or risk factors
- Pulmonary embolism: suspect in recent long-haul travel, usually sudden onset, pleuritic chest pain dizziness or syncope and risk factors for PE (see other sections)

Continue your closed questioning eliciting key features in the rest of the history. In the past medical history, ask about a history of previous TB, check for immunocompromise such as in HIV, malignancy, diabetes. Explore risk factors for HIV. Take a careful drug history, including intravenous drug use or others. Other medications such as phenytoin, warfarin and oestrogen containing pills that may interact with treatment. Smoking and alcohol history.

A careful systems review to identify other organ involvement:

- Neurological (meningeal TB): fever, headache, nausea, vomiting, neck stiffness and photophobia
- Genitourinary TB: frequency, dysuria, haematuria, loin pain
- Bone pain: bony lower back pain
- Skin: painful lower leg rash (erythema nodosum)

Explore concerns, ideas, and expectations

It is likely that the patient returning from areas with high incidences of tuberculosis and other diseases will have considered the possibility of such conditions. Ask the patient what concerns they have about their health.

What to tell the patient

'From the symptoms you are describing, my main worry would be you might have caught TB whilst you were abroad. Have you heard of TB or tuberculosis before?

'TB is a bacterial infection that anyone can catch and it is usually transmitted when infected people cough or sneeze. Most people become ill within a few weeks or months of breathing the bacteria and have active TB.

'Some people never become ill because their immune system gets rid of the bacteria. In other people the bacteria hide in the body at low level and the person does not get ill immediately but carries the infection and can become ill at a later stage. This is called latent TB.

'Active TB usually affects the lungs but can affect other body parts. Although you do not describe any other symptoms it is worth checking. To confirm the diagnosis you need to have some tests today, including a chest X-ray and sputum cultures. It is also important to check for certain viruses, such as the HIV virus, which sometimes pre-dispose or co-exist with TB.

'There is a cure for TB in the form of antibiotic treatment, which we should start before waiting for the results of the tests. The treatment duration is long, usually 6 months and it is very important you comply with treatment as it can cause serious consequences. Also you should not stop the treatment before it is fully complete even if you are feeling well, as you may still be infectious. I will provide further information about the side effects but it is important you have blood tests to check your liver tests every month. It is also important to prevent it from spreading to other people so we are obliged to screen any close contacts you may have had and offer them treatment too before they become ill. I will bring you in touch with a named nurse specialist whom you can contact if there are any problems at any stage.'

What to tell the examiner

Summarise the clinical case

'This young man with fever, haemoptysis and night sweats who has returned from an endemic area and has not previously been vaccinated with BCG is at high risk of respiratory TB. He does not give a history suggestive of other organ involvement. Although his risk factors for HIV are low I would ensure he has a test for HIV. I would proceed to some investigations and start management immediately. I would also inform the communicable diseases centre as TB is a notifiable disease.'

Investigations

To achieve a diagnosis of active pulmonary TB:

- Chest X-ray
- At least 3 sputum samples for TB microscopy and culture and prolonged incubation on Löwenstein–Jensen medium, before starting treatment or within 7 days of starting treatment
- Bronchoscopy and bronchoalveolar lavage if sputum unavailable
- In the presence of pleural effusion consider pelural tap (low glucose, ph < 7.3, high LDH and lymphocytosis)

Additional tests include:

- Pre treatment test colour vision as ethambutol may cause reversible ocular toxicity
- All patients with TB should have an HIV test as well as routine blood tests

Management

Remember communicable disease control notification and contact tracing and screening.

The standard recommended regimen for respiratory TB is:

- First 2 months: Rifampicin, isoniazid, pyrazinamide and ethambutol
- Next 4 months: Rifampicin, isoniazid

Be aware of deviations from the standard management in special circumstances such as meningeal TB and three times a week directly observed therapy in patients at high risk for non-adherence such as street or shelter dwelling homeless people, history of poor adherence or drug-resistant TB.

Avoid admission to hospital unless clinical or socio-economic need. If admission is necessary provide a negative pressure room or vented to the outside of the building. Patients can be discharged after 2 weeks of treatment if well and don't have MDR TB.

Assign a key worker to facilitate education, involvement and adherence. Measures may include health education counselling, home visits, patient diary, pill counts and random urine tests, social security benefits, housing and social services.

Consider factors that increase risk for drug resistance, such as:

- Previous TB
- Previous TB treatment failure
- Contact with known case of drug-resistant TB
- Birth in a foreign county with high incidence of TB
- HIV
- Resident in London
- Age 25–44 years
- Male

If resistance is suspected perform rifampicin resistance molecular tests on smear positive material or cultures. If these remain positive after 4 months of treatment, drug resistance should be suspected.

There is no routine follow-up after treatment completion. Follow-up for MDR TB for 12 months after completion.

> ### Screening for TB
>
> Diagnosing latent TB – Screen all household contacts and close non-household contacts with Mantoux testing and or interferon gamma test and chest X-ray. Mantoux negative results in household contacts who are previously unvaccinated should have interferon gamma testing 6 weeks after Mantoux. Offer BCG vaccination to contacts with negative Mantoux tests, no previous BCG vaccination and age < 35 years.
> Suspect latent in TB in patients with normal X-ray or with Mantoux results who are:
> - < 35 years old
> - HIV positive
> - Health workers
> - Mantoux positive > 6 mm without previous BCG
> - Mantoux positive > 15 mm, interferon gamma positive and previous BCG
>
> Treat for suspected latent TB in HIV positive patients who have come to close contact with smear positive TB patients. Latent TB treatment: 6 months isoniazid or 3 months isoniazid with rifampicin.

Further reading

National Institute for Health and Care Excellence (NICE) CG 117, Tuberculosis: Clinical diagnosis and management of tuberculosis, and measures for its prevention and control. London; NICE, 2011.

Case 148: Persistent cough or change in cough – investigation of cancer

Candidate information

Scenario

You are the medical registrar on call. A 78-year-old man has been referred by his GP for a persistent cough. The nurse in Accident and Emergency is concerned because she has seen the patient cough up some blood stained mucus. Additionally, she reports that the patient looks very emaciated. Please take a history from the patient, tell them what you think is wrong and discuss your findings with the examiner.

Actor information

You are a life-long smoker. You have been to see your GP a number of times for a cough. On the last occasion, you told the GP that you have lost two stone in weight over the past 3 months.

Prior to entering the room

Be careful before making assumptions with this scenario. Use it to form a preliminary differential but do not rush to exclude other causes. The scenario might be presented in such a way favouring one diagnosis but this may be misleading; an older, emaciated man coughing and put in isolation because of a presumed diagnosis of TB may actually be someone suffering with lung cancer.

The differential of persistent cough can be wide. In the absence of significant co-morbidity, an acute cough is normally benign and self-limiting. Apart from respiratory tract infection and inhalation of foreign body that are likely to be present with acute cough, most other causes are probably secondary to chronic causes. Consider productive and non-productive causes. Significant sputum production indicates primary lung pathology. Haemoptysis and weight loss will serve as differentiating factors. When cough is present with haemoptysis be sure to consider lung cancer, pulmonary embolus or TB.

On entering the room begin with open questioning

Attempt to explore the differential of cough, focusing on onset and duration, frequency, and quantity and appearance of sputum.

Screen for the characteristics of the cough. Is there diurnal variation and does it wake them up at night? Are there any triggers or aggravants? Where productive enquire as to the amount and character of sputum (serous, mucoid, purulent). Has there been haemoptysis? Is there associated chest pain and breathlessness?

Screen for systemic health. Has there been weight loss, general malaise and lethargy?

Narrow your differential

Causes of a productive cough include:

- Lung cancer-weight loss and haemoptysis (blood stained), breathlessness, chest pain from bony metastasis, long smoking history
- Pulmonary embolism-sudden onset breathlessness, pleuritic chest pain, recent long-haul travel, leg swelling or DVT

- TB-frank haemoptysis, cachexia, general malaise, weight loss, fever, cough, night sweats
- COPD-mucoid/purulent sputum
- Pulmonary oedema-pink/frothy sputum, breathlessness (worse in recumbent position), leg oedema

Causes of a non-productive cough include:

- Asthma-episodic, often seasonal wheezing and shortness of breath (see asthma section), nocturnal deterioration
- GORD-retrosternal burning pain, precipitated by posture change, worse after heavy meals
- Iatrogenic, e.g. ACE inhibitors

Open questioning suggests a diagnosis of lung carcinoma

With this diagnosis closed questioning should focus on the following

Continue closed questioning on past medical and social history. Be sure to take a thorough smoking history early in the encounter but avoid a punitive tone or judgmental approach.

Heavy smokers may have a previous diagnosis of COPD or chronic bronchitis. Ask about other previous respiratory, cardiac disease (also predisposes to cough) or history of lung cancer. Asbestos exposure significantly increases risk of neoplastic disease, thus screen for occupational history.

Consider extrapulmonary manifestations of bronchial carcinoma. Metastatic manifestations may include:

- Pancoast tumour may cause pain in the shoulder and inner arm and Horner's
- Horner's: unilateral papillary constriction, slight ptosis and loss of sweating when involving T1 root compression
- Left recurrent laryngeal involvement may present with voice hoarseness and bovine cough
- Bone pain and neurological symptoms such as seizures or focal neurology may point to metastatic disease
- Primaries in other sites that may spread to the lung – renal, prostate, breast, bone, gastrointestinal tract, cervical and ovarian

Non-metastatic manifestations may be endocrine, neurological, vascular, skeletal and/or cutaneous in nature:

- Ectopic secretion of ACTH, ADH, PTH-like peptide

- Myopathy, neuropathies, myasthenic syndrome, cerebellar degeneration
- Thrombophlebitis migrans, anaemia
- Hypertrophic pulmonary osteoarthropathy (clubbing, painful wrisits and ankles)
- Dermatomyositis, acanthosis nigricans

Explore concerns, ideas, and expectations

Summarising the case may focus attention on the likely diagnosis depending on the emphasis placed on smoking, or other risk factors, and a potential link with current symptoms. This may serve as a warning shot, preparing the patient for the discussion that will follow.

'So you have been smoking for most your life and have always had the occasional cough with sputum but recently you have developed a persistent cough for the last 8 weeks and it is gradually getting worse. You are concerned because recently you have started to cough up blood stained sputum and your wife thinks you have lost a lot of weight.

'What do you think may be causing your symptoms?'

'Have you considered the possibility of cancer?'

What to tell the patient

'I think it is important to run some tests to look closely at your lungs. A simple chest X-ray can be very informative but if it were normal it would be sensible to obtain a more detailed picture with a CT. This will look at your lungs in thin slices and we will be able pick up a wide range of information which will help us better understand the cause of your symptoms. It will be important to consider cancer as a potential diagnosis, and a CT will be useful in establishing this.

'Depending on our findings we can discuss treatment options. I do not want to rush ahead and talk to you about this without knowing with certainty what the underlying problem is but I will make sure we have plenty of time at your next appointment shortly after the scan to address all your questions.

'I can organise the chest X-ray today if it's ok with you and arrange for the CT scan in the next couple of days. Do you have any questions?'

What to tell the examiner

Summarise the clinical case

'This 70-year old man with a 45-pack per year smoking history has presented with an 8-week history of cough, haemoptysis and weight loss on a background of symptoms suggestive of chronic bronchitis. He is otherwise fit and healthy and has a good performance score. I would first like to exclude an underlying lung malignancy.'

Investigations

Examination may give clues as to the presence of significant masses or clinical signs related to associated pathology, commonly unilateral pleural effusions, or organomegaly/lymphadenopathy consistent with metastatic disease.

Imaging with chest X-ray looking for a hilar or peripheral mass, collapse or consolidation of the lung or pleural effusion (note that tumours need to be at least 1–2 cm to be visible on a plain radiograph).

'An abnormal or normal X-ray alone would not establish/refute the diagnosis. I would proceed to a staging CT scan to assess spread of the tumour, including liver and adrenal glands.' Abnormal CXR or CT should prompt urgent referral to chest MDT. Recent NICE guidelines recommend offering PET-CT, endobronchial ultrasound-guided TBNA or endoscopic ultrasound-guided FNA early in patients with intermediate probability of mediastinal malignancy on CT.

Tissue diagnosis should be made where possible. For peripheral tumours CT or US-guided needle biopsy. For central tumours, fibreoptic bronchoscopy enables sampling of nodes. Consider bronchoscopy to obtain biopsy or washings. Alternatively CT-guided fine needle aspiration or core biopsy from peripheral lesions if primary not accessible. Diagnostic pleural tap for cytology for malignant cells and biochemistry for exudates.

Depending on the history and examination findings you might want to investigate for paraneoplastic syndromes such as ACTH, Cushings, PTHr-peptide.

Management

Management depends on staging and patient suitability for major operation. Treatment and care should take into account patients' needs and preferences. Clinical nurse specialist should be involved in the early stages. The following management points are based on NICE guidelines (CG 121).

Non-small cell lung cancer (NSCLC):

- If medically fit may be a candidate for surgery, such as lobectomy or segmentectomy if complete resection can be achieved. Radical radiotherapy for patients with stage I, II or III NSCLC. All patients may be suitable for multimodal treatment with surgery, radiotherapy and chemotherapy. Involve a thoracic oncologist and thoracic surgeon early in the decision-making process and MDT.

Small-cell lung cancer (SCLC):

- For limited disease (T1-4, N0-3, M0) offer cisplatin based chemotherapy or carbopoatin in the presence of abnormal renal function. Consider concurrent radiotherapy if disease site can be encompassed in radiotherapy field and prophylactic cranial radiotherapy
- Surgery might be an option for T1-2, N0, M0 disease
- For extensive SCLC (T1-4, N0-3, M1) offer platinum-based chemotherapy. Thoracic radiotherapy after completion if response achieved

Palliative treatment:

- Palliative radiotherapy may help for symptoms control. Consider interventional endobronchial treatment for obstruction (endobronchial or SVC). Other palliative treatment would included malignant pleural effusion drainage, interventions for breathlessness, opioids, dexamethasone for symptomatic brain metastases
- Offer multi-disciplinary support for management of weight loss, loss of appetite, difficulty swallowing, fatigue and depression. Smoking cessation and nicotine replacement therapy is also important at any stage of treatment

- Offer counselling and support groups for both patient and family or carers. Consider general nursing issues. Home care or even placement for patients with high needs. Review with results to discuss management plan and address questions
- In general offer accurate and easy to understand information to patients and cares. Explain tests and treatment options including survival benefits

Prognosis:

- Depends on tumour type and staging
- Bronchial carcinoma is the commonest cancer in the west and leading cause of cancer death in women. 90% are caused by smoking. Only 5.5% are ever cured. It can be divided into small cell and non-small cell. The latter is subclassified into squamous (40%), large cell (25%), adenocarcinoma (10%) and alveolar cell (1–2%)
- Adenocarcinoma is common in non-smokers and is thought to be related to asbestos exposure. It occurs peripherally and may spread locally or distant. Squamous cell usually spreads locally and metastasizes late. Small cell (20–30%) arises from endocrine cells secreting polypeptide hormones. Paraneoplastic syndromes are common (ACTH and Cushing's). Small cell tumours metastasize early but respond to chemotherapy

Further reading

National Institute for Health and Care Excellence (NICE). CG121, The diagnosis and treatment of lung cancer. London; NICE, 2011.

Case 149: Change in bowel habit – malignancy

Candidate information

Scenario

You are the gastroenterology SHO. This 62-year-old man has presented to the outpatient clinic with a change in bowel habit, complaining of constipation for the last 6 months, now suffering from acute diarrhoea causing him significant embarrassment and distress. Recent blood tests by the GP have shown an iron-deficient anaemia. Please assess and offer advice on further management.

Actor information

You weren't particularly concerned when you noticed constipation a few months ago, but now you keep having episodes of diarrhoea. This has caused you considerable social embarrassment and resulted in prolonged time off work. Additionally, your GP has told you that you are anaemic, which you assume explains your lethargy, but you are unsure of the significance in relation to your other symptoms.

Prior to entering the room

Conceivably, scenarios revolving around an altered bowel habit could focus upon a variety of underlying aetiologies. The patient narrative and context of the symptoms will be all important in establishing the theme of the station and nature of the discussion. The possibilities range from young patients, in whom symptoms may prompt investigation of inflammatory bowel disease, to the older patient with red flag symptoms alerting to the possibility of a rectal mass, or where constipation and diarrhoea represent a feature of systemic disease or medication side effect. Employing a sensitive approach, to what are commonly distressing and embarrassing topics for patients to broach, will be vital.

On entering the room begin with open questioning

Establish the nature of the symptoms, the speed of onset and progression of the problem. Probe as to what the patient actually understands by the term constipation. Allow a full description of both new symptoms and what the patient would consider to be a normal bowel habit for them. Be sure to ask about frequency of defaecation, form of stool, the need for excessive straining and discomfort or pain on passing a motion, any sensation of incomplete evacuation or anorectal obstruction, and rectal bleeding. Recent or acute constipation is more likely suggestive of organic disease, whereas chronic symptoms, of several years, may point to functional problems.

The challenge in this scenario will be to discriminate between those cases requiring further, often invasive, investigation, and those where reassurance will suffice. Be alert to the likelihood of colorectal carcinoma with a tendency to looser or more frequent stools, progressing to constipation, and the possibility thereafter of overflow diarrhoea. Associated rectal bleeding without abdominal pain, symptomatic iron deficiency anaemia, weight loss, and general malaise represent red flag symptoms. Screen for symptoms suggestive of metastatic spread such as bone pain, breathlessness, or cough. Failure to pass wind/flatus may represent a progression to bowel obstruction, which in the presence of pain, bloating and vomiting would naturally require expedient escalation of treatment.

In considering the differential, remain open to the possibility of alternative causes of intraluminal obstruction or anal pathology, other than colorectal carcinoma, such as:

- Diverticular disease: recurrent episodes, left iliac fossa pain, often accompanied by low grade fever
- Stricturing on a background of inflammatory bowel disease, particularly with previous surgical intervention
- Fissure-in-ano or abscess: pain on defaecation and fresh rectal bleeding or pus
- Haemorrhoids: straining at stool, pain on defaecation, blood on wiping, lump protruding from anus

Be mindful of conditions associated with constipation including endocrine and neurological, such as:

- Hypothyroidism: cold intolerance, hair/skin changes, lethargy and proximal weakness, with weight gain
- Hypercalcaemia: nausea, vomiting, abdominal pain, mental disturbance
- Diabetes: polyuria, polydipsia, other autonomic disturbance
- Parkinson's: resting tremor, rigidity, bradykinesia, difficulty with manual tasks
- Spinal cord compression or demyelinating disease: urinary disturbance, sensory or motor lower leg neuropathy, sphincter dysfunction, perianal or perineal loss of sensation

Open questioning suggests a diagnosis of possible GI malignancy

With this diagnosis closed questioning should focus on the following

Appreciate the need to clarify the patient's past medical history to specifically rule out disease associations, such as those mentioned above. Thereafter, look to screen for alternative reasons for the onset of altered bowel habit, particularly a careful drug history.

Enquire as to the intiation of any new prescriptions and screen for medication with recognised associations with constipation and/ or gastrointestinal disturbance with blood loss and anaemia, such as:

- Tricyclic anti-depressants
- Anti-cholinergic medications
- Anti-convulsants
- Calcium-channel blockers
- Diuretics
- NSAIDs
- Immodium
- Opioids
- Iron supplementation

Enquire regarding a family history of cancer or other hereditary disease – HNPCC, polyposis coli, Peutz–Jeghers.

Considering the social history, smoking is associated with increased risk of colorectal cancer.

- Enquire about dietary change that might have contributed to change in bowel habit
- Be alert to behavioural factors: Poor bowel habit/lifestyle-ignoring desire to defaecate
- Anxiety and depression: anorexia nervosa, affective disorder

Explore concerns, ideas, and expectations

The patient may raise a wide range of concerns, such as the following. Give the patient a chance to verbalise thoughts in relation to colorectal cancer before you offer the idea in a completely unprepared patient. Alternatively, the patient may not be particularly concerned regarding the underlying cause, but primarily keen to resolve the symptoms, especially if, as in this case, hey are causing social embarrassment. In either case, warning shots are an important principle.

What to tell the patient

'I am concerned that your symptoms over the last 6 months may be linked. I am conscious of your anxiety in this regard but feel it important that we investigate further, as I am worried about a potential diagnosis of cancer. I would like to perform an examination today in clinic and arrange for a camera test to look at the bowels from the back passage. After the tests are completed I will organise an appointment for you to come back and discuss the results and potential treatment options.' Be prepared to answer questions relating to the details and practicalities of tests and investigations and the time to results.

What to tell the examiner

Summarise the clinical case

'This 62-year-old man complains of persistent change in bowel habit with looser stools and frequency up to 4 times a day over the last 8 weeks. There is associated rectal bleeding, mixed in with the stool and intermittent abdominal pain. He has also lost 3–4 kilos over the last 3 months.'

Investigations

- Digital rectal examination for palpable rectal mass or identification of rectal bleeding
- Blood tests to look for iron deficiency anaemia, tumour markers (CEA)
- If no major co-morbidity colonoscopy would be the gold standard for diagnosis with biopsies
- Flexible sigmoidoscopy with barium enema would be an alternative for patients with co-morbidities unlikely to tolerate or have a safe procedure
- CT colonoscopy is an alternative if there are facilities, especially in elderly patients or those with comorbidities or risk of perforation during colonoscopy
- Contrast-enhanced staging CT of the chest, abdomen and pelvis if colorectal cancer diagnosed

Management

Management of colorectal cancer depends on patient expectations, co-morbidities and staging and MDT decision. The following management points are based on NICE guidelines (CG 131).

Local colorectal tumours:

- Resectable primary rectal tumours: MRI for further characterisation followed by resection. Short course pre-operative radiotherapy for moderate risk tumours and pre-operative chemoradiotherapy for high risk tumours
- Unresectable colon or rectal tumours or borderline resectable: pre-oeprative chemoradiotherapy to allow for shrinkage and tumour response with high risk locally advanced tumours
- Laparoscopic or open surgery depending on the suitability for laparoscopic resection, the risks and benefits of both procedures, and the experience of surgeon

- Consider adjuvant chemotherapy after surgery for high-risk stage II/III colon cancer
- Advanced and metastatic colorectal tumours (metastatic or locally invasive and surgical excision with curative intent is unlikely):
- Hepatic metastases only – hepatobiliary MDT for decision regarding possible surgery
- Extra-hepatic metastases – MRI for suspected intracranial metastases and anatomic site-specific MDT and PET-CT scan for decision regarding radical surgery
- If both primary and metastatic tumours are deemed respectable – consideration of pre-operative chemotherapy and possibility of concomitant surgery for both tumours

Whenever surgical options are considered, a discussion about stomas will be required.

Screening for colorectal cancer
For average risk patients
< 50 years of age – no screening
> 50 years of age:
- Annual faecal occult blood test
- 5-yearly flexible sigmoidoscopy
- 10-yearly colonoscopy
For high risk patients:
Positive family history: if first or second degree relative with CRC or adenomas in relative < 60: annual faecal occult blood tests and 5-yearly flexible sigmoidoscopy, 10-yearly colonoscopy starting at age 40 years.
Genetic syndromes:

- Familial adenomatous polyposis: genetic testing for APC mutation at age 12 years. Yearly flexible sigmoidoscopy. In polyp identification full colonoscopy +/– prophylactic colectomy. Upper endoscopy surveillance recommended too
- Hereditary non-poluposis colorectal cancer: colonoscopic surveillance at 20–25 years as most tumours are right sided. Genetic testing for 1st degree relatives
- Peutz–Jegher's: 2-yearly upper and lower endoscopy, barium follow-through. Monitor for gonadal, breast and cervical cancer

Factors in past medical history:
- Polyps: surveillance colonoscopy for adenomas > 1 cm, villous or tubulovillous histology, multiple adenomas and dysplastic polyps. 3 yearly if colon cleared of polyps
- Colorectal cancer: 3–6 months after surgery surveillance colonoscopy for inspection of anastomotic site, at 1 year and 3–5 yearly thereafter
- Inflammatory bowel disease (see relevant case)
- Acromegaly: 3-yearly colonoscopy from age 40 years

Further reading

National Institute for Health and Care Excellence (NICE).CG131, Colorectal cancer: the diagnosis and management of colorectal cancer. London, NICE, 2011.

Case 150: Change in bowel habit – established inflammatory bowel disease

Candidate information

Scenario

As the SHO in the gastroenterology clinic you are asked to see a 35-year-old woman with a diagnosis of inflammatory bowel disease, attending for her annual review. Take a history from this patient and advise on any changes in management that may be necessary.

Actor information

Since you were last seen in the clinic, you have had 4 episodes where your symptoms have worsened, requiring steroid therapy. You wonder whether there are any other treatments available.

Prior to entering the room

In a patient with established IBD the aim of the history station would be to:

- Assess disease severity
- Identify any complications
- Identify side-effects from treatment
- Escalate management in chronic active disease

Complications to have in mind would include:

- Colorectal cancer
- Cholangicarcinoma
- Primary sclerosing cholangitis
- Ankylosing spondylitis/sacroilitis
- Strictures

On entering the room begin with open questioning

Screen for current symptoms, which may include bloody diarrhoea, pain, urgency or tenesmus. Establish the duration of the disease and extent of colitis – proctitis, left sided or more extensive (50% of patients have disease confined to colon/rectum, 30% beyond sigmoid, 20% pan-colitis). Attempt to gauge the level of control achieved with existing treatment and clarify the measures required to treat any flares since the last review.

> **Open questioning suggests a diagnosis of poorly controlled inflammatory bowel disease**

With this diagnosis closed questioning should focus on the following

Using closed questioning, establish disease severity and the presence of systemic disturbance to allow you to form an idea of how well controlled their disease is and if treatment escalation is advocated.

Highlight the importance of recent colonoscopy results if available in patients with long-standing disease that might require surveillance colonoscopies. Disease extending past the rectosigmoid is associated with higher risk for malignancy. Risk relates to duration, severity, and extent of disease.

Seek extra-intestinal manifestations of UC related to disease activity:

- Peripheral arthropathy
- Erythema nodosum
- Episcleritis or anterior uveitis
- Mouth ulcers
- Pyoderma

Other manifestations (unrelated to colitis) include:

- Ankylosing spondylitis
- Sacroilitis
- PSC

Important points in the past medical history include:

- Previous surgical intervention
- Previous polyps
- Falls and fractures in the context of nutritional deficiency and long-term steroid use

Enquire about smoking in the social history and any relation to flares. Be sure to take a family history focusing on auto-immune disorders and cancers.

Explore concerns, ideas, and expectations

Take time to explore what the individual patient considers to be the main issue. For example, are they keen to explore other treatment options?

What to tell the patient

'There is considerable scope for improvement in the control of your disease. I propose we make some changes to your current regime and consider the use of an immunosuppressant. I would hope that this improves day-to-day symptoms and reduces the number of flares. Additionally it would be sensible to arrange for a repeat sigmoidoscopy, or if tolerable a full screening colonscopy, to assess the current extent and severity of disease.'

What to tell the examiner

Summarise the clinical case

'The patient has an existing diagnosis of ulcerative colitis, identified at the age of 18-year-old. She has a limited colitis affecting the left sided colon and is usually maintained on oral mesalazine. Over the last year, she has had 4 flares, requiring oral steroids. Her father had colorectal cancer diagnosed at the age of 45 years which puts her at a higher risk of colorectal cancer development in the future although her colitis at present in limited to the left side. The frequency of her flares suggests her disease is not well-controlled and might require second line treatment with a steroid sparing agent.'

Investigations

Blood tests include ESR/CRP, FBC to look for anaemia of chronic disease or microcytic anaemia from chronic blood loss, iron studies to look for iron deficiency, and LFTs particularly in suspected PSC.

When considering systemic agents: TPMT before starting AZA as reduced enzyme activity is associated with higher incidence of myelosuppression and mercaptopurine may be indicated. FBC and LFTs before, and monthly after the initiation of treatment.

When suspecting a recent flare or active disease sigmoidoscopy should be sufficient. Colonoscopy for surveillance or more extensive colitis, but avoid in active flares as patient will be at higher risk of perforation (see below).

Management

Maintenance therapy includes: (see 'Further Reading' for reference)

- Mesalazine 1.2–2.4 g/day orally
- Topical mesalazine 1g daily for distal disease

For steroid-dependent disease, steroid-sparing agents should be considered:

- Azathioprine 2–2.5 mg/kg/day. The indications for azathioprine include: severe or frequent relapse; two or more steroid courses within 12 months; relapse at prednisolone doses < 15 mg; relapse within 6 weeks of stopping steroids
- Mercaptopurine 0.75–1.5 mg/kg/day
- Methotrexate possible alternative

- Ciclosporin reserved as salvage therapy for acute flares used for 3–6 months often as a bridge to azathioprine

Of proctitis:

- Topical mesalazine with/without oral preparations
- Add topical steroids if unresponsive
- Formulation: suppositories for rectosigmoid, foam liquid enemas for more proximal disease
- Add oral prednisolone if above fail
- Suppositories for rectosigmoid
- Non-stimulant osmotic laxatives if proximal faecal loading (PEG-based)

Of mild active left-sided colitis or more extensive disease:

- Oral mesalazine 2.4–4.8 g daily with/without topical mesalazine (needs monitoring as risk of interstitial nephritis)
- Prednisolone 20–40 mg reduced according to disease response over 4–8 weeks
- Confirm disease activity by sigmoidoscopy

Acute severe active colitis needs admission for intensive medical therapy, often intravenous steroids, and close monitoring for escalation of treatment with the possibility of surgical intervention where poor response to medical treatment or complications arise.

Further reading

Mowat C, Cole A, Windsor A, et al. Guidelines for the management of inflammatory bowel disease in adults. Gut 2011; 60:571–607.

Case 151: Difficulty in swallowing

Candidate information

Scenario

As the gastroenterology registrar you review an urgent referral in clinic from a GP for a 74-year-old man experiencing dysphagia. Please assess and advise regarding further management.

Actor information

You have been suffering from heartburn for many years but have managed it using over the counter antacids. Recently you have noticed that you have had difficulty in swallowing. You consulted your GP who has arranged for you to be seen today.

Prior to entering the room

In any dysphagia history you need to establish if the difficulty swallowing is associated with pain and whether it is limited to solids, liquids or both.

On entering the room begin with open questioning

Explore the nature of dysphagia, how long it has been present for, is the problem intermittent or constant, is the dysphagia worse for liquids than solids and what other symptoms they are experiencing.

Narrow your differential considering the causes of dysphagia:

In the wall

Gastrointestinal:

- Gastro-oesophageal reflux disease (GORD): intermittent, retrosternal burning pain, worse on lying, relieved on sitting forward, worse after meals, especially rich in fat. Long-standing symptoms may predispose to Barrett's or oesophageal cancer
- Achalasia: intermittent difficulty, worse for liquids than solids, associated food regurgitation and heartburn
- Oesophageal carcinoma: rapid onset and deterioration of symptoms. Dysphagia to solids first, then liquids. Haematemesis may be a feature. Associated anorexia, weight loss, symptoms of anaemia. Occasionally voice changes in vocal cord paralysis from tumour infiltration
- Plummer–Vinson syndrome: dysphagia with food sticking on upper part of oesophagus, middle aged female (web in upper oesophagus/post-cricoid web)

Infection:

- Chagas disease: recent travel in endemic areas (e.g. Brazil, Venezuela, Argentina) cardiac arrhythmias, gastrointestinal, respiratory and urinary symptoms

Autoimmune:

- Scleroderma

Outside the wall

- Pharyngeal pouch – elderly patients, regurgitation worse on lying down or coughing, food sticking behind manubrium, neck swelling, halitosis, aspiration pneumonia
- Mediastinal tumours/bronchial ca-haemoptysis, weight loss

- Enlarged left atrium in mitral stenosis
- Para-oesophageal hernia – intermittent dysphagia, worse after a big meal, associated hiccups

> ## Open questioning suggests a diagnosis of possible malignancy

With this diagnosis closed questioning should focus on the following

If considering a diagnosis of oesophageal cancer make sure you ask about symptoms suggestive of complications, such as:

- Pulmonary, hepatic, brain and bone metastases are common with SCC
- Adenocarcinoma spreads to regional and distant lymph nodes and liver
- Ask about breathlessness/haemoptysis, RUQ pain, confusion or headaches, and bone pain on systems review

Continue your closed questioning to complete your history. Establish any past medical history of conditions predisposing to oesophageal cancer such as achalasia, GORD/Barrett's and even previous malignancy – especially head and neck SCC. Exclude drugs that relax the lower oesophageal sphincter. Check whether there is a family history of achalasia or oesophageal cancer. Tobacco and alcohol history also important as they are both risk factors for the development of oesophageal carcinoma.

Barrett's oesophagus or columnar lined oesophagus is a precursor of development of oesophageal carcinoma. Its incidence has dramatically increased over the last years. Columnar lined epithelium may be a complication of long-standing gastro-oesophageal reflux disease. However, GORD may progress to adenocarcinoma without developing into Barrett's first making screening important in cases of long-standing, severe GORD.

Explore concerns, ideas, and expectations

Find out if they are suspecting what might be the problem first and whether they mention the possibility of a malignancy.

What to tell the patient

'I am worried that the symptoms you are describing are because of a blockage in the food pipe. I would recommend an urgent endoscopy, a test where a camera tube is passed from your mouth down into you stomach to establish what might be causing the blockage. Depending upon the findings we might be able to improve some of the blockage to relieve your symptoms at the time of the procedure. I will arrange a follow-up appointment soon after the procedure to discuss the results of biopsies if taken, and discuss treatment options.'

What to tell the examiner

Summarise the clinical case

'This man with a long-standing history of GORD who has never had a screening OGD complains of rapid onset dysphagia with associated odynophagia and weight loss. I am concerned there might be an underlying oesophageal malignancy and would like to refer him for urgent OGD and biopsy. In the meantime I would examine him to look for evidence of metastatic spread.' If you are confident enough you can expand upon the likely aetiology in view of long-standing GORD with a predisposition to adenocarcinoma rather than SCC, but that biopsy will aid confirmation.

Investigations

In the first instance organise the following blood tests: FBC may show anaemia of chronic disease or microcytic anaemia in which case iron studies may show a deficiency in the presence of chronic blood loss through a bleeding tumour. CRP is often elevated in malignancy. Renal function may be deranged in dehydration or protracted vomiting and albumin may be low because of malnutrition. Abnormal liver function may suggest metastatic disease. Hypercalcaemia may be seen in SCC secondary to PTH related peptide.

Other investigations would include:

- Plain chest radiograph: might pick up large tumours but also pulmonary spread
- OGD: gold-standard for diagnosis and option for therapeutic dilatation. May show tumour in the oesophagus, or the presence of pre-malignant Barrett's oesophagus. Biopsies are essential. Therapeutic dilatation is a treatment option for patients with obstructing tumours or structuring disease
- CT for staging

Management

Management of oesophageal cancer is via an MDT approach. The exact management approach depends on staging. In general, curative surgery may be an option in early stages with/without adjuvant chemoradiotherapy. Therapeutic dilatation and stenting can be offered for palliation.

Case 152: Cirrhotic liver disease

Candidate information

Scenario

You are the gastroenterology registrar. A 60-year-old man with jaundice has been referred to the outpatient clinic with suspected cirrhosis by the GP after routine blood tests showed abnormal LFTs and a cirrhotic liver on ultrasound. Please take a history from the patient and tell him about any further investigations and/or treatments that are necessary.

Actor information

You saw your GP last month because your family commented on a yellowed appearance of your eyes. As explored by your GP in the community, you drink approximately one bottle of red wine each evening after work. You drink more at the weekends. If the candidate asks you directly, you will admit that you are worried by your drinking habits and are keen to seek help to cut down.

Prior to entering the room

When you are dealing with such a scenario there are many things to consider. Abnormal LFTs, jaundice and a cirrhotic liver probably give you the diagnosis of cirrhosis. Your job is to try to establish the cause of liver disease, make an educated guess as to how advanced the disease is and if there is evidence of decompensation or complications and of course provide a sound management plan that might prevent progression to cirrhosis or prevent/reverse decompensation.

On entering the room, begin with open questioning

Let the patient guide you at first by asking open questions to find out how long they have been symptomatic (if at all), what prompted investigation in the first place and about the general state of their health.

> **Open questioning suggests a diagnosis of chronic liver disease**

With this diagnosis closed questioning should focus on the following

Try to identify points in the history which suggest the cause of their liver disease:

- Exposure to hepatitis B or C (e.g. previous blood transfusion, haemodialysis, maternal infection, needle exposure) or HIV
- A history of other auto-immune conditions, bowel pathology such as IBD
- Careful drug history, recreational drugs, intravenous drug abuse, over the counter or herbal. Drug history should ask specifically about use of NSAIDs, opiates, statins, aminoglycosides that may cause worse hepatic function or predispose to bleeding. Take a careful vaccination history especially for hepatitis B
- Alcohol history, focusing on type of alcohol and frequency of consumption, duration and pattern of drinking
- Recent travel history: job and occupational exposure, especially healthcare workers, sex workers
- Sexual history for identification of risk factors of sexually transmitted disease including Hepatitis and HIV
- Family history of auto-immune disease, genetic disease, diabetes

- Others including haemochromatosis, with a history of diabetes, cardiomyopathy, hypogonadism, skin pigmentation, and arthritis, or α_1-antitrypsin with cirrhosis and emphysema

Next assess for history of complications of cirrhosis, such as:

- Variceal bleeding: upper GI bleeding, haematemesis, malaenia, epigastric pain
- Ascites
- Hepatic encephalopathy
- Hepatocellular carcinoma (especially in the context of hepatits C)
- Malnurishment
- Infection/SBP
- Osteoporosis: check for low impact or spontaneous fractures

The presence of Jaundice, encephalopathy or ascites indicates decompensated cirrhosis. If the patient is describing such symptoms try to establish the cause:

- Natural disease progression
- Recent alcohol binge/alcoholic hepatitis
- Concomitant infection with hepatitis virus, e.g. A
- Infection/SBP: abdominal pain, distension, fever
- Upper GI bleeding: malaena, haematemesis, epigastric pain
- Dehydration: excessive vomiting, malnutrition, decreased or concentrated urinary output
- Constipation: may lead to encephalopathy
- Drugs: new or hepatotoxic
- Portal vein thrombosis: abdominal pain, fever, mesenteric infarction
- Budd–Chiari: abdominal pain, ascites, hepatomegaly over several months
- HCC: recent weight loss or abdominal pain

Explore concerns, ideas, and expectations

It is likely that any discussion surrounding the patients concerns will be primarily directed towards alcohol use and dependency.

What to tell the patient

'I suspect that all the problems we have discussed today are related to damage to liver caused by excessive alcohol over the years. Alcoholic liver disease may be asymptomatic for long periods. By the time it is identified, usually on routine blood tests it means that the liver is already damaged, which seems to have happened in this case. The liver is a complex organ and among other things it helps filtering toxins from the blood, regulates cholesterol levels and helps fight infection. All of these functions are impaired when damage occurs and ultimately prolonged alcohol misuse can seriously damage the liver irreversibly and even lead to death. Cirrhosis is the final stage of alcoholic liver disease. The damage is irreversible but stopping alcohol immediately prevents any further damage and can lead to gradual recovery of liver function. The treatment options depend on you and whether you are prepared to stop drinking.

'In the meantime I need to organise some tests to assess the degree of damage to your liver and rule out any other causes of liver disease.'

What to tell the examiner

Summarise the clinical case

'This 60-year-old man referred by his GP with jaundice, abnormal LFTs and ultrasound evidence of cirrhosis gives a history suggestive of decompensated liver disease with jaundice and ascites following a recent alcohol binge accompanied by a recent short history of melaena and haematemesis indicating probable variceal disease. Alcohol induced liver disease is most likely implicated, however, I wish to exclude other causes, such as hepatitis C infection.'

Investigations

The investigative strategy in this patient would include the following:

- Full liver screen including: liver function tests, GGT, AST, hepatitis A, B and C, HIV, serum copper levels, ferritin, α_1-antitrypsin
- FBC to look for anaemia, renal profile for signs of dehydration/hyponatraemia/renal failure/hepatorenal syndrome, and clotting screen which is likely to be derange due to altered liver synthetic function
- Alpha-fetoprotein for suspected hepatocellular carcinoma
- US liver and Doppler study to assess hepatic portal veins

Management

When there is evidence of decompensation, admit the patient for further tests and treatment. Monitor closely for complications including infection. Correct electrolyte disturbance and provide nutritional support. Unless faced with acute bleeding, consider routine OGD to look for varices and banding. Prophylactic propranolol may be considered for prevention of variceal bleeding. Therapeutic drainage of ascites may be considered in symptomatic patients.

Case 153: Previous renal transplant

Candidate information

Scenario

As the renal SHO, you have been asked to assess a 61-year-old man who has been referred by his GP with abnormal renal function tests and decreasing urine output. He has previously been a renal transplant recipient. Please take a history and discuss your findings with the patient. A discussion with the examiner will follow.

Actor information

You have been sent to the renal clinic because your GP has noticed that your renal function tests have been deteriorating. Despite being asymptomatic, you are concerned that your transplanted kidney may be failing.

Prior to entering the room

Decreasing urinary output and abnormal renal function indicate a failing graft. In general, most complications related to renal transplants will be secondary to infection or graft rejection but you should bear in mind all complications associated with renal transplants, namely opportunistic infection secondary to immunosuppression, hypertension, hyperlipidaemia, cardiovascular disease (increased 10-fold compared to the general population), diabetes mellitus (pre-transplantion but also new onset secondary to corticosteroids), tumours or disease recurrence. Recurrent renal disease accounts for fewer than 4% of graft failures. The degree of immunosuppression is also directly linked with the development of certain complications, as subtherapeutic levels will lead to higher incidence of and rejection whereas toxic levels may have a direct nephrotoxic effect. Immunosuppressants alone will lead to a higher rate of opportunistic infections and malignant transformation due to immune suppression. In addition, graft rejection may be difficult to clinically distinguish from infection, as the former may also present in a similar fashion or the two may co-exist.

The most important aid in scenarios involving renal transplantation is to establish early on the length of time after transplantation; the type of complications is directly associated to the length of time post transplant.

On entering the room begin with open questioning

Open questioning can be very informative as most patients with renal transplants and their relatives will be very knowledgeable about their condition. Do not underestimate the patient and their ideas about the cause of their symptoms.

Find out why and when they had their transplant and if the source was cadaveric or from a living donor. Cadaveric transplants are associated with more episodes of rejection, infection and are associated with a lower survival rate (81% at 5 years compared to 91% in living donor). Was it a pre-emptive transplant and had they received renal replacement therapy beforehand. Find out if there have been previous episodes of rejection or infection and subsequent changes to medication. The immunosuppressive regime should be established early on in the history as well as any recent medication changes and overall compliance with treatment.

> ## Open questioning suggests a diagnosis of deranged function in a renal transplant

With this diagnosis closed questioning should focus on the following

Complication of renal transplantation giving rise to refection.

Rejection

Graft failure may be completely asymptomatic but may also present with decreasing urinary output, hypertension and discomfort around the transplant site. Needless to say you should enquire about any symptoms consistent with infection including fever, respiratory, urinary and bowel symptoms.

- Hyperacute rejection usually occurs intra-operatively due to ABO or HLA class I incompatibility.
- Acute rejection in the first 6 months from surgery occurs in 15% cases and often patients have recurrent episodes of rejection. Presents as fever and graft pain
- Late rejection after 6 months, usually a result of immunosuppressive withdrawal after 6 months
- Chronic rejection after 1 year usually manifests as progressive loss of renal function and proteinuria

Infection

Patients who have experienced previous episodes of rejection may require high dose immunosuppression with a resultant susceptibility to infection and resultant complications. Expect a history of fever, contact with ill patients and/or mucocutaneous, respiratory, urinary, bowel symptoms.

Consider opportunistic infections during the 1st month post transplant and up to 6 months when immunosuppression reaches its peak levels.

- Early: during the first month, usually related to peri-operative pathogens and localise in urinary tract (*E. coli*), line infections (*Staphylococcus aureus* or *Streptococcus viridans*), wound (*Streptococcus viridans*, *Staphylococcus aureus*) and respiratory (*Streptococcus pneumoniae*)
- Intermediate: during the first 6 months expect opportunistic infections. Fever, general malaise, arhthralgia, myalgia. Most common pathogens: CMV, PCP, *Candida*, *Listeria*, *Aspergillus*. High fever, derraged LFTs and leukopenia are often seen in CMV disease
- Late: after 6 months. The type of infection depends on general health. If graft failure is normal and on low dose immunosuppression expect infections similar to the general population. In patients with poor functioning grafts, recurrent rejection episodes or high dose immunosuppression expect chronic and opportunistic infections. Consider infections with latent viruses such as CMV, VZV, EBV and hepatitis

Cardiac/vascular

Cardiovascular complications are commoner in pre-existing cardiac disease, hypertension, steroids, diabetes, smoking and previous episodes of rejection. Hypertension may be a result of native kidney disease, graft dysfunction or immunosuppressant. Most cases occur in the first 12 weeks from surgery.

- Renal artery thrombosis: usually presents in the immediate post-transplant period. Sudden cessation of urine output
- Renal vein thrombosis: early complication, decreasing urinary output, haematuria, pain and swelling over graft site
- Renal artery stenosis: later. Uncontrolled blood pressure, peripheral oedema

Urinary leak

Common around 2 months: fever, abdominal swelling and graft dysfunction.

Malignancy

Usually secondary to chronic immunosuppression and viruses with malignant potential such as EBV, HBV and HHV8. Kidney transplant patients are particularly at risk of non-melanoma skin cancer, kidney, non-Hodgkins, and gynaecological cancer related to HPV infection (cervix, vulvovaginal) but in general higher incidence of most cancers including lung, colon, bladder, prostate testis.

Drug nephrotocixity

Although non-compliance is the commonest cause of late acute rejection, ciclosporin and tacrolimus are directly nephrotoxic and hence tight level control is warranted.

Drug interactions are very important too when considering levels especially the P450 enzymes.

- Increased ciclosporin levels: calcium channel blockers such as diltiazem, antibiotics such as erythromycin
- Decreased levels: antibiotics such as isoniazid, rifampicin (anti-TB prophylaxis is very common in the transplant population), anti-epileptics
- Others: amphotericin, aciclovir, NSAIDs have a synergistic nephrotoxic effect (without affecting levels)

Recurrent renal disease

Focal segmental glomerulosclerosis, HUS, oxalosis, and membranoproliferative glomerulonephritis are considered high risk for transplant loss.

Explore concerns, ideas, and expectations

Many patients with renal transplantation have a wide range of knowledge surrounding their condition and may be 'medicalised'. Therefore, afford them the time to voice any concerns as they feel appropriate.

What to tell the patient

'The obvious concern is one of potential transplant rejection. In order to better appreciate the current situation we will perform repeat blood testing and arrange for an ultrasound before reviewing the current management and exploring potential options.'

What to tell the examiner

Summarise the clinical case

The case is one of a pre-emptive cadaveric kidney transplant 6-months ago presenting with decreasing urine output in the context of abnormal renal function indicative of a failing graft. The most common causes of graft failure at 6-month include rejection and opportunistic infection. The history is not suggestive of an infectious cause although immunosuppressants can mask symptoms. I would proceed with a full work-up to rule out infection and other causes of graft failure.

Investigations

Explain you would firstly examine the patient fully for signs of sepsis, volume status and careful examination of transplanted kidney. You would record the temperature, blood pressure and body weight as well as urinalysis. White cells are present in infection and obstruction, where as red cells may point to glomerulonephritis.

Baseline blood tests should include inflammatory markers and FBC to look for evidence of sepsis (leucocytosis, raised CRP), serum urea and creatinine which will be elevated in the context of a failing graft (a 20% rise in serum creatinine defines graft failure) and very importantly immunosuppressive levels (ciclosporin or tacrolimus usually) to rule out toxic or subtherapeutic levels.

Full septic screen including blood, urine cultures and stool cultures as well as chest

X-ray. Ultrasound scan to look for obstruction or perinephric collection and colour-flow Doppler of the renal transplant to look at vasculature and perfusion. Finally a graft biopsy may provide a definitive diagnosis.

Management

Management depends on the underlying cause of transplant dysfunction. Treat reversible causes such as infection, electrolyte disturbance and volume abnormalities. Patients in severe acute renal failure might even require haemodialysis.

Optimise immunosuppression and drug regime. In suspected drug-related nephrotoxicity, if a trial of dose reduction does not result in improved serum creatinine proceed to biopsy. Consider corticosteroids in the context of rejection.

Other considerations include:

- If blood transfusion is required, CMV negative irradiated blood should be used.
- Intravenous hydrocortisone often used in patients on long-term steroids at risk of adrenal insufficiency
- Maintain a patient-centered focused approach, re-assuring the patient but at the same time alert them to impending graft failure and the possibility of graft loss
- Other general tips to consider: screening for malignancy at regular intervals, tight diabetic, hypertensive, lipidaemia control for optimal cardiovascular state

Additional themes worth considering

Assessment prior to renal transplantation
- Careful history for pre-exisisting cardiovascular disease, CMV, HBV, TB and other chronic infections. EBV negative patients receiving EBV positive transplant have an increased risk of post-transplant lymphoproliferative disorder (7-fold). In cases of previous malignancy a window

period of 2–5 years disease free should be allowed before transplantation
- ABO blood group and HLA typing, CMV, EBV, VZV, hepatitis B, hepatitis C and HIV tests
- Immunisation to HepB
- Full cardiovascular work-up and screening for cardiovascular disease. Patients with the following should have cardiac stress tests: Age > 49, diabetes, abnormal resting ECG and history of ischaemic cardiac or cerebrovascular disease. Coronary angiography or stress echocardiography is recommended for further testing in abnormal results

Types of graft: living related donor, live unrelated donor, cadaveric grafts from brainstem dead donor.

Note that simultaneous kidney – pancreas transplantation would be the treatment of choice for patients with type 1 diabetes mellitus, chronic renal failure including predictive date of requiring dialysis within 6 months or on dialysis

Pre-transplantation counselling including potential risk of recurrent disease (accounts for 5% of allograft loss secondary to primary focal segmental glomerulosclerosis, IgA nephropathy, mesangiocapillary glomerulonephritis); smoking cessation advice as there is evidence that quitting smoking pre-transplant reduces the relative risk of graft failure.

- Contraindications to renal transplantation: Absolute contraindications include: active infection or systemic disease or metastatic cancer, cancer, severe untreated heart disease, liver insufficiency and HIV (unless CD4 count > 200 for more than 6 months and undetectable viral load on stable antiretroviral therapy for more than 3 months and no major infectious or neoplastic complications)
- Relative contraindications include: HCV, HBV, morbid obesity, atherosclerosis, cardiac disease, uncontrolled hypertension, smoking, unresolved psychosocial issues

Case 154: Headache

Candidate information

Scenario

You are the SHO in the neurology clinic. This 27-year-old female nurse has been experiencing headaches of increasing frequency and severity. Please take a history from the patient. Inform the patient of your findings and inform them of your management plan.

Actor information

You started to have headaches a couple of months ago. You have seen your GP four times with the same complaint. Additionally, you presented to Accident and Emergency one evening with a particularly severe headache. You are concerned that you may have a brain tumour. You had been using over the counter painkillers but despite taking the maximum doses the headaches have persisted and so in addition began using medication from hospital supplied on prescription by one of the doctors from the ward.

Prior to entering the room

Headache is one of the most common clinical presentations in general medicine and frequently encountered in the PACES exam. Often the diagnosis is a clinical one and investigation, which is often extensive and invasive, should be reserved for cases where suspicion exists of a worrying underlying pathology. It is the responsibility of the clinician to discriminate between benign and sinister features, reassuring where necessary. Often the need to implement trial management with analgesia or lifestyle modification, and arrange review as a safety net, is a prudent approach.

On entering the room begin with open questioning

Allow the patient to fully voice her concerns and offer an account of her symptoms. Prompt the patient where necessary to establish onset, duration, frequency and character.

Be prepared for the 'emotional patient' where the symptoms have caused significant distress, disruption to daily living and previous management from the GP has been unsuccessful. In such cases it will be necessary to demonstrate sufficient empathy to gain trust and allow a fresh review of symptoms to facilitate joint management decisions. Alternatively, it may be necessary to deal with pre-conceived ideas as to the agenda for the consultation. Patients may have been referred with the false promise of neuro-imaging or the prescription of stronger analgaesia. In such situations it is important to reassure the patient, consider appropriate testing or treatment if the history warrants it, but in all likelihood, some negotiation will be required.

Attempt to organise the symptoms and stratify using the framework of primary versus secondary headaches. Making use of such definitions will aid an organised approach to a symptom with a wide and varied differential diagnosis. It may be that in the first instance a candidate will exclude the features of common primary headaches before going on to ask closed questions in respect of a secondary cause.

Primary disorders are those not associated with an underlying pathology and commonly include migraine, tension-type, and cluster headache.

Secondary disorders – headache attributed to an underlying pathological condition. Includes any head pain of infectious, neoplastic, vascular or drug-induced origin.

It is also useful to think about acute versus chronic in terms of an objective measure. While you are unlikely to encounter an acute headache caused by a bleed or infection be precise when attributing chronicity to a headache.

Narrow the differential and think about patterns of symptoms associated with headaches.

Primary headaches

Migraine

Frequently unilateral and pulsating, with an insidious onset lasting up to 72 hours. Commonly associated with aura, nausea, and sensitivity to light and tinnitus or sensitivity to sound. Worse with activity, preference to lie in the dark, resolution with sleep. Recurrent episodes aggravated by routine physical exertion, with chronic history. Look for a family history.

Tension-type headache

Frequent or continuous, mild to moderate in

severity, and importantly bilateral. May be described as band or vice-like, occipital or frontal pain that spreads to the entire head that is often worst at the end of the day.

Cluster headache

Rapid onset of severe headaches, lasting from 15 minutes to 3 hours. Commonly multiple attacks on the same day. Prominent unilateral orbitotemporal focus and may have trigeminal involvement with lacrimation or flushing.

Secondary headaches

Regarding secondary headaches consider the diagnosis of secondary headache in patients presenting with new onset headache or headache that differs from their usual headache. In order of importance in this setting:

Analgesia headache

Remains a diagnosis of exclusion but requires a clear history of significant analgesia use. This should be excluded in all patients with chronic headache, as defined above.

Benign intracranial hypertension

This is a key diagnosis to consider where the scenario is with a young woman as there is a predilection for young woman in the third decade. There is a migraine-like headache, but it is associated with diplopia, pulsatile tinnitus, and loss of peripheral vision. Be alert to risk factors, classically obesity and medication such as the oral contraceptive. There is some evidence of a link to demyelinating disease and lupus and this may be a consideration. With a similar risk factor profile, and in pregnancy, also consider venous thrombosis.

Infection

Infection is worth excluding and may include sinusitis or dental problems. Sinusitis is likely with positional facial (on leaning forward – 'like a bowling ball') or tooth pain accompanied by a clear history of illness, fever, or rhinorrhea. Dental abscess occurs on a background of poor dentition, aggravated by mastication. Often it causes pain that is sharp and shooting in nature, with pain referral to the ear or temple.

Acute angle-closure glaucoma

Unilateral: Halos around lights, decreased visual acuity, conjunctival injection, vomiting.

Giant cell arteritis

Unilateral throbbing pain: Exacerbated by touch often described as pain when combing hair. Associated with visual disturbances and jaw claudication.

Mass effect – neoplastic

While the most common cause of early morning headaches is in fact migraine, classically this will raise alarm bells to the possibility of mass effect. Seek to elicit evidence of diplopia, particularly on looking laterally (false localising sign). Pain aggravated by postural changes, straining, or coughing. Altered behaviour where frontal lobe involvement. New onset seizures possible. Vomiting or focal neurologic deficits with significant mass effect. This may be what the patient is most worried about and may be the elephant in the room. Be prepared to raise the topic, even where the symptoms may not warrant it.

Where there is a history of HIV or cancer the threshold for further investigating a headache is lower, thus ensure you ask the patient about any known diagnosis or consider screening for symptoms suggesting their involvement.

> ## Open questioning suggests a diagnosis of headache due to persistent analgesia

With this diagnosis closed questioning should focus on the following

Be clear as to the exact analgaesia used. Attempt to build up a timeline with the patient, establishing at what point different medication were trialed, in what strength and quantities. Not only will this be crucial to any potential diagnosis but it may prove insightful for the patient and aid comprehension of subsequent discussions.

Explore concerns, ideas, and expectations

- What does the patient attribute the headaches to? Be prepared to discuss cancer and think carefully as to the language used
- Pay particular attention to the social history and identify areas of stress
- Explore substance misuse. Does she believe that the use of too many pain killers could cause her symptoms or represent a problem in relation to substance misuse?
- Screen for symptoms of depression, which may contribute to the presentation as a source of headache and negatively impact upon the perception of symptoms and ability to cope

What to tell the patient

Be guided by the content in the history to inform the patient as to what you think the underlying diagnosis is, what investigations may be necessary and any management options that may be used.

In this case, the patient has been using opiate-based analgesia and will need to stop such medications given the likely diagnosis of headache due to overuse of analgesia.

Arrange a shared plan with the patient either to review results or to return (to this case to her GP, but in other situations a repeat clinic review) to assess progress.

What to tell the examiner

Summarise the clinical case

'The patient has a recent history of headaches, without red flag symptoms, which has continued in the setting of persistent opiate use and in the absence of symptoms of another diagnosis.'

Investigations

Full neurological examination, fundoscopy and blood pressure check are indicated.

Neuroimaging is not indicated in patients with a clear history of primary headache; without red flag features of a potential secondary headache; and a normal neurological examination.

In settings where imaging with CT or MRI is agreed, it is important to counsel the patient with regard to what you are looking to exclude and warn them that such investigations may demonstrate incidental findings not related to their symptoms that may warrant further investigation in of themselves.

Management

Assess analgesia prescribing using the WHO pain ladder, advising the patient to avoid opiate-based analgesia. The treatment of analgesia headaches should be with abrupt withdrawal in the case of simple analgesia or triptans, or gradual withdrawal of opiates. Headaches are likely to initially worsen. Prophylactic medication may be of some benefit.

The management of other types of headache is discussed below:

- Acute management of migraine involves simple analgesia and the use of tryptans. Subsequent management involves the avoidance of precipitants and, if necessary, the use of prophylactic medications. Importantly women with migraine associated with aura, or over 35 years and without aura, should not use a combined oral contraceptive pill due to increased relative risk of stroke
- Benign intracranial hypertension should be investigated with CT and lumbar puncture. Management is weight loss and stopping of medication thought to be causing symptoms. Diuretics or steroids may be useful and surgical treatment can be considered, where there is concern about eyesight, with optic nerve sheath fenestration and shunting
- Giant cell arteritis investigated with ESR and CRP, biopsy, occasionally imaging with angiography and treatment predominantly with steroids
- Headaches in pregnancy should be treated in the first instance with paracetamol. MRI with contrast venography should be considered where concern relates to potential venous thrombosis

Case 155: Visual disturbance

Candidate information

Scenario

As the registrar in the rapid-access TIA clinic, you are asked to see a 73-year-old man who has been referred by Accident and Emergency overnight having presented with an episode of acute visual loss. Please take a history from the patient. Inform the patient of your findings and inform them of your management plan.

Actor information

Last night you noted deterioration in your vision that occurred suddenly. You promptly presented to Accident and Emergency where you were reviewed by a doctor who indicated you might have suffered a 'mini-stroke'.

Prior to entering the room

The history of acute visual disturbance may involve the discussion of a plethora of symptoms ranging from flashing lights and floaters to blurring, disturbance of colour, or loss of vision. While the nature of the visual disturbance will doubtless provide sufficient grounds for discussion in of itself, be aware that the underlying aetiology is likely to prompt discussion of larger themes in medical practice such as diabetes, transient ischaemic attacks and stroke, or conditions predisposing to vascular occlusions such as sickle cell disease. Thus, be sure to take cues from the station information and the patient in tailoring your approach to the discussion. The strong candidate will succinctly gather details of the visual disturbance before considering information relevant to the context, such as risk stratification of cerbrovascular disease, or diabetes control, for instance.

On entering the room, begin with open questioning

Allow the patient to describe their symptoms, initially without prompting, but be sure to establish key features that will enable the differential to be narrowed. In all cases of visual loss, establish the following features:

- Painful or painless
- Monocular or binocular visual loss – although important, recognise the limitations

of establishing this in retrospect without the luxury of examination when symptomatic.

- Partial or total
- Transient or persistent – establish the duration of the episode
- Sudden or gradual in onset

Discriminating between monocular and binocular visual loss can be invaluable in considering the underlying cause. Monocular visual loss implies a disorder anterior to the optic chiasm, likely affecting the structure of the eye or the optic nerve. Transient binocular visual loss suggests a more posterior process, involving the optic chiasm, tracts, or radiations, or the visual cortex.

Thereafter, consider – partial versus total and acute versus gradual visual loss.

Partial versus total visual loss

Causes of partial visual disturbance include:

- Stroke – homonymous hemianopia
- Pituitary tumour – bitemporal hemianopia
- Retinal vascular occlusion – horizontal
- Glaucoma – peripheral field loss
- Macular degeneration – central field loss
- Migraine

Causes of total visual loss include:
Acute:
- Amaurosis fugax
- Temporal arteritis
- Optic neuritis
- Central retinal vein/artery occlusion
- Papilloedema – raised ICP

Gradual:
- Cataract
- Glaucoma
- Diabetic retinopathy

A typical history of painless monocular, transient, total visual loss is consistent with amaurosis fugax and transient ischaemic attack. The patient may describe the classical 'curtain descending across the visual field'. The symptoms should satisfy the criteria of TIA, lasting typically for a period of minutes, and resolving completely within 24 hours. Where symptoms last more than 24 hours with no residual disability, consider the diagnosis of a non-disabling stroke.

Open questioning suggests a transient ischaemic attack

With this diagnosis closed questioning should focus on the following

Seek further evidence of carotid territory attacks including hemiparaesis, hemisensory loss, or dysphasia.
Clarify:

- Whether aspirin was given at the time of the symptoms
- Identify whether previous episodes possible. Importantly, two or more TIAs in a week constitute crescendo TIAs and correlates to a higher risk of stroke
- Establish ABCD2 risk of stroke

Explore concerns, ideas, and expectations

Visual loss is a concerning symptom. The patient may know the relevance of TIAs in relation to stroke risk and may be concerned about the implications in relation to future disease.

What to tell the patient

'I suspect you have had a transient ischaemic attack. The risk of stroke after a TIA in the first 5 years is approximately 7% per annum. It is important to treat your modifiable risk factors, such as treating hypertension, stopping smoking and reducing your cholesterol, to prevent a stroke from happening in the future. I would like to organise some investigation today in our clinic to rule out common sources of problems that we may be able to treat and reduce your overall risk.'

What to tell the examiner

Summarise the clinical case

'This patient describes symptoms consistent with a transient ischaemic attack. I would examine the patient in full, looking for any evidence of neurologic deficit but also perform ophthalmoscopy to look for cholesterol emboli and auscultate for carotid bruits.'

Investigations

Investigations are preferably performed within 1 week of symptoms. The ABCD2 score, if high, may mandate inpatient investigations.

- If high risk (ABCD2 score > or crescendo TIA in whom vascular territory is uncertain) diffusion-weighted MRI head
- Carotid Doppler to look for atherosclerotic plaques
- Blood pressure
- Risk stratification tests including fasting lipids and glucose
- ECG and Holter monitor to look for atrial fibrillation and echocardiogram to rule out cardiac thrombus

Management

Management aspects include lifestyle modification:

- Wight loss
- Stop smoking
- Exercise

Further reading

Johnston SC, Rothwell PM, Nguyen-Huynh MN, et al. Validation and refinement of scores to predict very early stroke risk after transient ischaemic attack. Lancet 2007; 369:283–292.
Ferguson GG, Eliasziw M, Barr HW, et al. The North American Symptomatic Carotid Endarterectomy Trial: surgical results in 1415 patients. Stroke 1999; 30:1751–1758.
European Carotid Surgery Trialists' Collaborative Group.Randomised trial of endarterectomy for recently symptomatic carotid stenosis: final results of the MRC European Carotid Surgery Trial (ECST). Lancet 1998; 351:1379–1387.

Case 156: Tremor

Candidate information

Scenario

You are the registrar in the general medical clinic. You are asked to see a 68-year-old retired university lecturer who is attending for a review following a recent hospital admission. An accompanying letter from his General Practitioner raises concerns over a tremor that has been present for the last 18 months. Last month a fall resulted in a minor head injury necessitating a short stay for observation, although the discharge summary made no reference to the tremor. Please take a history from the patient. Inform the patient of your findings and inform them of your management plan.

Actor information

Your GP has referred you to the medical clinic because of a tremor that has become apparent over the past year and a half. Your wife has also noted that you have been getting more forgetful over a similar period.

Prior to entering the room

In assessing tremor as a presenting complaint, be mindful that the most common tremors encountered in clinical practice are essential tremor and those related to Parkinsonism. The strong candidate will take cues from the scenario in considering the latter but not rush to a presumptive diagnosis. The key to this station will be to evaluate the tremor leading to a larger diagnosis and gauge the patient's insight and readiness for such news, employing warning shots where possible and arranging for further investigation or review to ensure a safety net.

On entering the room begin with open questioning

For all tremors, consider categorising based on those occurring at rest, related to posture, or related to movement/intention. This will itself discriminate between a wide range of causes. Thereafter, consider a general review of symptoms and evaluate:

- Duration of symptoms and acuity of onset – insidious or abrupt. In any case of abrupt onset tremor, exclude drugs, toxins or trauma as a cause.
- Body parts affected – predominantly upper/lower limbs, but also consider the face
- Alleviating or exacerbating factors such as caffeine and alcohol

Narrow the list of differential diagnoses based on the character of the tremor.

Resting tremor, occurring with the limb supported from gravity:

- Parkinson's disease – low frequency, 'pill rolling', unilateral classically of the hand
- Drug-induced Parkinsonism

Postural tremor, with the limb maintained in a position against gravity:

- Essential – slow, coarse or fine, symmetrical tremor, usually involving the upper limbs but often also the head and voice
- Dystonic
- Drug induced
- Alcohol or drug withdrawal – associated with diaphoretic symptoms and hallucinations
- Hyperthyroidism
- Decompensated liver disease or renal failure – often in the context of encephalopathy
- Physiological – fine, rapid tremor occurring in healthy individuals commonly alleviated or suppressed by alcohol

Intention tremor, during purposeful voluntary movement:

- Cerebellar pathology – alcohol/demyelinating disease/CVA

> **Open questioning suggests a diagnosis of parkinsonism**

With this diagnosis closed questioning should focus on the following

The Parkinson's tremor classically manifests as an insidious onset, over a period of months, usually after the age of 60 years, of a hand at rest. The legs, chin, lips and trunk may also be affected. Typically described as 'pill-rolling', a coarse tremor at a frequency of 5–7 Hz, in a unilateral distribution. Symptoms may progress, with time, to become bilateral and may disappear with action.

Complete the diagnostic triad by enquiring specifically about concomitant bradykinesia and rigidity. Rigidity often precedes tremor in many patients. Look for functional difficulties such as changes in co-ordination relating to problems with every day tasks like buttoning shirtsleeves or tasks requiring a finer degree of manual dexterity.

Ask about balance impairment and changes in gate, posture, or recurrent falls. Commonly falls occur when attempting to turn quickly or with unexpected loss of sure footing with an inability to react due to loss of postural reflexes.

A collateral history will be invaluable, particularly in relation to signs of dementia. Family members or friends might have commented on the patient's facial expression (hypomimia) and flat mood or signs of depression. Interestingly, sleep problems may be an early sign of Parkinson's disease, even before motor symptoms have begun. Some of the common sleep problems for Parkinson's patients include:

- Insomnia
- Nightmares
- REM sleep behavior disorder – acting out dreams during sleep
- Restless leg syndrome
- Sleep apnoea

Review the patient's medications and exclude neuroleptics and anti-emetics that may cause akinetic–rigid syndrome, mimicking the early signs of bradykinesia in Parkinson's disease.

Be sure to get a feel for the social history and the patient's functional capacity as previously alluded to. Ask about the patient's ability to carry out activities of daily living unaided – establish the home set-up, support network and any pre-existing level of care package. It is important that you are seen to assess, the functional and psychosocial effects of the tremor.

Spend time discussing alcohol intake and its relation to symptoms. Also review smoking history and pack years in view of the established inverse association with Parkinson's.

Explore concerns, ideas, and expectations

Allow the patient to express their ideas and concerns as to the potential diagnosis. Prepare for a variety of responses from the patient that could conceivably develop themes of denial, worry and suspicion, or the pragmatic approach.

'I don't mind the tremor; I think it is just my nerves. My leg shook like that for years. My fall was just a silly lack of concentration crossing the street. Surely they have nothing to do with each other. There's nothing serious going on is there doctor?'

'My father experienced something very similar, as a family we never talked about it and I hoped it wouldn't happen to me but I fear the worst doctor.'

'Is this Parkinson's doctor? I have done plenty of reading around the subject but I am confused as to how you can confirm the diagnosis. What do we need to do? I am keen to start treatment early if it will make things better.'

What to tell the patient

'Your symptoms are suggestive of Parkinson's disease, a type of degenerative disease that affects the movement pathways in the brain and typically gives rise to the kind of tremor you describe. Its treatment can be difficult and the disease tends to progress with time. I will give you some more information to read about the disease and its complications and bring you back to discuss all this at length.'

Where appropriate discuss falls prevention and consider an early discussion about cognitive decline, personality changes, depression, lethargy and fatigue, financial planning, insurance, and disability applications.

What to tell the examiner

Summarise the clinical case

'This patient describes symptoms consistent with an akinetic–rigid syndrome, with unilateral hand tremor, rigidity and bradykinesia, all suggestive of Parkinson's disease. Diagnosis is predominantly clinical. Tremor without other characteristic Parkinson's symptoms suggests either early disease or the potential for an alternative diagnosis.'

Investigations

Differentiating between Parkinson's disease and Parkinsonism is largely clinical, assessing the relative importance of drugs or family history and balancing the context of examination findings.

Neuroimaging can be of limited use:

- MRI brain to look for cerebrovascular disease, multiple infarcts and presence of Lewy bodies (if Lewy body dementia is suspected)

- SPECT scan in cases of uncertain Parkinsonism to differentiate between Parkinson's disease and atypical parkinsonisms such as multiple system atrophy and progressive supranuclear palsy and other causes (unassociated with loss of dopaminergic neurons) such as essential or dystonic tremor, medication induced Parkinsonism or tremor.

Management

- Levodopa is the gold standard for motor symptoms used with a peripheral DOPA decarboxylase inhibitor such as carbidopa. Long-term therapy may lead to reduced efficacy, on-off (fluctuations) and dyskinesias.
- MAO-B inhibitors (selegiline) as monotherapy or adjuncts for early onset motor fluctuations

- COMT inhibitors (entacapone)-blocks L dopa metabolism
- Dopamine receptor agonists (pramipexole and ropinirole)
- Apomorphine pump

Patients may require anti-emetics for nausea, atypical neuroleptics and even cholinesterase inhibitors for cognitive impairment or hallucinations.

Further discussion around 'Parkinson-plus' syndromes is possible. These include:

- Multiple system atrophy – extra pyramidal symptoms and autonomic failure
- Progressive supra nuclear palsy – extra pyramidal symptoms, postural instability, falls from failure of downward gaze and dementia
- Lewy body dementia – Parkinsonian features with dementia

Case 157: Established multiple sclerosis

Candidate information

Scenario

A 40-year-old woman with known multiple sclerosis attends the neurology clinic for review. As the SHO covering the clinic you have been asked to take a history from the patient before reviewing the case with your consultant. The patient has been attending the clinic for many years and is keen to hear your opinion on her case. Summarise your understanding and offer a management plan.

Actor information

You have presented for your yearly review.

Prior to entering the room

Chronic disease, diagnosed early in life, predisposes to a multitude of problems. Be prepared to encounter issues relating to disease progression and treatment, often complicated by anxiety and depression. Reviews in clinic represent an important link to the healthcare team, offering patients an opportunity to talk openly about their condition, seek reassurance, and gain support for often seemingly insurmountable challenges. Aim to cover a review of symptoms, an assessment of disease progression, evaluation of any response to treatment and challenges related to side effects.

On entering the room begin with open questioning

It can be useful in such a scenario, where the patient returns on a regular basis, to enquire as to their health and circumstances since the last review. This will encourage the discussion to develop around themes driven by the patient. That said, all patients with chronic disease, and particularly those with MS where the diagnosis is typically made early in the third or fourth decade, develop close relationships with their healthcare team. Thus, consider introducing yourself as a new member of the team, and asking them to give you a summary of their case.

Attempt to explore the details surrounding their diagnosis, including symptoms, tests and results as the patient understands them.

Establish the type of MS, and in doing so, clearly demonstrate to the examiner an understanding of the distinction between relapsing–remitting and progressive disease:

- Complete or near-complete resolution of symptoms between attacks: relapsing–remitting MS
- Development of steady progression without resolution between exacerbations after an initial course of relapsing–remitting disease: secondary progressive MS
- Steady progression without resolution of symptoms between exacerbations: primary progressive disease

Attempt to highlight the variation in symptoms between attacks, consistent with indiscriminate demyelination throughout the central nervous system. Patients are likely to have experienced a range of symptoms, albeit subtle in many cases, but commonly one or more of:

- Visual disturbance associated with optic neuritis, often pain and partial loss of vision of one eye
- Blurred vision or monocular blindness due to ocular palsy/inter-nuclear ophthalmoplegia
- Loss of colour vision
- Sensorimotor disturbance
- Assymetrical spastic paraparesis
- Paraesthesia
- Dysaesthesia of limbs
- Thermal dysaesthesia

Enquire as to the effect of hot weather, hot baths or saunas on symptoms as related to Uhthoff's phenomenon.

Open questioning suggests a diagnosis of multiple sclerosis

With this diagnosis closed questioning should focus on the following

There is likely to be a central theme that will become the focus of the discussion in this scenario. Moving from open to closed questioning will require tact given the sensitive nature of themes that will range from pregnancy or self catheterisation in young women to worsening symptoms with poor prognosis and disease progression in the older patient.

Enquire specifically about current symptoms and resultant level of disability, commonly:

- Visual problems such as eye movement trouble, diplopia or oscillopsia
- Spasticity and/or tremor with mobility issues
- Pain and paroxysmal features
- Bladder disturbance including urgency, retention and recurrent UTIs
- Impotence
- Fatigue
- Depression
- Memory and thinking

Screen past medical history, specifically asking the patient if they ever experienced seizures or have a pre-existing diagnosis of epilepsy. Clarify current medication and treatments. Be sure to gather a focused social history including assessment of the patients support network, package of care, and coping strategies. Screen for signs of depression where appropriate, even if thought unlikely. Be alert to excessive alcohol use.

Explore concerns, ideas, and expectations

Be prepared for varying themes, introduced by the patient, which may change the direction of the consultation. Three common examples are discussed here: childbearing, urinary problems and treatment issues.

'My partner and I are keen to start a family'; MS commonly affects young women of child bearing age necessitating clear information from the candidate surrounding pregnancy related questions:

- MS should not prohibit patients from becoming pregnant
- There is no evidence that MS is inherited
- Symptoms may in fact improve during pregnancy in some patients however there is thought to be a high risk of relapse postnatally
- Current recommendations relating to disease modifying drugs such as α-interferon suggest stopping prior to conception where possible.

'I can't seem to pass enough urine, constantly feel like I want to go, and keep suffering from infections. A friend from my support group self-catheterises, but I'm just not sure that I could cope with that'. Involvement of the spinal column often results in bladder dysfunction, ranging from mild urgency or hesitancy, to partial retention or incontinence, and frank incontinence in advanced disease. Treatment of recurrent infections due to retention is not uncommon and can have a significant bearing on quality of life, including sexual appetite and wellbeing. Self-catheterisation can offer patients control and reduce infections when used with appropriate antibiotic cover. Self-care can be facilitated through specialist nurses and community teams to offer guidance and support initially.

Poor response to treatment: 'I feel like things are just getting worse, are there other treatments that might help?' Be sure to consider not only disease modifying drugs and the use of steroids for acute flares, but also treatment of symptoms in of themselves and, importantly, depression. This may necessitate a discussion of management with the patient other than predominantly with the examiner – see below.

What to tell the patient

The discussion with the patient will very much depend upon the themes that form the focus of the history. Naturally, where there is any doubt as to the established diagnosis then this should be reflected in the proposal of further investigation, although this would be more likely in an appropriate scenario of new diagnosis. Be mindful that diagnosis relies on a thorough history to establish discrete neurological manifestations, which, in the first instance, are often subtle. Thereafter, MRI brain and spinal cord to demonstrate plaques consistent with MS. Where there is doubt, evoked potentials and/or cerbrospinal fluid testing for oligoclonal bands is prudent.

A hollistic approach to the ongoing management will be key. The strong candidate will try to offer a plan going forward that will incorporate specialist referrals where necessary, community support from specialist nursing teams, adequate information re support groups and sources of additional information, and timely subsequent clinic review. Changes to, or initiation of, drug treatment should not distract from the wealth of alternative discussion points.

What to tell the examiner
Summarise the clinical case

Succinct summary of the patient's diagnosis, profile of symptoms and frequency of relapses, current management and ongoing issues. Thereafter, targeted discussion of salient features from the history. Try to steer the discussion towards topics of interest, such as novel treatments, or focus on specific symptoms that were most troublesome to the patient.

Investigations

The diagnosis of multiple sclerosis is predominantly a clinical one. However imaging and investigations can be used to support the diagnosis, in line with the McDonald criteria.

A diagnosis can be made on the basis of 2 or more relapses and 2 or more objective clinical lesions.

- MRI – evidence of cerebral, classically periventricular, or cord plaques. There is no consensus on the role for serial imaging with MRI to monitor the response to treatment or progression of disease
- Evoked potentials relate to electrical signals generated in the central nervous system in response to sensory stimulation of peripheral nerves. Visual evoked potentials are slowed
- Lumbar puncture with CSF analysis – oligoclonal IgG bands

Management

Be clear as to the rationale for treatment of acute flares versus disease modifying drugs and treatment of specific symptoms.

Acute relapses:

- Steroids – used to reduce severity and length of acute relapse.

Disease modifying drugs:

- Beta interferon – decreases the frequency of relapses and delays disability but does not alter disease progression. No role in progressive disease
- Glatiramer – analogue of a component of myelin basic protein thought to act as a decoy for the immune system
- Mitoxantrone – immunosuppressant used in progressive disease
- Natalizumab – monoclonal antibody, directed against adhesion molecule α_4-integrin, reducing leukocyte passage across the blood–brain barrier

Symptom control:

- Spasticity – baclofen or dantrolene, botulinum toxin and physiotherapy
- Tremor – clonazepam, gabapentin
- Fatigue – amantadine, selegiline
- Bladder disturbance – anti-cholinergics, e.g. oxybutinin or tolterodine, intermittent self-catheterisation or it may be that the switch from self-catheterisation to long-term or supraprubic catheterisation is necessary

- Impotence – sildenafil
- Depression – tricyclic or SSRI, consider counselling referral
- Pain and paroxysmal features – carbamazepine, gabapentin
- Visual problems – ophthalmology referral (exclude acute flare)

- Neuropsychological referral

Multi-disciplinary team involvement is important and may require input from a wide range of healthcare professionals (neurologist, GP, specialist nurse, occupational therapy, physiotherapy, counselling team).

Case 158: Fever in the returning traveller

Candidate information

Scenario

You are the medical registrar on call. This 40-year-old man has presented to Accident and Emergency with febrile illness for the last 3 weeks and has been referred for further investigation. Please take a history from the patient. Inform the patient of your findings and management plan.

Actor information

You have recently returned from an extended trip to Zambia and have been feeling unwell since your arrival back in the UK. You did not take malaria prophylaxis.

Prior to entering the room

Definitions for pyrexia of unknown origin (PUO) vary, but it refers to a fever, persistent for a number of weeks with the cause not found despite appropriate initial investigations.
Consider the differential diagnosis:

- Malaria
- Enteric fever (typhoid/paratyphoid)
- Viral hepatitis
- Ricketsia
- Dengue

The most common causes of PUO are:

- Malignancy
- TB
- Endocarditis
- Gallbladder disease
- HIV infection
- Auto-immune disorders

On entering the room begin with open questioning

Explore the patient's symptoms and establish the onset and duration of symptoms in relation to travel history. Prompt the history where appropriate with a generalised review of symptoms.
Take a full travel history including short stays and airport transfers considering the possible infections associated with different areas:

- Tropics or sub-Saharan Africa (malaria)
- Africa (rickettsia, ameobiasis, katayama, visceral leishmaniasis)
- South/Southeast Asia (enteric fever)
- Middle East (brucellosis)
- Others (leptospirosis, trypanosomisasis and viral hemorrhagic fever)

Enquire about associated symptoms:

- Fever with rash (dengue, HIV, ricketsia, schistosomiasis)
- Fever with jaundice (leptospirosis, viral hepatitis, yellow fever)
- Fever, headache, myalgia, arthralgia and malaise (malaria)
- Constipation/diarrhoea, dry cough (enteric fever)
- Rash, night sweats, weight loss, diarrhoea (often seen in HIV)

Ask about accommodation, confirming whether it was rural or urban. Go on to enquire about the activities undertaken, with associated risk in mind, including sexual encounters, drug use and exposure to foreign healthcare systems.

Open questioning suggests a diagnosis of malaria

With this diagnosis closed questioning should focus on the following

Establish pre-travel precautions, such as anti-malaria prophylaxis (note that correct prophylaxis with full adherence does not exclude malaria), and the use, if any, of a mosquito net or insect repellents.

Exclude complications:

- Confusion, seizures or a reduction in Glasgow coma scale: cerebral malaria
- Dark red or black urine: blackwater fever

Explore concerns, ideas, and expectations

If the patient has traveled to an endemic area (or if they know people who have had the condition) they may be concerned about malaria. Allow them to vocalise their concerns and address these appropriately.

What to tell the patient

'I suspect the symptoms you are describing may be related to an infection you might have caught whilst abroad, namely malaria. It is a tropical disease that is transmitted by mosquitoes through bites. You can become sick very quickly but it is entirely treatable. We can confirm the diagnosis with blood tests, which will also direct the appropriate treatment. However it is safer for you to be admitted to hospital to undergo the investigations and receive the correct treatment and we can monitor you for any complications such as breathing problems or liver problems. Do you have any questions?'

What to tell the examiner

Summarise the clinical case

'This patient gives a history suggestive of malaria. The main differential would be enteric fever (although he has not returned from an endemic area), HIV seroconversion and viral hepatitis. I would proceed to a full examination, to look for evidence rash, eschar, hepatosplenomegaly, lymphadenopathy or jaundice although examination findings might be non-specific.'

Investigations

Investigations would include:

- Blood film and rapid diagnostic test for malaria (regardless of whether or not malaria prophylaxis has been taken)
- FBC – lymphopenia common in viral infection and typhoid, eosinophilia often seen in parasitic or fungal infection, and thrombocytopenia in malaria, dengue, acute HIV, typhoid
- Serum save
- HIV testing in all patients
- Hepatitis A,B,C
- Urinalysis: haemoglobinuria in malaria, proteinuria and haematuria in leptospirosis
- Blood cultures
- Stool and urine cultures
- G6PD (especially before primaquine treatment)

Management

The management of malaria depends on whether the causative parasite is falciparum or non-falciparum. Chloroquine followed by primaquine for non-falciparum. Quinine and doxycycline for uncomplicated falciparum.

Case 159: Sore, stiff hands

Candidate information

Scenario

You are the registrar in rheumatology clinic. This 40-year old woman has been referred by her GP with a history of sore, stiff hands. Please take a history from the patient. Inform the patient of your findings and your management plan.

Actor information

You have been referred to clinic with worsening pain and stiffness in your hands. This is affecting your ability to carry out simple tasks such as opening jars.

Prior to entering the room

Consider the differential diagnosis of sore, stiff hands:

- Arthritis
  - Rheumatoid
  - Osteoarthritis
  - Psoriatic
- SLE
- Crystal Arthropathy – Gout

On entering the room begin with open questioning

'I understand from your GP you have been troubled with stiff hands. Could you tell me about the problems that you are experiencing?'

Screen for a rheumatological history. Establish the nature of pain, stiffness, swelling, deformity, disability and systemic illness. Be clear in relation to the onset, duration and timing of symptoms, particularly early morning stiffness.

Unless already covered, enquire about: Other joint involvement:

- Symmetrical PIP, MCP, wrist, knee, ankle, MTPs – commonly seen in RA
- C-spine, thoracolumbar, first CMC, DIP, patellofemoral – commonest in OA
- First MTP – commonest in gout

Associated joint symptoms

- Stiffness, especially morning stiffness
- Swelling
- Deformity

Systemic features

- Fever
- Weight loss
- Tiredness
- Breathlessness

Open questioning suggests a diagnosis of rheumatoid arthritis

With this diagnosis closed questioning should focus on the following

Important negatives include:

- Psoriatic arthritis: rash
- Reiter's syndrome: urethritis, conjunctivitis
- Reactive arthritis: post dysentery
- Ankylosing spondylitis: low back pain and stiffness, asymmetrical peripheral arthritis (hips, knees, shoulders)
- Gout: mono-articular arthritis, usually big toe or knee

Establish current medication. Is there relief from NSAIDs suggestive of inflammatory arthritis? Does the patient take any diuretics, especially thiazides, which may precipitate gout?

Ask about extra-articular manifestations:

Eyes

- Keratoconjunctivitis sicca
- Scleritis: painful red eye
- Episcleritis: uncomfortable red eye

Cardioplumonary

- Pericarditis
- Pleuritic chest pain or shortness of breath
- Interstitial fibrosis

Neurological

- Carpal tunnel
- Peripheral neuropathy

Explore concerns, ideas, and expectations

Are they particularly concerned about the lack of function? The patient's job is of particular importance given the relative dependence on manual dexterity in both the work place and activities of daily living.

What to tell the patient

'I suspect you have a condition called rheumatoid arthritis, an inflammatory disease that affects the joints. I need to examine you and organise some tests to confirm the diagnosis. Depending on the tests and your symptoms we will discuss treatment which often involves painkillers and often disease-modifying drugs to suppress disease activity.'

What to tell the examiner

Summarise the clinical case

'The patient gives a history suggestive of rheumatoid arthritis as evidenced by morning stiffness lasting more than 30 minutes for more than 6 weeks, involving 3 joint areas, including both wrists.'

Mention if there is evidence of extra-articular manifestations.

'I would examine all the joints, looking for boggy synovial thickening and joint effusions as well as rheumatoid nodules.'

Investigations

An appropriate investigative strategy would include:

- Rheumatoid factor
- Anti-CCP antibodies
- FBC-normocytic anaemia, raised WCC and raised platelets with acute phase response)
- ESR may be elevated
- Plain radiographs for diagnosis of erosions. Radiological changes in affected joints are loss of bone density on either side of the joint, soft tissue swelling, erosions, loss of joint space, deformity (subluxation or complete dislocation)
- Synovial fluid aspiration: straw coloured with raised WCC (not done routinely)

Management

Important points in the patient's management include:

- Symptomatic relief with adequate pain relief, reduction of stiffness and swelling
- Early referral to the multi-disciplinary team
- DMARDs within 12 weeks of disease onset – methotrexate remains first line
- Biological medications such as infliximab or etanercept

Case 160: Back pain

Candidate information

Scenario

You are the SHO in the rheumatology clinic. A 30-year-old man has been referred with insidious onset lower back pain and stiffness. Please take a history from the patient and discuss a relevant management plan.

Actor information

You have noted lowed back pain and stiffness, which has been worsening recently. You cannot remember any accidents or trauma that could have caused the back pain.

Prior to entering the room

Consider the differential diagnosis of back pain, which includes:

- Traumatic
- Infective – osteomyelitis, TB
- Inflammatory – ankylosing spondylitis, discitis
- Neoplastic
- Metabolic – osteoporosis, osteomalacia
- Degenerative – osteoarthritis
- Vascular – aortic aneurysm/dissection

On entering the room begin with open questioning

Ask about the onset of the pain. Sudden onset back pain can be trauma-related, due to disc lesions or pathological fracture. Gradual pain may suggest degenerative disease.

Consider exacerbating/relieving factors, such as:

- Aggravation on movement/relief by rest in mechanical
- Worst after rest: inflammatory
- Worse on cough/strain: intervertebral disc prolapse
- Morning stiffness: ankylosing spondylitis

Consider the patient's age as a predictor of likely aetiology:

- 15–30: traumatic, ankylosing spondylitis (especially in males)
- 30–50: degenerative, prolapsed disc, malignancy
- >50: degenerative, osteoporosis, myeloma
- Older women: osteoporosis

Screen for associated symptoms:

- Abdominal pain, dysuria, menorrhagia
- Night sweats, fever in infective
- Sensorimotor symptoms/bladder involvement (degenerative/cord compression)
- Sciatica (degenerative)

The past medical history may offer important context for current symptoms:

- Malignancy
- Menopause (osteoporosis)
- Gastrectomy (osteomalacia)
- Diabetes (infective)
- Immunosuppression (infective)

Open questioning suggests a diagnosis of ankylosing spondylitis

With this diagnosis closed questioning should focus on the following

Systems review should include questions about extra-articular manifestations/complications:

- Iritis
- Plantar fasciitis
- Hip/knee involvement
- Crohn's/UC
- Rashes: psoriasiform dermatitis
- Peri-/myocarditis

Consider Red Flag symptoms, including:

- <20 years or >55 years
- Weight loss
- Pyrexia
- Painful spine in all movements
- Localised bony tenderness
- Continuous non-mechanical pain

The patient is young and male and has no red-flag symptoms. The pain is worse in the morning. The most likely diagnosis is ankylosing spondylitis.

Explore concerns, ideas, and expectations

This young man has potentially debilitating symptoms, which have been chronic. Explore functional limitations and impact with potential disability.

What to tell the patient

'From what you tell me, I suspect your back pain is caused by a condition called ankylosing spondylitis, where there is inflammation in the spine. We will need to carry out some investigations to confirm the diagnosis. Once the investigations are done we will see you again in clinic to advise on specific treatment options.' In the interim I would like to offer you suitable analgaesia and make a pre-emptive referral to physiotherapy.'

What to tell the examiner
Summarise the clinical case

'I suspect the diagnosis is ankylosing spondylitis, given the young age of the male patient, sacroiliac joint involvement and stiffness. I would complete my diagnosis after examination to look for features of ankylosing spondylitis such as exaggerated thoracic kyphosis, compensatory hyperextension of neck, loss of lumbar lordosis, fixed flexion of knees, compensatory flexion of knees.'

Investigations

- FBC: normochromic, normocytic anaemia
- ESR: may be elevated
- Rheumatoid factor: negative
- Radiology: spinal radiographs may show: sacroilitis, squaring of lumbar vertebrae, bamboo spine. Further imaging may be required

Management

Principles of management include:

- Conservative and symptomatic
- Exercise, analgesia
- DMARDs for peripheral, but not axial symptoms
- Biological therapy

Case 161: Established diabetes

Candidate information

Scenario

You are the endocrinology SHO. This 60-year-old woman is attending the diabetes clinic for annual review of her type-2 diabetes. Please take a history from the patient. Discuss any concerns in relation to current disease control, explaining any proposed changes to her management.

Actor information

You were diagnosed with type 2 diabetes 10 years ago. You have come to clinic today for your annual review. Despite an absence of symptoms, your GP tells you that the blood tests you have had done recently mean that you need tablets to 'control the sugar levels'. You were started on medication 1 year ago and had another tablet added 2 months ago.

Prior to entering the room

In a patient with established diabetes, seek to:

- Optimise glycaemic control
- Assess modifiable risk factors
- Screen for complications

On entering the room, begin with open questioning

Explore the diagnosis, clarifying the initial symptoms and subsequent management. Be clear on the progress of the disease and reasons necessitating changes to medication and control of current symptoms. Attempt to gauge compliance not only with medication but with modifiable risk factors relevant to tight glycaemic control including diet, alcohol intake, and exercise.

> **Open questioning suggests a diagnosis of poorly controlled and/or complicated diabetes**

With this diagnosis closed questioning should focus on the following

Closed questioning should focus on symptoms relating to diabetic control, complications of diabetes and side effects of current medications.

Diabetic control

- HbA1c levels and home fingerprick glucose levels
- History of hypoglycaemia attacks: frequency, severity and awareness
- Hyperosmolar hyperglycaemic state (HHS)
- Weight and trend of weight loss or gain

Complications of diabetes

Vascular disease

- Exertional angina or breathlessness
- Intermittent claudication
- Cardiovascular disease may be clinically silent

Kidneys

- Known microalbuminuria/proteinuria
- Haematuria or other urinary symptoms/retention

Retinopathy

- Visual disturbance
- Last retinal screening
- Any retinal laser phototherapy

Neuropathy

- Sensorimotor neuropathy: numbness, tingling and burning. Include issues relating to diabetic feet such as non-healing minor injuries, painless ulceration, deformity requiring podiatry input
- Mononeuritis multiplex: III, VI nerve involvement
- Amyotrophy: painful, wasted quadriceps or pelvifemoral muscles. Ask for difficulty climbing stairs
- Autonomic neuropathy: orthostatic hypotension, urine retention, erectile dysfunction

Ask about the drug history including the current diabetes regimen. Is the patient having any side-effects from their medications? Are they on appropriate medications to lower their cardiovascular risk, such as aspirin, ACE inhibitors and statin medications?

The social history should include an assessment of the patient's smoking history. It is also important to clarify their driving status.

Explore concerns, ideas, and expectations

This is the patient's annual review. Have there been any new developments in the past year that the patient is concerned about? Are there any ongoing and/or unresolved issues from previous clinical reviews?

What to tell the patient

Where concern relates to poor glycaemic control, explain 'I see you have had diabetes for quite a while now. I am concerned that your diabetes is not well-controlled as you seem to be developing some of the recognised complications. It is important to try to achieve consistent sugar control to prevent these complications from progressing further. Therefore, I would like to proceed to examining you and then organise some tests. My impression is you might need to go to the next step of treatment, with the consideration of insulin. In the interim, I cannot stress the importance of helping yourself by being more physically active, losing weight, eating a healthy diet and stopping smoking. It is very important to tell you doctor or GP if you start developing hypoglycaemic symptoms, these might interfere with your ability to drive.'

What to tell the examiner

Summarise the clinical case

'This patient seems to have poorly controlled diabetes on two oral anti-diabetic agents and seems to be developing peripheral neuropathy. I would like to perform a full body examination, including a formal neurological examination.'

Investigations

Appropriate investigations include:

- Bed side tests: blood pressure, urinary dipstick for proteinuria/microalbuminuria
- Blood tests – HbA1c, renal profile, liver function (look for raised transaminases which may suggest non-alcoholic fatty liver disease) and a fasting lipid profile
- Urine protein:creatinine ratio to assess for proteinuria
- Fundoscopy

Management

The management of patients with diabetes is provided through a multi-disciplinary approach.

General health promotion in diabetes includes promoting exercise, weight loss, a balanced diet, and good glycaemic control.

Regarding glycaemic control, if the patient is already established on metformin and sulfonylurea, consideration of a third oral agent (thiazolidinedione or dipeptidyl peptidase 4 inhibitor) is possible or injectable agents (insulin or GLP-1 receptor agonists).

Ensure the patient is on appropriate anti-hypertensive medications, such as ACE inhibitor or ARB.

Case 162: Heat intolerance and weight loss

Candidate information

Scenario

You are the SHO in the endocrinology clinic. This 45-year-old woman presents with heat intolerance and weight loss over the past 5 months. Please take a history from the patient. Inform the patient of your findings and inform them of your management plan.

Actor information

You have become concerned that you have lost weight recently. Through the winter you found yourself wearing very few clothes even when others were wrapping up. Although you are happy that you are saving on central heating you are concerned because your GP told you they think you may have some problems with your thyroid.

Prior to entering the room

Consider the differential diagnosis of weight loss, which includes, but is not restricted to, the following:

- Malignancy, cardiac failure, respiratory disease, malabsorption, renal or liver failure

- Hyperthyroidism, diabetes, Addison's disease
- TB/HIV
- Depression, anorexia

On entering the room begin with open questioning

The patient gives you a 5-month history of weight loss of 2 stone. She has a good appetite and a good dietary intake. She also describes heat intolerance, sweating but no night sweats.

> **Open questioning suggests a diagnosis of hyperthyroidism**

With this diagnosis closed questioning should focus on the following

Screen for systemic manifestations of hyperthyroidism:

- Tremor
- Palpitations, dyspnoea, angina
- Diarrhoea
- Hair loss
- Menstrual irregularity
- Anxiety, insomnia
- Dysphagia, dyspnoea, hoarseness: invasion of malignant lesion

Important negatives:

- Polydypsia and polyuria in diabetes
- Anorexia, malaise, nausea and vomiting, diarrhoea in Addison's (usually cold intolerance)
- Change in bowel habit, PR blood in GI malignancy
- Episodic chest tightness, pins an needles, sweating, abdominal pain, vomiting, syncope in phaeochromocytoma

Past medical history:

- Cardiorespiratory disease, renal or liver failure may all lead to weight loss
- Other auto-immune conditions: Addison's, diabetes, pernicious anaemia, vitiligo: may point to polyendocrine syndrome or autoimmunity

Drug history:

- Lithium and amiodarone may precipitate thyroid disease
- Radiation exposure is a risk factor for benign and malignant thyroid disease
- Self-medication

Is there a family history of auto-immune thyroiditis? Is there a history of medullary thyroid cancer that might raise your suspicions of MEN2?

Systems review:

- Cardiorespiratory: symptoms of heart failure in thyrotoxic cardiomyopathy, angina, atrial fibrillation
- Ophthalmology: visual acuity, colour vision loss
- Skin: pre-tibial myxoedema, onycholysis, vitiligo

Explore concerns, ideas, and expectations

Allow the patient time to inform you of any particular concerns they have. Is there one particular symptom that is worrying them more than others? For example, tremor, which may be considered as relatively minor, may be considered by the patient to be the most debilitating.

What to tell the patient

'Your symptoms are suggestive of an over-active thyroid gland. There can be many causes, although the commonest is antibodies that you have made against your thyroid. I would like to examine you next and order some tests to help establish the diagnosis before I propose treatment.'

What to tell the examiner

Summarise the clinical case

'I suspect this patient has hyperthyroidism. I would proceed to examine her and look for evidence of hyperthyroidism such as goitre, fine tremor, atrial fibrillation and associated features such as ophthalmopathy.'

Investigations

Investigations would include:

- Thyroid function tests: In hyperthyroidism one would expect an undetectable TSH with elevated free T3 and T4
- Antithyroid peroxidise and TSH receptor antibodies
- Technetium-99 radioisotope scan to differentiate Graves from nodular goitre in appropriate cases

Management

Treatment options in hyperthyroidism include:

- Symptom control: propranolol

- Thyroid suppression: Carbimazole (side effects: agranulocytosis, headache, rash, alopecia) or propylthiouracil
- Partial thyroidectomy
- Radioiodine

Case 163: Diabetes insipidus

Candidate information

Scenario

As the endocrinology registrar you have been asked to review a 47-year-old man referred by his GP with with polyuria and polydipsia. When assessed by his GP in the community, he also mentioned problems with his vision and you note that he has also been referred to the neurology clinic for this complaint. Please take a history from the patient. Inform the patient of your findings and discuss your management plan with the examiner.

Actor information

You have been experiencing worrying symptoms recently, including increased thirst and blurred vision. You are concerned because your job as an accountant requires extended periods of concentration, however you have been suffering from a lack of sleep due to the need to pass urine during the night, and are consequently struggling during the day and falling behind with clients and deadlines.

Prior to entering the room

Consider the differential diagnosis of polyuria and polydipsia:

- Diabetes mellitus
- Diabetes insipidus
  - Cranial
    - Idiopathic (ADH deficiency production)
    - Posterior pituitary lesions (craniopharyngioma/pineal gland tumours)
    - Cranial surgery
    - Head trauma
  - Nephrogenic
    - Chronic kidney disease
    - Drugs (lithium, demeclocycline)
      - Hypokalaemia
      - Hypercalcaemia
      - Tubulo-interstitial disease
  - Hereditary (X-linked)
- Excessive fluid intake
  - Psychogenic
  - Drug-induced from anticholingergics
- Drugs, such as diuretics

On entering the room begin with open questioning

The patient is likely to complain of excessive urine production often accompanied by frequency of micturition and excessive thirst, feeling dry no matter how much fluid intake they have. This may disrupt their daily routine and lead to irritability, feeling run down and generally unwell.

Is there a diurnal pattern to the excessive urination? While prostatic disease is relatively unlikely in a 47-year-old man, all things being equal it is important to screen for prostatic symptoms.

> ### Open questioning suggests a diagnosis of diabetes insipidus

With this diagnosis closed questioning should focus on the following

Check for visual symptoms in pituitary tumours or evidence of anterior pituitary hormonal imbalance such as symptoms of thyroid, endocrine, or menstrual problems.

Past medical history:

- Head trauma, head surgery, brain tumours
- Diabetes
- Chronic kidney disease, recent hospital admission with sepsis and haemorrhage all predispose to ATN

- Malignancy and hyperparathyroidism cause chronic hypercalcaemia which can cause polyuria (nephrogenic diabetes insipidus)
- Cardiac history: may implicate fluid balance management and preclude use of vasopressin in treatment

Drug history: Drugs to specifically ask about in the drug history include:

- Therapeutic diuretics
- Opiates (inhibit ADH secretion)
- Lithium/demeclocycline
- Anti-cholingergics (stimulate thirst)
- Nephrotoxic drugs (may precipitate tubular necrosis which can result in severe polyuria)

Take a full family history. Nephrogenic diabetes insipidus is rarely inherited.

Explore concerns, ideas, and expectations

From the candidate instruction it is impossible to tell what the patient's particular concerns (if any) will be. The polyuria and polydipsia may be of secondary importance to him that the visual symptoms. The impact upon his ability to work is likely to be of significance and demand discussion in relation to speed of treatment and possible options to improve symptoms. He may also be concerned in relation to his ability to drive due to the deterioration in his vision.

What to tell the patient

'Your symptoms are compatible with a condition called diabetes insipidus, which is very different from diabetes mellitus, the common form of diabetes. It results from a deregulation in the water level system. If it is left untreated it can lead to severe dehydration and shock. We need to run some more tests to confirm the diagnosis and provide treatment according to the cause.'

What to tell the examiner

Summarise the clinical case

'The patient gives a history of recent onset polyuria and polydipsia with symptoms of dehydration on a background of visual disturbance suggesting central diabetes insipidus possibly from a pituitary tumour such as a craniopharingioma.'

Investigations

Investigations would include:

- Blood tests:
  - Renal function and electrolytes for renal failure, hypernatraemia or hypokalaemia
  - Glucose
  - Paired urine and serum osmolality (also seen the urine for urinary sodium and specific gravity)
- If the biochemical picture suggestive of diabetes insipidus (urine specific gravity < 1.005 with urine osmolality < 200 mOsm/kg, random plasma osmolality > 287) then proceed to a water deprivation test. In diabetes insipidus water deprivation increases plasma osmolality and sodium with no change in urine osmolality. In central diabetes insipidus. Exogenous ADH increases urine osmolality > 50%. In nephrogenic diabetes insipidus exogenous ADH has little or no effect
- MRI brain to look at the pituitary gland

Management

Management of central diabetes insipidus includes:

- Treat the underlying cause
- Medication:
  - Hormonal: desmopressin or vasopressin (avoid the latter in coronary artery disease or give nifedipine)
  - Nonhormonal agents: chlorpropamide, carbamazepine, clofibrate, diuretics (thiazides), and NSAIDs (indomethacin though limited efficacy)

Management of nephrogenic diabetes insipidus includes:

- Conservative management: normal thirst mechanism can self-regulate. Withdraw offending drugs. Optimise renal impairment
- Medication: non-hormonal agents

In an emergency:

- Replace urinary losses with dextrose and water or other hypo-osmolar fluid
- Avoid hyperglycaemia
- Avoid volume overload
- Avoid rapid correction of hypernatraemia. Reduce Na by 0.5 mmol/L every hour

Case 164: Weight gain

Candidate information

Scenario

You are the registrar in endocrinology clinic. A 65-year-old woman has been referred by her GP with concerns relating to weight gain. She is well known to the respiratory service with chronic restrictive airways disease but recently missed her annual review, although she was seen in the cardiology clinic 1-month prior. Please obtain a history, an examination is not required, and discuss your thoughts with the patient including plans for further investigation or management.

Actor information

You were diagnosed at the age of 45 years with idiopathic pulmonary fibrosis. Treatment has proved problematic and you have required long periods of high-dose steroids, which have offered significant benefit and reduced symptoms of breathlessness. Your most recent cardiology review was reassuring with no evidence of heart failure. The weight gain has been progressively worsening over 3 months and is particularly noticeable around your tummy. In fact your legs are very thin. You have also noted your skin to be of poor quality despite liberal use of moisturiser and you have developed prominent 'stretch marks'. While you are not so concerned with regard to your appearance, worryingly your exercise tolerance has been impacted. The GP first referred you to a cardiologist fearing that it may be 'fluid retention' but the doctor who reviewed you in clinic seemed more concerned about your steroids.

Prior to entering the room

Patients with chronic diseases often pose particular challenges, for a number of reasons. The history can often be extensive, demanding an ability to steer the conversation in order to obtain the most relevant information. Achieving this without seeming dismissive of information upon which the patient places great emphasis, but which in reality is of limited value, can be difficult. The potential for complications and side effects increases complicating the case further. The relative increase in exposure to medical professionals will also likely empower the patient to take control of consultations, and become more demanding. Often patients will be very well informed and in possession of vast mounts of detailed knowledge pertaining to their disease. As such you must be clear on the scope of the history and attempt to establish a shared understanding with the patient as to the limitations of time and prioritise the aspects of the case that require more detailed discussion from the outset.

On entering the room begin with open questioning

Invite the patient to give you an overview of her recent symptoms. Where appropriate use the patient information to open up details of the case while maintaining an open approach 'I understand that you are normally reviewed in the respiratory clinic, can you tell me more about that'. Place the symptoms in context of the past medical history.

Seek to quantify the weight gain. Screen for additional symptoms and attempt to narrow the differential. Common causes of weight gain, and associated symptoms, include:

Endocrine

- Cushing's – hirsutism, acne, stretch marks, thin skin, depression, easy bruising, impotence, muscle weakness
- Hypothyroidism – tiredness and lethargy, weakness, cold intolerance, anorexia, dry skin, constipation, menorrhagia
- Polycystic ovarian syndrome – hirsutism, obesity, irregular menses, diabetes

Fluid retention

- Cardiac failure – exertional symptoms including chest pain and breathlessness, peripheral oedema, orthopnoea, and paroxysmal nocturnal dyspnoea
- Renal failure – polyuria, lethargy, peripheral oedema
- Liver disease – ascites

Physiological

- Increased intake with reduced exercise
- Pregnancy – amenorrhoea, nausea, urinary frequency, breast tenderness

Take a detailed drug history paying particular attention to exogenous steroid. Be sure to remain flexible with regard to the differential diagnosis and be seen to screen for other medication with the potential for weight gain:

- Lithium and amiodarone, may cause hypothyroidism
- Calcium channel blockers may lead to peripheral oedema
- Anabolic steroids, growth hormone
- Anti-psychotics such as olanzapine which commonly increases appetite

> ## Open questioning suggests a diagnosis of corticosteroid excess

With this diagnosis closed questioning should focus on the following

Screen for the full constellation of signs and symptoms commonly associated with Cushing's syndrome, including:

- Cushingoid or 'moon' facies
- Centripetal adiposity
- Intra-scapular fat pad – 'buffalo hump'
- Thin atrophic skin
- Poor wound healing and easy bruising
- Abdominal striae
- Weakness with evidence of proximal myopathy

Consider the potential for conditions commonly associated with prolonged exposure to raised levels of corticosteroid include:

- Hypertension
- Insulin resistance or diabetes
- Recurrent infections
- Osteoporosis
- Mental disturbance including low mood and depression

Despite the likelihood of an iatrogenic cause, consider signs and symptoms that might suggest a pituitary adenoma including headaches and visual disturbance which is classically a bitemporal hemianopia. Polyuria and galactorrhoea may also be seen.

Explore concerns, ideas, and expectations

Be prepared to consider different themes introduced by the patient.

'The GP mentioned the possibility of side effects from steroids but was reluctant to change my medication due to the nature and severity of the fibrosis and current breathlessness:

- 'Does this mean I need to stop steroids, and if so how will that impact upon my fibrosis?'
- 'If I stop the steroid, will the weight gain be reversible or can I expect symptoms to continue to get worse?'

What to tell the patient

'From what you tell me, I suspect that the weight gain you have experienced is due to a condition called Cushing's syndrome, caused by the steroid used to treat your fibrosis. I would like to arrange for some tests to confirm the diagnosis. It will be important to get the input of the respiratory team in making adjustments to your medication and consider alternative management options.'

What to tell the examiner

Summarise the clinical case

Demonstrate an understanding of the potential causes of Cushing's syndrome, other than exogenous steroid. Be clear in relation to Cushing's disease, causing Cushing's syndrome as the result of excess pituitary production of ACTH, usually secondary to a pituitary tumour. Re-iterate that the patient did not complain of symptoms of raised intracranial pressure of visual disturbance to offer clinical context.

Investigations

In suspected Cushing's syndrome investigations seek to confirm the diagnosis, rule out significant complications, and distinguish between the potential causes.

The diagnosis is largely clinical but it is useful to confirm raised cortisol levels with random testing and 24-hour urinary collection measuring free cortisol.

Urine dipstick can be useful in assessing for glycosuria and excluding hypokalaemia on blood testing would be prudent.

Dexamethasone testing and ACTH measurement:

- Low dose dexamethasone suppression testing demonstrates a failure to suppress cortisol levels
- Where the low dose dexamethasone test is positive ACTH is measured. ACTH levels

will be undetectable in primary adrenal disorders, whereas ACTH will be high if the cause is either Cushing's disease or an ectopic ACTH producing tumour

- Where the low dose dexamethasone test is positive and the ACTH is raised, performing a 48-hour dexamethasone test will confirm Cushing's disease as evidenced by a partial suppression of cortisol. Imaging will then be required with CT or MRI brain for pituitary disease

Management

- Management depends on the underlying cause
- Metyrapone can be used to decrease plasma cortisol levels
- Surgery can be considered for adrenal adenomas, pituitary tumours, or tumours with evidence of ectopic ACTH production

Chapter 7

Communication skills and ethical scenarios (station 4)

Case 165: Informed consent for an invasive investigation or procedure – chest drain insertion

Candidate information

Scenario

You are the medical registrar on call. A 68-year-old man has presented with a large unilateral pleural effusion. Your task is to consent the patient for chest drain insertion. You do not have to take a detailed history.

Actor information

You have been experiencing worsening breathlessness for a few months now. It is affecting how far you can walk. You presented to your GP today who has sent you up to hospital for urgent assessment. You have been told you have 'fluid on the lung' that needs to be removed. The candidate will explain the procedure to you and seek your consent. Underlying concerns relate to a previous smoking history, recent weight loss and change in cough with blood in your sputum. Your father passed away from lung cancer and you have refused to seek medical attention sooner due to apprehension surrounding the suspected diagnosis.

Approach to the case

When seeking consent for an invasive investigation or procedure in PACES, several principles apply:

The procedure should be necessary. Obtain a brief history, confirming current symptoms or previous investigation and results that are consistent with a need for the investigation or procedure that you are consenting for.

The patient should have capacity to give consent for the procedure. Assessing the patient's ability to understand and make a decision based on the information provided in your discussion is important. Formal capacity assessment may be required where there is doubt based on your interaction.

Explain the need for the investigation or procedure. 'The reason why we wish to insert a chest drain today is because the symptoms and previous tests you have had suggest that the breathlessness you are experiencing is due to a collection of fluid in the chest. By carrying out this procedure we aim to drain off the fluid, resulting in both an improvement in your symptoms and allowing for analysis to suggest the likely cause of the fluid accumulation.' By doing this, you have also explained the benefit of the procedure, an important part of any consent form.

Explain, in terms understandable to the patient, what will happen during the procedure. 'Firstly, we will mark a suitable entry point using an ultrasound probe. Then, using sterile technique and local anaesthetic, a needle will be inserted through the skin and chest wall into the fluid-filled chest cavity. A tube is then placed into the chest, which will drain into a bottle by the side of the bed. The tube will be stitched securely into place and covered with a sterile dressing.'

Explain the risks. GMC guidance states that the discussion of risks will usually involve discussion of:

- Side effects
- Complications
- Failure of intervention to meet its desired aim

It is convenient to start any conversation about procedural risk with the statement 'Every procedure has risks.' Then go on to discuss both the serious and common risks. You are not expected to know every risk for every medical procedure, but you should be familiar with common invasive investigations and procedures that are considered to be common competencies of a medical registrar.

> ### Common competencies
>
> Examples of procedures with which candidates should be comfortable consenting for include:
> - Abdominal paracentesis
> - DC cardioversion
> - Knee aspiration
> - Chest drain insertion with ultrasound guidance – effusion versus pneumothorax
> - Central line insertion
> - Lumbar puncture

Summarise what has been said and ask the patient if there is anything they want further explained and if they have any other questions. If the patient is happy to consent, tell them that you will fill out the consent form and ask them to sign it.

Where the patient has capacity, and refuses to consent based on inadequate information relating to either the indication for, or the practical steps involved with, the procedure, seek to provide further sources of information. If practical, allowing a period of contemplation with access to material such as pamphlets, internet sites, nursing or senior colleagues is appropriate. Signposting to support groups may also be worthwhile.

Be prepared for a discussion of the wider condition, such as:

- Causes of the effusion – 'is this cancer doctor?'
- Recurrent effusions – failure of treatment of the underlying disease
- Duration of drain and need for inpatient stay

GMC guidance

'You must work in partnership with your patients. You should discuss with them their condition and treatment options in a way they can understand, and respect their right to make decisions about their care. You should see getting their consent as an important part of the process of discussion and decision-making, rather than as something that happens in isolation.'

Additional themes worth consideration:

- The anxious patient where reassurance fails, overriding concern regards risk, and consent is not obtained
- The confused patient where capacity to consent is in doubt requiring a formal capacity assessment
- The skeptical patient who has experienced complications in the past
- 'I want general anaesthetic; I don't want to be awake for any of it.' Explaining safe sedation and anaesthesia

Further reading

General Medical Council (GMC). Consent: patients and doctors making decisions together. London; GMC, 2008.

Case 166: The patient refusing to consent

Candidate information

Scenario

You are the gastroenterology SHO. You have been asked to consent a 67-year-old woman for upper and lower GI endoscopies to investigate iron-deficiency anaemia in the context of significant weight loss. Please obtain this patient's consent.

Actor information

You are a 67-year-old woman who has been investigated by her GP for weight loss. You have lost approximately 7 kg in weight in the last 6 months (dropping two dress sizes). Your GP sent you for blood tests and told you that you were anaemic. They also tested some of your stool and told you there was blood in it. You have had a change in bowel habit recently, tending towards constipation. You are aware that your GP is concerned about cancer, but are unwilling to undergo endoscopy, as you are concerned that the discomfort will be intolerable. Despite any reassurances given to you, you will refuse endoscopy, but are willing to consider alternative investigations.

Approach to the case

Introduce yourself to the patient and build a rapport with the patient. What does the patient understand to be the purpose of today's visit? Explain to her what having an upper and lower GI endoscopy entails and explain the risks and benefits. Her consent should be sought: In this scenario the patient will refuse consent.

Explore the patient's reasons for withholding consent, bearing in mind that patients with capacity do not actually need to give a reason to withhold consent.

Assess the patient's capacity by explaining to her the indications for the investigations and the potential implications of late diagnosis of a GI cancer. It should be ensured that she understands, retains, and weighs up the information given to her. Ensure that she can communicate back her refusal and reasons for doing so.

If the patient has capacity (and we must assume she does unless we have evidence to the contrary) she cannot be forced to have the endoscopy.

The strong candidate will go on to seek to find alternative ways to investigate the patient's anaemia. Discuss with the patient other potential investigation modalities including capsule endoscopy and CT colonography. The patient should be invited to have a conversation with the consultant, avoiding the impression of punitive consequences to her refusal, stressing the need to identify an alternate plan of investigation. Reassure her that she will not be forced to undergo any investigations or treatments with which she is uncomfortable, and where possible alternative approaches will be explored. The fundamental premise of the case is the underlying suspicion of cancer and the need to establish a diagnosis to facilitate treatment.

Case 167: Consenting for a clinical trial

Candidate information

Scenario

This 60-year-old woman has recently suffered an ST-elevation myocardial infarction. As the cardiology registrar, you have been asked to consent her for a double-blind, randomised control trial for a new anti-lipid drug. The primary end point is reduced mortality over 5 years. The protocol states that should she consent, she would receive either the trial drug or placebo once daily for the 5 years of the study. The drug is to be added to her current medication. Side effects in phase 2 trials included headaches and occasional gastrointestinal upset. Your task is to discuss participation in the trial with the patient and seek her consent for involvement in the trial.

Actor information

You have recently been hospitalised for a heart attack. You have been asked to meet with the doctor to discuss taking a new medication as part of a trial. You are not sure what this will involve and would like some further information. Assuming all your concerns are addressed, you are happy to participate in the trial.

Approach to the case

Introduce yourself to the patient and inform them of the purpose of the consultation. 'As the Cardiology registrar I have been asked to meet with you today to discuss the possibility of you participating in a clinical trial for a new medication to treat high cholesterol in patients who have recently had a heart attack. I would like to tell you a bit about the drug and the trial to see if you would be interested in taking part. If you have any questions or concerns at any stage, please feel to interrupt me'.

Make an early statement that reassures the patient that there is no obligation for her to participate. 'Let me say from the outset, that participation in this study is entirely voluntary and if, at any stage, you decide that you do not want to take part that will be absolutely fine. Let me also reassure you that if you decide not to consent to participation in the trial it will have absolutely no effect on your care and you will still receive the best medical treatment we can provide.'

Provide the patient with some background information regarding the medication and the condition it is designed to prevent/treat. 'There is a constant desire to develop new drugs to treat and prevent heart attacks more effectively and therefore help people to live longer. We know that having higher cholesterol puts people at higher risk of heart attack and there are several drugs that help to lower cholesterol. These have been shown to help in patients who have had heart attacks by reducing the risk of further heart attacks and death.'

Inform the patient of the aim(s) of the trial (primary end-point). 'We know that the drug reduces cholesterol so now we want to see if it has a beneficial effect on life-expectancy. You would take tablets every day for 5 years, coming to see us in the clinic every few months for check ups.'

Explain the structure of the trial. 'Should you agree to participate, you will be given tablets to take every day. These will either be the trial drug or a placebo (a tablet which has no medication in it whatsoever). The study is known as a double-blind, randomised control trial. The double blind bit means that neither you nor I will know whether you are taking the actual drug or the placebo. The randomised bit means that the decision whether you get the actual drug or the placebo is entirely random, thus preventing any bias coming into selection.'

Explain the potential benefits. 'The potential benefit to you is that you have a 50:50 chance of taking a drug which we believe will have a positive effect on your cholesterol and therefore on your life-expectancy.'

Clearly lay out any potential draw-backs and include a discussion of side-effects. 'There is also a 50:50 chance that you will be taking an extra tablet every day which contains no drug. We know from previous research on this drug that people taking it can experience headaches, joint pains, or abnormalities in liver function. As with any drug, there is also the possibility that someone taking it may have a side-effect that has not been noted before.'

Re-iterate to the patient that, if they decide not to consent to involvement in the trial, such a decision will have no effect whatsoever on their current and future care. It is vitally important that patients understand this, otherwise they may feel they are being pressurised into participation.

Summarise to the patient the information that has been covered. They should go on to ask them if they have any further questions or concerns.

Ask the patient if they consent to being involved in the trial. Whatever their decision, the candidate should repeat their decision back to them and tell the patient that this will be documented in their notes. This acts as a safety net so all parties can be sure of the decisions that have been made. 'Thank you for consenting to participate in the clinical trial. I will document your decision to give consent in your notes.' If required or requested, a period of contemplation should be offered.

Conclude by asking the patient to sign the trial consent form and offer the patient written information on the trial.

Additional themes worth consideration:

- The patient in whom issues arise surrounding suitability. For instance concerns surrounding compliance with current medication and as such potential for non-adherence with trial
- Patient refusal on the grounds of concerns in relation to side effects from medication
- The patient propositioning to ensure placement in the treatment arm of the trial and related ethical dilemmas

Case 168: Assessing capacity

Candidate information

Scenario

You are the on-call SHO for the medical wards. You have been asked by the nurse in charge of the Care of the Elderly ward to review an 82-year-old man, who is refusing antibiotics to treat a lower leg cellulitis. Please speak to the patient, assess his capacity to refuse treatment, and seek to resolve the situation.

Actor information

You have been admitted for cellulitis of your right leg. You are refusing to accept your intravenous antibiotics, which were started 5 days ago. Your reasoning being that the intravenous access through which the antibiotics are being given has required frequent replacement (only disclose this if asked directly why you are refusing antibiotics). You are not confused.

Approaching the case

Although this case is primarily about assessing capacity, there are also several other important elements that will be assessed, including communication skills and consideration of causes of potential confusion. The key principles in approaching scenarios of this kind are discussed below within an appropriate method of how to approach the case.

Introduce yourself to the patient and explain your role and the reason for your interaction. 'I have been asked by the nurse in charge to have a chat with you about the antibiotics you have been prescribed. Would that be acceptable?'

Summarise the situation, as you understand it. 'I've been told that you do not want your intravenous antibiotics. Is that correct?' The patient will respond in the affirmative.

An assessment of the patient's capacity is key. 'The reason why we would like you to take the antibiotics is to treat the infection you have in your leg. Without the antibiotics, the infection will may not get better and indeed is likely to get much worse. Do you understand such reasons for concern?' The patient will respond that he does understand. He realises the importance of the antibiotics. At this stage the candidate can now say that the patient has met the first

two criteria for having capacity – an ability to understand the information they are given and the ability to weigh it up.

> ### Criteria for capacity
>
> For a person to have capacity to make decisions regarding their own care, the following four criteria must be met: The patient must be able to understand the information they are given, retain that information, weigh up the information and communicate their decision back to the clinician. Always bear in mind that paragraph 64 of the GMC guidance on capacity (2008) states that: 'You must work on the presumption that every adult patient has the capacity to make decisions about their care...'

It is important to understand why the patient is refusing treatment. Ask the patient directly why, despite understanding the importance of the antibiotics, he is still refusing to accept them. He will reply that the recurrent need to insert new cannulae is causing him considerable distress. It is important to elicit this piece of information as it now affords the candidate several options for resolution of the scenario, as discussed later in the case.

Do not forget to screen for reversible causes for confusion. It will be prudent to request the patient's notes, observation charts and most recent blood results.

Check that the patient has retained the information that was previously given to him. 'Forgive me for asking again, but may I check that you are clear as to the reasons why we are prescribing you intravenous antibiotics, can you repeat my explanation back to me?' He will give a suitably accurate account. With this, the patient meets the third criterion for possessing capacity – the ability to retain information.

Ask the patient if, despite you explaining the need for intravenous antibiotics, he still refuses to receive them. By his response, he meets the final criterion for having capacity – the ability to communicate one's decision.

After having decided that the patient does indeed have capacity to refuse treatment, your task then changes to how to resolve the situation. There can be no hard and fast rules with this, but suitable tactics could include:

- Reassurance with regard to further cannula insertion. Discussion with regard to an appropriate choice of anatomical site in addition to options for securing the access or protecting it with bandaging. Involvement of the nursing staff to demonstrate a concerted effort within the team to promote longevity of the access and reduce the need for replacement would be sensible. Offer your services as a senior member within the team with relative skill and experience as compared with junior doctors, nursing staff or phlebotomist, should this be an issue with the patient

- Alternatively, offer an assessment of his current progress including an examination, review of observation chart and blood tests, and consider the potential for conversion to oral antibiotics

Stress to the patient that the final decision in relation to his treatment lies with him. The patient will state that he is happy to receive oral antibiotics.

Additional themes worth consideration:

- The confused patient – acute confused state, delirium, secondary to infection/sepsis
- The confused patient – co-morbidity of advanced dementia

Case 169: The patient who lacks capacity

Candidate information

Scenario

One of the patients on your ward has been admitted with a non-resolving diabetic ulcer on his heel, which has failed to respond to several courses of intravenous antibiotics. The advice of the vascular MDT meeting has been that an amputation is the most appropriate intervention in this case. As well as other co-morbidities, the patient has a history of vascular dementia. It has been judged by your consultant that the patient lacks capacity to make decisions regarding his own care. Please discuss the plan of action with the patient's next of kin.

Actor information

You are the wife of a 60-year-old man who has had diabetes for many years. He has had a problem with an ulcer on his foot for the past 18 months and has been in hospital four times for prolonged courses of intravenous antibiotics. He has been diagnosed with vascular dementia and requires considerable care and supervision. The doctor will inform you that they feel the best course of action is for an amputation of the affected foot. Initially you are against this plan due to concerns about whether your husband would want it. Underlying concerns relate to

dissatisfaction with the current package of care received, and the consequence of mobility issues on the ability of your husband to return home. You have been considering the option of a nursing home and this deterioration in his health has highlighted your inability to cope.

Approach to the case

Important principles to remember when dealing with a patient who lacks capacity are:

- Decisions should be made that serve to act in the patient's best interests
- Treatment initiated in the patient's best interests must be the 'least restrictive'
- It is important to keep lines of communication open with the patient's next of kin. This acts both to reduce the likelihood of conflict and also to give an idea of what the patient's wishes may have been, had they possessed capacity
- Ensure that if any legal documentation exists, in the form of an advance directive or relating to power of attorney, these are given due consideration

To commence the consultation, introduce yourself to the patient's relative. They should confirm their name and their relationship to the patient. Clarify their status as the next of kin.

Ask the patient's relative what they understand the current situation to be. This is an effective tactic in all communication situations as it gives you an idea of what level of understanding the patient/relative has of the scenario and allows the candidate to judge how much information is required and at what level to pitch it at.

Establish a joint understanding of the seriousness of the situation and the current thinking in relations to management options. Explain that, due to the persistence of the infection in the heel ulcer, demonstrated by both recurrent admissions and poor response to treatment, there is significant concern that it will be impossible to eradicate the infection with antibiotics alone. There is additional concern in relation to the potential for complications, primarily sepsis, and that such an eventuality would likely carry a poor prognosis, even death.

Go on to explain that a meeting of a range of specialists involved in the patients care have come to a joint decision that the best treatment option would be to perform an amputation of the foot. The benefits of this would be to remove all of the infected and necrotic tissue as a means of eradicating the infection. It would be hoped that the stump and scar would subsequently heal. At this stage pause and ask if the patient's relative has any questions.

Explain that all the team realise that amputation is a major step and that it would not be considered if it was not felt to be a necessary step to manage a difficult and serious situation. Seek to identify and address the relative's views now that the aspects of the case above have been discussed with them.

Below are some additional points for consideration, which may form part of a discussion with the examiner:

- Ethics committee: In most PACES scenarios, any conflict will be resolved in the course of the discussion. In the event of persistent disagreement, suggestion to the examiner of referral to the hospital's clinical ethics committee is a sensible plan
- Be clear that the relative is unable to refuse the treatment suggested. It would be a misunderstanding of the candidate instructions to think that the point of the station is to seek the relative's consent. As the patient has been judged to be incapacitated, any interventions that are carried out on his behalf are done so in what is deemed to be his best interests, as decided by the medical team. The candidate is trying to foster agreement with his relatives and defuse any conflict, but is not seeking their consent
- Is amputation the 'least restrictive' intervention? The candidate information is deliberately ambiguous. Based solely on the information provided, one could argue that options, which are least restrictive, include further courses of intravenous antibiotics, or to perform limited tissue debridement. This is obviously a complex case that provides plenty of scope for discussion between the candidate and the examiner

> ### Mental Capacity Act 2005 (England and Wales)
>
> The following points are adapted from the GMC guidance (2008) on the Mental Capacity Act. This states that actions taken under the act must abide by several principles:
>
> - Unless it has been established otherwise, the patient should be assumed to have capacity
> - 'All practicable steps' should be taken to aid a patient to become able to make a decision on their own care
> - Just because a person makes unwise decisions does not make them unable to make decisions on their own care
> - Any action or decision made under the remit of the Mental Capacity Act 2005 must be done in the patient's best interests
> - The action taken must be considered to be the 'least restrictive' on the patient's rights and freedom of action.

Further reading

General Medical Council (GMC). Consent: patients and doctors making decisions together. London; GMC, 2008.

Department of Constitutional Affairs. Mental Capacity Act 2005. Code of practice. London; The Stationary Office, 2007.

Case 170: Breaking bad news to a relative

Candidate information

Scenario

You are the cardiology registrar. You have been asked to meet the wife of a 70-year-old man who was admitted with an extensive anterior STEMI. His background includes active metastatic prostate cancer, which has so far been refractory to treatment, and vascular dementia with a background MMSE of 19/30. He has had all appropriate treatments but is in severe cardiac failure and is not expected to survive his current hospital stay. Please talk with his wife and inform her of the prognosis.

Actor information

Your husband was admitted after having an episode of chest pain at home. He has dementia and has been unwell for an extended period of time with prostate cancer, for which he has been told the treatment is not working. You are concerned about your husband's chances of surviving his heart attack but are prepared for the worst. Your children both live overseas and they are unable to travel home for another few days but are hopeful that they will be able to say goodbye and are looking for such an assurance from the doctor.

Approach to the case

Breaking bad news often arises in the context of a discussion with the next of kin. In the majority of cases this will involve a patient in whom the prognosis is poor or indeed is dying. Often the initial consideration is one of confidentiality in that the discussion with the relative may occur where the patient is incapacitated and as such cannot consent to disclosure of information. The basic premise is that it is in the patient's best interest to discuss the case openly with appropriate members of his family. An appreciation of confidentiality should be made clear however, to satisfy the examiners expectations – a statement along the lines of 'Your husband is very ill, and while ordinarily I would look for his consent to discuss the details of the case with you, I think it would be in his best interests for you to understand the situation he is in to make decisions and support him at this time.'

Establish the relative's current understanding of the patient's current condition. Be prepared to fill gaps or clarify statements that are either incorrect or lack appropriate detail but avoid overloading them with information. Gauge what they want and need to know. Often it is best to impart small amounts of key information repeatedly to ensure mutual understanding as to the severity of the situation. Where necessary employ the use of 'warning shots' to prepare a relative for bad news – often indicated by non-verbal cues.

Summarise the situation and attempt to 'paint the picture' of what is an irretrievable situation. It should be stated very clearly that it is the opinion of the medical team that the patient will not survive this current admission. Pause. It is essential that the patient's relative is given time to absorb the information. Often, an uncomfortable but necessary silence will ensue, demanding the confidence not to talk or continue the discussion too hastily.

Do not be afraid to encourage the relative to discuss how they are feeling and express their emotions.

Encourage questions relating to what happens next. Gauge the ability of the relative in any given scenario to continue with difficult discussions, which may include:

- The decision to resuscitate
- Withdrawing care
- Brainstem death testing
- Organ harvesting
- Requesting a postmortem

Look to give some form of indication as to prognosis and the expected speed of deterioration but avoid committing to specifics. The relative may be keen to resuscitate or escalate care until her children have arrived. The discussion will require an emphasis on the patient's best interests and focus on developing hope tempered with realism. Her husband may survive long enough for her children to see him but that if he does not, then this is something they should prepare for and an emphasis on quality of life is prudent.

Summarise, check understanding and offer to see her again with her children or other relatives if they would find it useful. Offer your condolences where appropriate.

Additional themes worth considering:

- The relative that demands more be done to treat the patient. Difficulties establishing a ceiling of care and managing expectations
- Chronic conditions where death is not imminent but there is likely steady decline without the potential for improvement or reversibility

Case 171: The decision to resuscitate

Candidate information

Scenario

You are the general medical SHO working in the team responsible for the care of an 80-year-old man with a background of Alzheimer's dementia, chronic kidney disease and ischaemic heart disease. He is dependent on care for all activities of daily living and lives in a nursing home. He suffered an ischaemic stroke 7 days ago and subsequently developed a severe hospital-acquired pneumonia. He is not expected to survive this admission and over the past 24 hours has experienced a significant deterioration. Your consultant has asked you to talk to the next of kin about his decision, taken during the morning ward round, to sign a 'Do Not Attempt Resuscitation' form.

Actor information

You are the patient's daughter and next of kin. You are aware of the stroke but until today you were unaware of the severity of the pneumonia and are concerned that he appears much worse than when you last visited. The most important aspect of his care from your perspective is that he does not suffer, having had a difficult and traumatic experience of prolonged end of life care leading up to the death of your mother. The doctor will discuss with you the current prognosis and explain the decision in relation to resuscitation, with which you agree, but you are concerned about a lack of palliative care involvement in the case. Based on your experience with your mother in the same hospital, your knowledge of the system appears to be greater than that of the doctor you are speaking to and this is a source of frustration and worry if not openly acknowledged.

Approach to the case

Introduce yourself and confirm that the woman to whom you are speaking is the patient's next of kin.

Explore her current understanding of his underlying state of health, recent events and current condition.

Thereafter, having gauged the daughter's level of insight, succinctly summarise the case for her. Attempt to mirror some of her statements.

Incorporating her terminology may engage her in discussion and help build a rapport.

It should be made clear that, given the patient's weight of co-morbidities and his current poor condition, the consultant in charge of his care and the rest of the medical team are all in agreement that, in the event of the patient's heart stopping it would not be in her father's best interests to try and revive him.

Be clear that despite the best possible medical care, her father is not expected to survive and that the end could come soon. However, although a DNAR has been put in place, treatment is still ongoing.

Official guidance for resuscitation decision making

In 2007, a joint statement was released by the British Medical Association, the Resuscitation Council (UK), and the Royal College of Nursing. Entitled 'Decisions Relating to Cardiopulmonary Resuscitation' it addresses various issues surrounding resuscitation. The document notes that 'Healthcare professionals have an important role in helping patients to participate in making appropriate plans for future care in a sensitive but realistic manner, making clear whether or not attempted CPR could be successful. Helping patients to reach a clear decision about their wishes ... should be regarded as a marker of good practice ...' The joint statement notes that decisions made regarding resuscitation must comply with the Human Rights Act 1998. When discussing the communication of DNAR decisions to patients, the joint statement remarks that clinicians should 'Offer patients as much information as they want, provide information in a manner and format which patients can understand, answer questions honestly and explain the aims of treatment'.

With tact and compassion, you must explain that in this case, given the extensive co-morbidities and limited functional reserve, CPR is not considered to be in the best interests of the patient and would therefore be inappropriate. It would be prudent to further discuss ceilings of care and clarify while treatment is ongoing, any further requirement such as respiratory support would only be considered, at most, in the context of the ward environment, and not with an admission to

HDU or ITU. This is likely to prompt discussion in this case of end-of-life care.

The involvement of relatives/friends in resuscitation decisions

When considering the discussion of DNAR decisions with relatives or those close to the patients, note that the joint statement says that this is 'not only good practice but is also likely to be a requirement of the Human Rights Act (Articles 8 and 10) [and] the Mental Capacity Act 2005 (England and Wales)'. Section 9.2 of the Joint Statement deals with 'Adults who lack capacity, have neither an attorney nor an advance decision but do have family or friends.' The statement notes that the final decision rests with the senior clinician in charge of the case (the patient's consultant). It goes on to say that 'the views of those close to the patient should be sought ... to determine any previously expressed wishes.'

In some cases, the patient's relative may try to insist that the patient receives CPR in the event of a cardiac arrest. This changes the focus of the consultation. In such cases, you must be clear that while you are seeking to explain the rational for a DNAR, and hoping for agreement, you are not seeking the next of kin's consent.

Attempt to incorporate an explanation that CPR is classified under law as a medical intervention, and as such, the final decision regarding its use lies with the medical team. Even in scenarios where disputes arise, it is important to be seen by the examiner to be putting yourself on the side of the patient and working with the next of kin to reach agreement. Remember, the solution is not to argue with the next of kin, it is to educate them on why CPR is inappropriate in the given situation.

If any disagreement persists, offer to arrange a meeting with the consultant in charge of the patient's care and be seen to involve the palliative care team and senior nursing staff on the ward. Often the matron on the ward is a useful link to services available and in coordinating care.

Close the scenario by briefly summarising what has been discussed to ensure shared understanding.

Further reading

Decisions relating to cardiopulmonary resuscitation. A joint statement from the British Medical Association, the Resuscitation Council (UK) and the Royal College of Nursing. J Med Ethics. 2001; 27:310–316.

Case 172: Withdrawing (life-dependent) care

Candidate information

Scenario

As the on-call registrar, you received handover prior to the weekend that a 92-year-old patient on the care of the elderly ward had been deteriorating over a period of weeks. The consultant responsible for management set the ceiling of care as 'ward-based management'. On review there is evidence of multi-organ failure as a result of advanced chest sepsis that has failed to respond to intravenous antibiotics. Currently she is in pulmonary oedema with hypoxia and hypotension. She is anuric with evidence of acute kidney injury. Her inflammatory markers are worsening and she has become confused and drowsy. You feel that continuing treatment is not in her best interests given the irretrievable situation. The patient's co-morbidities include dementia, chronic airways disease and heart failure. You have been asked to discuss withdrawing care with her son.

Actor information

Your mother has been in hospital for the last 3 weeks with a chest infection that 'never really got better'. The nurses called you this afternoon to tell you that her condition has worsened and that you should come to the hospital. Your understanding is that she is close to death. You wish to ensure that she does not suffer in any way however you are anxious about withdrawing care. Your mother has always been a 'fighter' and would be reluctant to 'give up' albeit her quality of life has been poor since her dementia and heart failure worsened.

Approach to the case

Introduce yourself and confirm the identity of the patient's relative and their relationship to the patient including status as next of kin. Explore the level of understanding of his mother's current illness and progress. This will give an indication as to whether he has insight into the seriousness of the situation. Summarise the case as appropriate.

It should be explained to the patient's son that given the number of problems affecting his mother and the number of organs that aren't working properly, the medical team feel that this is an illness from which the patient will not recover. Time should be afforded to absorb such information, check for understanding, and invite questions to aid clarification.

Proceed to tell the son that the medical team feels that, given the current clinical condition and the poor response, continuing current treatment is inappropriate. Ask the son how he feels about what has been said. The purpose of such a discussion is not to seek consent but to establish from him, and the wider family, what the patient's wishes might have been.

If the son asks why his mother has not been moved to intensive care, take the time to explain that given her frail condition and concomitant health problems, it is unlikely that a stay in intensive care would benefit her. The concept of a lack of functional reserve is a useful one, explaining that the patient is unable to mount a sufficient response, and that this is the reason for a lack of recovery as opposed to a failure of treatment per se. As such it would be expected that intensive care might prolong life, but not aid recovery and ultimately not be in the best interests of the patient.

In the event of conflict, the appropriate course of action would be to contact the consultant on-call for the weekend and arrange for the relative to meet them to discuss the case. The principle to focus upon when the patient lacks capacity is the medical team's responsibility to act in what they perceive to be the patients best interests, taking into account any advanced directives and the relative's view on what they understand the patient would have wanted.

The case should conclude by discussing the role of palliative medicine and end-of-life care with the aim of making the patient as comfortable as possible.

Case 173: Brainstem death testing

Candidate information

Scenario

You are the intensive care SHO. A 30-year-old man is currently a patient in your unit after being hit by a motor vehicle a week ago. He has suffered severe diffuse traumatic brain injury and is on a ventilator. He is not expected to survive and the team is preparing to carry out brainstem testing. You have been asked to discuss with the patient's next of kin, his mother, the details of brainstem testing.

Actor information

You are the mother of a 30-year-old who sustained severe head injuries after being hit by a car last week. He has been in the intensive care unit on 'life support' ever since. From the outset things did not look good and you are aware of the grave prognosis. Over the past 24 hours the consultant has informed you that they do not think your son will recover. They have told you they will be doing some tests on his brain (brainstem testing), which are expected to show his dependence upon machines. You have had limited access to the consultant in charge of your son's care and have found a large amount of the information relayed by the SHO thus far to be technically complicated and in language that you struggle to understand. You are seeking a clear explanation of your son's clinical state and what brainstem testing actually means.

Approach to the case

Relatives will often struggle to come to terms with the loss of a loved one where the removal of care is required, instead clinging to the possibility of recovery. Individual cases will vary with content and emphasis, but the general key for success in this scenario is to use knowledge of the principles of brainstem death, combined with effective communication skills, to explain what can be a complicated concept.

What is brainstem death?

Brainstem death is a clinical state where there is total loss of brainstem function, resulting in an apnoeic coma that, without artificial ventilation, would result in death.

How do we test for brainstem death?

Given that the diagnosis of brainstem death is a life-ending episode, it is not surprising that there are specific rules regarding testing for it. These are laid out clearly in 'A Code of Practice for the Diagnosis and Confirmation of Death' (Academy of Medical Royal Colleges, 2008). A general algorithm for diagnosing brainstem death includes:

- Identify coma
- Exclude possible reversible factors (hypothermia, disturbances in metabolism, drugs)
- Testing is done by two clinicians, both of who are 5 or more years post-full registration with the General Medical Council and one of whom is a consultant. The length of time between the two episodes of testing is regarded as a matter of clinical judgement
- Pupillary light reflex, corneal reflex (take care not to damage the cornea as it may be used in transplant), and vestibulo-ocular reflexes are absent
- Absent motor response 'within the cranial nerve distribution [due to] stimulation of any somatic area' in combination with 'No limb response to supraorbital pressure' and an absent gag reflex are compatible with brainstem death

- Assess response to apnoea testing. Apnoea is confirmed when there are no spontaneous respiratory movements when the patient is disconnected from the ventilator and the $PaCO_2$ is allowed to reach 6.65 kPa measured by arterial blood gas testing

Brain stem death: time of death

One potentially confusing aspect of brainstem death, and therefore one which will require careful explanation is the time of death once brainstem testing is completed. Although the patient is technically still alive until the conclusion of the second repeat testing, upon reaching a diagnosis of brainstem death, the time of death is considered as the time of conclusion of the first test.

Definition of death

There is no legal definition of death in the UK. *A Code of Practice for the Diagnosis and Confirmation of Death* recommends that death should be defined as the 'irreversible loss of the capacity for consciousness, combined with irreversible loss of the capacity to breathe.' The document argues that since brainstem death produces the clinical state set out above, brainstem death equates to the death of the patient.

The following are conditions under which the diagnosis of brainstem death should be considered:

- The patient's condition is due to irreversible brain damage for which the cause is known
- The patient is deeply unconscious
- Not influenced by drugs (medications or otherwise)
- Not due to primary hypothermia
- Not due to reversible endocrine, metabolic or circulatory factors
- Mechanical ventilation is necessary due to inadequate/absent spontaneous ventilation

Be aware that where brainstem function remains intact, despite loss of cortical function, a diagnosis of persistent vegetative state is made.

Further reading

Academy of Medical Royal Colleges. A Code of Practice for the Diagnosis and confirmation of death. London: Academy of Medical Royal Colleges, 2008

Candidate information

Scenario

You are the intensive care SHO. A 30-year-old man is currently a patient in your unit after being hit by a motor vehicle a week ago. He has suffered severe diffuse traumatic brain injury and is on a ventilator. He is not expected to survive and the team is preparing to carry out brainstem testing. The patient does not carry a donor card and is not on the organ donor register. He does not have an advance directive. You have been asked to talk with the patient's next of kin, his mother, with a view to obtaining consent for organ harvesting. You do not need to discuss the details of brainstem testing.

Actor information

You are the mother of a 30-year-old who sustained severe head injuries after being hit by a car last week. He has been in the intensive care unit on 'life support' ever since. From the outset things did not look good and you are aware of the grave prognosis. Over the past 24 hours the consultant has informed you that they do not think your son will recover. They have told you they will be doing some tests on his brain (brainstem testing), which are expected to show his dependence upon machines. The doctor will ask you for consent for organ harvesting. Your son had never expressed a view on organ donation but you think he would have been in favour of it. Before you give consent you have some concerns. As long as the doctor answers these concerns appropriately, you will give consent.

Approach to the case

Ask the patient's mother what has been discussed with her in the last 24 hours to confirm that she understands that brainstem testing is about to happen and is likely to confirm brainstem death.

A discussion on organ harvesting should be instigated with a statement such as: 'I know it is a difficult topic to talk about, but whenever a patient is considered as unwell as your son, we are obliged to talk to their relatives about the possibility of organ donation. Do you feel in a position to talk about this now?' A statement such as this will quickly identify those relatives for whom organ donation is a 'non-starter,' but for those who will consider giving consent, will act as a gentle introduction to the subject. Where there is reluctance to engage in discussion, the challenge will be to impress upon the relative the time sensitive nature of the matter.

The relative should be asked whether, to the best of their knowledge, the patient had ever expressed any views on organ donation and if so, what were they?

Explain the process of organ donation. If the relatives were to give consent, after death was confirmed with brainstem testing, they would be given a short time to spend with him, and then he would be taken to the operating theatre for harvesting/recovery of organs. Organs, ranging from his heart, lungs, liver, kidney and corneas could be used. His body would then be returned to the family for burial.

Questions the relative may ask include:

- Will the body be disfigured? There will be scars, but they will not be visible with the body presented in the standard way by the undertakers (with a shroud)
- Will it delay the funeral? No. The process of harvesting should not ordinarily delay any funeral arrangements
- Will all his organs be used? Organs will be harvested and decisions on their suitability for transplant will be taken on an individual basis
- He was a smoker; does that mean he can't donate his organs? Not necessarily. Of course, it may be that organ damage from smoking may preclude transplantation of some organs, most obviously the lungs in a heavy smoker. It is unlikely, however that a 30-year-old would have such significant smoking damage that would prevent lung transplantation
- Will we get to know about who gets the organs? Relatives are given a limited amount of information about the recipient: age (by decade), gender, and the outcome of the transplant

Additional themes worth consideration:

- Possession of a donor card or member of the organ donation register yet the relative is refusing consent. The current position, which many would argue is unsatisfactory, is that even if the patient is in possession of a donor card or has signed the organ donation register or has expressed wishes to donate their organs, if the next of kin refuses consent, organ donation often does not occur. Candidates should note, however, that the Human Tissue Act 2004 contains provisions that make it 'lawful to take organs for transplantation where the deceased consented before his death.' However it does note that good practice dictates that relatives are consulted

- Next of kin refusing to accept death and unwilling to discuss organ donation where

the patient in whom death has occurred has an advance directive indicating their wish for organ donation. Advance directives are legally binding

Further reading

NHS Blood and Transplant (NHSBT) and the British Transplant Society (BTS). Guidelines for consent for solid organ transplantation in adults. Cheshire; NHSBT and BTS, 2011.

Case 175: Requesting a hospital postmortem

Candidate information

Scenario

You are the general medical SHO. A 68-year-old woman was admitted on Friday evening with a history of significant weight loss and confusion. The impression on the post-admission ward round was of likely malignancy with unknown primary. On the ward round a plan was made for various investigations to take place after the weekend. On Sunday evening, 48 hours after admission, the patient suffered a cardiac arrest and died. In the context of a sudden deterioration without a firm diagnosis, the consultant in charge has advised that a postmortem would be advisable to identify the cause of death. You have been asked to speak to the patient's son to obtain consent.

Actor information

Your mother had been complaining of weight loss for approximately 3 months. You took her to see her GP last Friday as she had become increasingly confused. The GP sent her up to the hospital where you were told she required admission for further investigation. On Sunday evening you received a telephone call from the nurse in charge of the ward to let you know that she had passed away suddenly. Nobody has been able to tell you exactly what she has died of, but you overheard the nursing staff mentioning cancer when they were turning

down her bed. When the doctor raises the possibility of a postmortem you are reluctant. You don't want your dead mother 'cut into'. Ask the doctor about what exactly the postmortem entails. You are also concerned about the funeral arrangements, as you are unsure how a postmortem will affect these. Providing the doctor addresses your concerns appropriately, you will give consent for a postmortem.

Approach to the case

Introduce yourself and begin by offering your condolences.

Ask the patient's relative what they understand to be the recent course of events. If necessary, they should be informed of any details they may not know/understand. Explain that due to uncertainty regarding the exact cause of death of their mother, the consultant in charge of her care feels that a post-mortem would provide invaluable information as to the cause of death.

Discuss with them any questions they may have about postmortems. Once the discussion is complete, the relative should be asked a very clear question whether they consent to a postmortem.

Areas for discussion relevant to postmortems:

- 'Why do you need to do a postmortem? It won't make any difference to the fact my mother is dead, will it?' It is important to answer this question frankly and accept the relative's point that it will not change the fact that his mother had died. It may however, help give 'closure' if they know exactly why she died. Much more a secondary consideration is that a postmortem may shed light on a particular condition and thus potentially provide information to the medical profession to help other patients in the future

- 'Will the scars disfigure her?' A useful way of answering this question is to tell the relative that scars from the postmortem will not be visible with the body dressed in a funeral shroud. You can then ask the relative if they want to know further details about the incisions (many will not). If they do, tell them that there is an incision made in the front to allow access to the chest and abdominal organs. To examine the brain, a scalp incision is made at the back, again, not visible with the body on its back

- 'What about the funeral arrangements?' A postmortem typical takes place within 2 or 3 days, after which the body is released to the funeral director. Thus, there should not be a significant delay to the funeral (bear in mind that different religions have specific beliefs about funerals regarding timing so be careful not to be blasé about 'significant delays')

- 'I have read about scandals where hospitals have kept people's organs. How can I be sure this won't happen to my mum?' If this question is raised, it is important to accept that, yes, there have been problems with this in the past, but after extensive investigation, strict rules and regulations have been put in place to ensure it does not happen again. Unless the relative is specifically asked for permission, no organs will be retained. After examination, they will be returned to the body. It may be that a request is made ahead of the postmortem for an organ to be retained. This may for various reasons, either because it is thought to be relevant to the cause of death, of for relevant research. Written consent would be sought before the event. There is a 'half-way house' in which consent may be sought to keep the organ for a limited period, after which it would either be returned to the patient's next of kin or disposed of by the hospital

Mandatory postmortems

Consent for a postmortem is not required when a coroner orders one to be carried out. Examples of such scenarios are when the death is sudden or unexpected; if there are suspicious circumstances; or if their doctor had not seen the deceased in the 14 days preceding their death.

Case 176: Driving with disease

Candidate information

Scenario

A 48-year-old man with type 2 diabetes has recently had changes to his medication. Please discuss the implications of the addition of insulin to his current driving status.

Actor information

You have had type 2 diabetes for 3 years and despite weight loss, diet modification and treatment with tablets your control has remained poor. The doctor who reviewed you clinic 4 months ago was concerned about the effects on your eyes and kidneys and started you on insulin twice a day. Since then your blood sugar has been improving but you have experienced two hypoglycaemic episodes, with symptoms of profuse sweating and feeling faint, without warning, attributed to difficulty managing your insulin requirements. Despite being informed of your obligation to inform the Driver and Vehicle Licensing Agency (DVLA) of a change in circumstances you have not done so and have continued to commute to work – 40 miles from your home, including stretches of motorway.

Approach to the case

When faced with a communication station case based on the topic of driving regulations, several key principles apply:

- Knowledge of driving regulations. The DVLA website provides information on a wide range of conditions via an A–Z list
- The three main conditions to know about are diabetes, epilepsy, and coronary artery disease. A fundamental understanding of the main factors of each condition prohibiting driving is important. However, the full guidance is often complicated and detailed thus it is always sensible to caveat any discussion with a patient by stating that you will give them clear written advice
- The way in which information is projected is important. You should remember to remove yourself from the driving regulations. You are not telling that patient that they cannot drive; rather that you are duty bound to inform them that the DVLA is telling them that they cannot drive – this is not just semantics
- Do not let the patient leave the station thinking you have made a judgment on their driving. The message is not that people with any given condition are bad drivers. Instead, the message is that there is an inherent danger, totally independent of the patient's driving ability, due to the nature of the condition or possible complications of treatment, that give rise to the potential for serious harm to themselves and/or others
- Be sure to clarify the patient's occupation and relate this to either dependency upon travel or a group 2 license (see below)
- Take the time to explore the patient's concerns and questions

Be clear that the rules for individual medical conditions vary depending on whether the patient holds a group 1 (car or motorbike) or group 2 (heavy goods vehicle) license.

Group 1 – diabetes

To qualify for a group 1 license, insulin-dependent patients must demonstrate:

- Awareness of hypoglycaemic episodes
- Less than 1 hypoglycaemic episode over the previous 12 months (where they were dependent upon others for their wellbeing)
- Willingness to perform blood glucose monitoring 2 hours prior to driving and every 2 hours thereafter
- Normal standards for visual acuity, without diplopia or visual field defects

Where criteria are met, a 1, 2, or 3-year license may be issued.

The same rules apply to non-insulin dependent diabetic patients, only where there is use of oral medication with known risk of hypoglycaemia, or where episodes of hypoglycaemia have occurred.

In all cases of diabetes, the DVLA must be informed if the patient does not have awareness of hypoglycaemic episodes.

Group 2 – diabetes

To qualify for a group 2 license, insulin-dependent patients must demonstrate:

- Full awareness of hypoglycaemic episodes and understanding of risks involved in relation to driving
- No hypoglycaemic episodes over the previous 12 months (where they were dependent upon others for their wellbeing)
- Willingness to perform blood glucose monitoring 2 hours prior to driving and every 2 hours thereafter. Regular blood glucose monitoring should be performed using a glucometer with a memory function allowing review of a 3-month period during assessment with an independent specialist on an annual basis

Where criteria are met, a 1-year license may be issued.

The same rules apply to non-insulin dependent diabetic patients only where there is use of oral medication with known risk of hypoglycaemia, or where episodes of hypoglycaemia have occurred. That said, all diabetics must inform the DVLA and undergo regular medical review. Non-insulin dependent patients may be issued a license for 1, 2, or 3-year periods.

Group 1 – epilepsy

Isolated seizure, which refers to a single seizure or multiple seizures within a 24-hour period, having never suffered a seizure previously, requires a 6-month period off driving.

A formal diagnosis of epilepsy under group 1 licensing is considered by the DVLA as two seizures within a 5-year period. To qualify for a license the patient must be seizure free with or without medication for a period of 1 year. Exceptions to this include:

- Pattern over 1 year, exclusively of sleep seizures – full license granted even if sleep seizures continue
- Likewise, seizures where consciousness and ability to control a vehicle are not impaired demonstrated for 1 year

- Having been seizure free for a period of 1 year on medication, and where agreed with a medical practitioner to come off medication, breakthrough seizures may occur. If a breakthrough seizure occurs, a seizure free period of 6 months is required on the same medication to regain license.

Group 2 – epilepsy

A formal diagnosis of epilepsy under group 2 licensing is considered by the DVLA as 2 seizures within a 10-year period. To qualify for a license patients must be seizure free for 10 years without medication.

Following an isolated seizure a patient is required to adhere to 5 years off driving from the date of the seizure.

Where a seizure is thought to be provoked by an event, which is unlikely to occur again, such as head injury, the DVLA may consider this an exceptional circumstance. Importantly, seizures in the context of alcohol, drug misuse, sleep deprivation or medication changes are not usually considered to be provoked. Each case is considered on an individual basis. This applies to group 1 licenses also.

Group 1 – acute coronary syndrome and coronary intervention

Following coronary angioplasty a period of 1 week off driving must be adhered to. A return to driving is then possible provided there are no plans for further intervention within a 4-week period, the LV ejection fraction is >40%, and there are no other disqualifying conditions.

A period of 4 weeks off driving is required following CABG.

Group 2 – acute coronary syndrome and coronary intervention

Following coronary angioplasty a period of 6 weeks off driving must be adhered to. A return to driving is based on an ability to satisfy functional/exercise testing and where no other disqualifying conditions exist.

Breaking confidentiality and informing the DVLA

One aspect that may come up in the examination is the scenario where the patient refuses to stop driving. Reasons given for this may include livelihood or other need to drive (hence importance of addressing this). It may be possible to negotiate with the patient by informing them that many employers will allow the patient to retrain or move to a different part of the workforce. In such a situation where the patient informs the candidate that they will continue to drive despite being advised of the DVLA rules, the strategy should include the following:

- Confirm that the patient understands the information they have been given
- Re-advise them of the legal requirements

If they still refuse to stop driving, demonstrate to the examiner, that you are aware of all the appropriate steps that should be taken, including:

- Seek the help of a senior doctor (registrar or, preferably, consultant)
- Assuming no senior is available, the patient should be informed that in a situation such as this, both the DVLA and the patient's GP will be informed. In addition to this, the patient will receive a letter documenting the medical advice and what actions the medical team have taken to inform the DVLA
- It should be confirmed with the patient that they understand what they have been told

Other themes worth consideration:

- Other conditions that may arise include transient ischaemic attacks, stroke, and arrhythmias
- Patients working as taxi drivers can be particularly challenging. Often, local authorities require group 2 licenses, muddying the waters somewhat
- Vehicles that do not require a license – forklift trucks, farm vehicles and sit-on lawn mowers. The Health and Safety Executive advises that the standards for operating these vehicles should be similar to that of comparative road vehicles. Employers are required to satisfy health and safety regulations
- Electric wheelchairs and mobility scooters are not considered vehicles, but if they are used on the road then an application must be made to the DVLA
- The impact upon insurance premiums will also be impacted and patients should be made aware of this

Further reading

Driver and Vehicle Licensing Agency. At a glance guide to the current medical standards of fitness to drive. For medical practitioners. Swansea: Driver and Vehicle Licensing Agency, 2014

Case 177: Genetic counselling

Candidate information

Scenario

A 26-year-old man has been referred by his GP. The patient's father has recently been diagnosed with Huntington's disease and as such the GP is requesting genetic counselling. As the neurology registrar you are asked to review the case, provide appropriate information and discuss the potential implications.

Actor information

You are a 26-year-old married man with two young children. You have a poor relationship with your father who has been suffering with severe depression complicated by psychosis for many years. His physical health started to deteriorate, to the best of your knowledge this year, but you are unaware of the nature of the symptoms. The diagnosis of Huntington's disease is a recent one and you know nothing about the condition other than it is inherited. You were reluctant to attend because you don't understand the need given that you have no symptoms and are in excellent health. You are worried about the potential for developing similar mental health problems as your father but will only discuss this if asked directly and with some persistence.

Approach to the case

Introduce yourself and clarify your role. Explore the patient's understanding and expectations of the referral from his GP. Attempt to manage expectations from the outset, in that you are not in a position to offer formal genetic counselling nor test the patient, but rather offer information surrounding the condition to allow the patient to make a decision on whether he wishes to pursue formal testing.

Allow the patient to talk openly with regard to his father's disease, exploring his initial presentation and current symptoms. Attempt to gauge the patient's current level of understanding of Huntington's disease, pitching the subsequent interaction at a level that will be easily understood. Remain flexible with your approach, clearly demonstrating compassion and empathy in relation to both the father's current mental and physical health and the impact upon the patient's relationship with him.

Summarise your understanding of the patients knowledge and outline the areas that you wish to discuss in more detail, including:

- Clinical features of Huntington's disease and age of onset of symptoms
- Basic genetics and mode of inheritance with consideration of the implications on the patient and his family
- Options with regard to genetic testing and how such a service is accessed

Clinical features

Onset is usually during middle age, between 30 and 50 years of age.

Symptoms are usually insidious and relate to dementia or psychiatric disturbance, highlighting the importance of the father's mental health history in the vignette, and movement disorders.

Abnormal movements include chorea, myoclonic jerks, ataxia and gait disturbance.

Be clear as to the untreatable nature of the disease with a poor prognosis. Life expectancy is approximately 10–15 years from onset of symptoms with considerable associated morbidity.

Genetics and mode of inheritance

Huntington's has autosomal dominant inheritance.

Explain in simple terminology that the disease is related to inheritance of abnormal genetic code – excessive CAG repeats of the Huntingtin gene (HTT). HTT is passed from affected parent to child and that, given the mixing of genetic material between father and mother, he has a 50% chance of inheriting the disease.

- If he has inherited HTT with excessive CAG repeats, then he will develop Huntington's, linked to high penetrance
- If he has not inherited his father's HTT, then he will definitely not develop Huntington's

Usually asymptomatic until after middle age so the patient may already have children, as in this case.

If he does not have the abnormal genetic code, there will be no need to test his children. If he does, then they would require testing, as they would have the same 50% chance of inheritance.

Be sure to pause and ensure adequate understanding of the details discussed. When explaining inheritance of disease to patients who have no prior knowledge of genetics, a simple family tree diagram will help to visually describe the pattern of inheritance.

The patient's understanding of the content of the conversation should be checked. If he seems to be struggling with the information, take the time to go back over the basics. If he is judged to have a good understanding and he has no specific questions, then the principle of anticipation should be covered. This is the phenomenon by which Huntington's tends to display more severe symptoms earlier in the life of successive generations. It is un-necessary to go into the details of expansion of trinucleotide repeats with the patient; however, this may form the basis of a discussion with the examiner.

Genetic testing

Formal genetic counselling and testing can be accessed with a referral to specialist services, however the examiner may require evidence of an understanding of the principles involved:

- Consent for testing requires that the patient understands the nature of the disease being tested for, underpinning the importance of the conversation outlined above
- The indications for testing must be understood. The implication of a positive result must be fully appreciated by the patient and linked to predictive versus diagnostic testing. Importantly with Huntington's disease, a positive result indicates a sufficiently long CAG repeat which predicts likelihood of onset of disease provided the patient lives long enough. As such a positive result is considered predictive, while symptoms onset would be diagnostic. For other conditions genetic testing may in fact be used for risk profiling (e.g. BRCA testing in breast cancer or familial adenomatous polyposis), identifying carrier status (e.g. cystic fibrosis), or prenatal testing (e.g. trisomy 21)
- Clearly identify the benefit of testing. This is often linked to the mode of inheritance or to the ability to initiate treatment and improve outcomes. In Huntington's disease, where no treatment is available the benefit of testing centres upon informed decision making in relation to family planning
- The accuracy of testing should be understood. Where there is likely to be a degree of uncertainty, due to limitations

of testing, this should be made clear to the patient prior
- Privacy and confidentiality should be considered, particularly in relation to disclosure to third parties, which may include family members, who may also require testing, employers, and insurance companies. Consider the Huntington's patient in whom they refuse to disclose a positive test result to their children
- The risks of testing also need to be made clear, albeit applicable predominantly to prenatal testing and risk to pregnancy

Hypothetical discussion of a positive test may ensue. If the patient were to test positive, themes for further discussion would likely focus upon the implication of the result and ensuring that the patient understands the disease. Thereafter, it is possible that issues of confidentiality may arise – it is prudent to consider situations such as a reluctance to inform family members and the refusal of wider family testing. While confidentiality must be maintained, encouraging an open attitude with full disclosure to those closest to the patient will be important, albeit a challenge demanding great skill and tact. Indeed, this highlights the importance of pre-testing discussion with family members, with joint decision-making, and is a vital point to stress with the examiner, as a means to avoid such a situation.

Where the patient has not yet started a family, a discussion in relation to assisted conception with in vitro fertilisation and pre-implantation testing, or pre-natal testing, may arise.

Genetic testing and insurance

The British Government and the Association of British Insurers set out in the document 'Concordat and Moratorium on Genetics and Insurance' in 2001 that anyone who has had a predictive test to assess their susceptibility to genetic conditions can take out significant insurance cover without disclosing the results. This agreement has been extended to 2017 with the next review due in 2014.

At the end of the consultation, revise the basic information with the patient to be sure that he is going away with the right factual understanding. Refer to support groups for the disease. Offer a further clinic appointment, and the opportunity to return with family members if desirable.

Additional themes worth consideration:

- Genetic cases may be used by examiners in the context of breaking bad news to patients. Consider situations requiring the explanation of investigation results, confirming a diagnosis such as cystic fibrosis or multiple sclerosis, and related discussion

Further reading

Association of British Insurers. Concordat and Moratorium on Genetics and Insurance. London: UK Government & Association of British Insurers, 2011

Case 178: Percutaneous endoscopic gastrostomy feeding

Candidate information

Scenario

A 60-year-old man with head and neck cancer attends the gastroenterology clinic for pre-assessment. He is due to undergo chemoradiotherapy and as a result will be unable to tolerate food and drink for an extended period of time. Please counsel him about the need for PEG feeding.

Actor information

You have recently been diagnosed with a head and neck cancer. You have been told that you will need a feeding tube put into the stomach while you are having your treatment. You are due to meet the doctor today to discuss the details. While apprehensive about the procedure you are hoping to understand the practicalities of placement and want to be clear on the possible risks and associated complications.

Approach to the case

Introduce yourself and explain the purpose of the consultation. The patient should be asked about what has happened thus far, what he understands of his diagnosis, proposed treatment and need for PEG feeding. An open approach will allow you to judge his level of knowledge and help build up a rapport but beware spending a disproportionate amount of time on history taking. Attempt to focus swiftly on to the topic of PEG feeding.

It should be explained to the patient that due to the intensive treatment given to head and neck oncology patients, it is unlikely he will be

able to tolerate fluids or oral foods. He should be informed in simple language that the standard management is to insert a PEG tube to ensure he meets his nutritional requirements during this period.

At this point, the patient may or may not have any idea about what a PEG is. As with all explanations to patients in MRCP PACES, this must be explained in a manner that:

- Contains no medical jargon: 'A PEG is a tube that is inserted through the skin into the stomach. The medical abbreviation stands for percutaneous endoscopic gastrostomy'
- Is alert to the patient's sensitivities
- Addresses what you understand to be the patient's concerns

Explain to the patient, in basic terms, the technique of PEG insertion, involving upper GI endoscopy, and then an incision in the skin to insert the tube into the stomach. Discuss the need for light sedation, often with midazolam, or simply lidocaine throat spray. Most patients tolerate it well although it can be an uncomfortable and distressing experience in a minority. As with all procedures, inform the patient of the common and serious complications, but at the same time explain that the balance of risk and benefit lies strongly towards benefit. Complications can be divided into those related to the PEG insertion and those related to feeding via a PEG

Complications related to PEG insertion include:

- Peritonitis is a rare but serious complication. It can occur due to leakage of the stomach contents into the peritoneum via the iatrogenic defect in the stomach wall.

This is a life-threatening complication requiring urgent surgical intervention
- Wound site infection. There is evidence to show that the risk of wound site infection is significantly reduced by use of prophylactic antibiotics at the time of PEG insertion

Complications related to feeding via the PEG include:

- Irritation of the surrounding skin (due to leakage of gastric contents)
- Blocked PEG tube
- The PEG tube can fall out, requiring replacement
- The tube and its buffers can be internalised, drawn into the skin due to raised tension

Allow the patient time to ask any questions they have. If they have any specific questions that exceed your knowledge base, the patient should be told that the question will be discussed with either a member of the oncology team (for cancer-related questions) or the gastroenterology consultant or PEG nurse (for PEG insertion-related questions) and the answer relayed back to the patient. Avoid ambiguity if uncertain and do not feel embarrassed to admit to not knowing an answer.

As the consultation nears its close, ask the patient if they think they are happy to go ahead with the PEG. The majority of patients will say yes. In this case a date can be arranged. If they say no, they can be offered a discussion with one of the gastroenterologists to seek to assuage their concerns. The patient should be offered some information sheets to take home with them and signposted to relevant websites or online resources.

Additional themes worth consideration:

- Alternative situations in which PEG feeding is commonly encountered such as stroke rehabilitation, where it has been demonstrated to be highly beneficial and improve prognosis, and dementia, where its value remains controversial
- Situations where families either insist on PEG feeding, where it is not in the patient's best interests, or alternatively where they resist, and are not in agreement despite potential benefit. Be prepared to compare PEG feeding with alternatives such as short term nasogastric tub feeding, or total parenteral nutrition. Such cases may have an increased focus towards capacity, consent and the incapacitated patient

Further reading

Nicholson FB, Korman MG, Richardson MA. Percutaneous endoscopic gastrostomy: a review of indications, complications and outcome. J Gastroenterol Hepatol 2000; 15:21–25
Jain NK, Larson DE, Schroeder KW, et al. Antibiotic prophylaxis for percutaneous endoscopic gastrostomy. A prospective, randomized, double-blind clinical trial. Ann Intern Med 1987; 107: 824–828.

Case 179: HIV testing – recent unprotected sex

Candidate information

Scenario

A 29-year-old woman is attending the GUM clinic, concerned about the risk associated with recent unprotected sexual intercourse, requesting medication. Assess the case and advise the patient on an appropriate course of action.

Actor information

You are in a long-term relationship with your boyfriend however recently you have been experiencing difficulties. 48 hours prior you were on a night out with your girlfriends and consumed an excessive amount of alcohol. You had sexual intercourse with a man that you had met for the first time in a club. Due to intoxication you cannot recall the full details of the encounter and are unclear as to the use of protection. Concerns relate primarily to the risk of HIV transmission.

Approach to the case

Encouraging an open discussion relies upon making the patient comfortable and ensuring a non-judgmental approach to what are often embarrassing and difficult topics to articulate. A matter of fact attitude can be useful but risks the impression of being cold and uncaring. Often, reassurance is all that is required.

Sexual health history taking

A brief history is a useful place to start. Avoid overcomplicating such an approach, but the basic content of a sexual health history may offer the platform on which to develop the relevant themes of the scenario.

Allow the patient to explain her reason for attending and express her concerns. Attempt to understand:

- Date of last sexual contact and the number of partners in the last 3 months
- Establish the gender of the partners – more relevant with men who have sex with men (MSM) but also women who may have bisexual partners
- Nature of intercourse by anatomical site – vaginal, anal and oral
- Use of protection
- Suspicion of previous or current infection by symptoms or confirmed diagnosis
- Existing diagnosis of blood borne virus and history of previous HIV/hepatitis testing

Understanding HIV and AIDS

Where the patient raises concerns or worries in relation to transmission of HIV establish what they understand of the disease. Clarify and summarise the salient points as necessary.

Attempt to gauge the validity of concerns in relation to HIV exposure. Establish whether there is evidence to suggest that the sexual contact has a confirmed diagnosis of HIV. For instance have they been contacted with information to that effect? Indeed, has the partner disclosed recent blood testing, including viral load and details of current treatment? While such a situation may seem implausible, it is the first step in moving the conversation towards a consideration of relative risk.

Risk of transmission related to exposure, need for testing, and consideration of post exposure prophylaxis

The concept of risk needs to be introduced. While statistics are rarely welcomed in such a scenario, often with anxious patients fearing the worst, they can be used to offer context. It is not recommended to rote learn figures, but useful to employ something along the lines of:

'In the highest risk groups, men who have sex with men, engaging in unprotected anal intercourse the risk of transmission, where HIV status is unknown, is less than 1 in 1000, increasing to approximately 1 in 100 if known HIV positive. Your risk is considerably less than this. As a heterosexual engaging in unprotected vaginal intercourse, the risk is likely between 1 in 30,000 and 1 in 200,000'. Avoid focusing on absolute numbers, conscious that they will vary with time and between populations, the point here is that the relative risk may in fact be quite low.

However, as alluded to, risk may be increased by certain factors. Most importantly, where possible it needs to be established as to whether the sexual contact is known to be HIV positive. Thereafter, consideration is given to the nature of the sexual intercourse in relation to acts performed, ejaculation, and the possibility of trauma and exposure to blood.

In reality, such information is usually obtained in clinic and referenced to a pro-forma to risk stratify patients. For the purposes of MRCP PACES, be mindful that the most important features pertaining to high-risk encounters include:

- Known HIV positive partner (in which case establishing the viral load would be paramount)
- Unprotected intercourse
- Receptive, greater than insertive, anal intercourse
- Trauma

It should be made clear that testing can and should be offered regardless of perceived risk. Testing may be routine blood tests or potentially more expedient point of care testing. A repeat test is always required 12 weeks later (newer antigen testing may be feasible at 4 weeks).

Where exposure is considered highrisk, testing should be performed and post exposure prophylaxis (PEP) offered provided presentation is within 72 hours. Counselling should include:

- An understanding that regardless of whether the baseline test is negative continued compliance with a 4-week course of antiviral medication is required
- The need to have a second HIV test 12 weeks post completion of PEP
- The side-effects of the drugs and the support available in the clinic and in the community to help adherence
- Promotion of safer sex, particularly over the initial 4-month period

- Issues around disclosure and confidentiality (see below)
- Psychological support as necessary, often relating to high-risk behaviour complicated by substance misuse or the impact of potential infection

In the first instance a starter pack is often made available, containing a combination of anti-viral medication in addition to medication to aid tolerance such as anti-emetic and anti-diarrhoeal medication, which will last the patient up to 5 days. Review thereafter in the GUM clinic allows for review and potential alteration of the regime based on further information, which may have been obtained in the interim.

Principles of confidentiality and information sharing in sexual health

Routinely, the attendance at, and results from, sexual health clinics are not shared with other medical health professionals, including a patient's GP. Exceptions to this include where the patient was in fact referred in by their GP or where the patient consents to sharing of the information, often to allow continuity of care, particularly where conditions are chronic and may impact upon other health issues for which the GP is responsible.

There are certain instances where confidentiality cannot be maintained and sharing of information is required, including:

- In response to a court order
- Notifiable diseases (Health Protection Agency) and situations where there is deemed considerable risk to others
- Where there are concerns about safeguarding vulnerable adults or children

The intention to share information should be discussed with the patient first, unless prohibited by a court order.

Other infections associated with high risk behaviour

Where concern exists with regard to HIV infection, screening should also be performed for commonly encountered sexually transmitted infections including hepatitis.

Conclude by checking understanding with the patient. Reiterate the salient points of the discussion, particularly the need for compliance with medication if prescribed and the need for a repeat test at 12 weeks.

The method of communicating results to the patient should be agreed, either with a planned return visit to the clinic or by text message. It is good practice for the clinic to deliver the results directly and never via a third party.

Additional themes worth consideration include:

- The patient who requests PEP but does not wish to be tested for HIV. HIV testing is mandatory for all patients receiving PEP
- Drug resistance in HIV positive individuals may influence the choice of PEP in patients who are concerned about exposure and risk of transmission from that person. This should not delay start PEP where indicated but may result in modification of the regime at a later date when details of resistance available
- The pregnant patient. Pregnancy is not a contraindication for PEP but expert advice should be sought
- Individuals with repeated high-risk exposure. Repeated exposure should be considered as cumulative risk when making a decision to prescribe PEP. When exposed repeatedly during a period of PEP, the medication does not need to be extended beyond the existing 28-day course
- The individual in whom PEP has been started but noncompliance has proven troublesome
- A patient demanding PEP when it is not indicated. There is often a public perception of a right to medication. This scenario challenges the candidate to explain the risk versus benefit principle of antiviral medication, often best centred upon the potential adverse side effects of medication

Further reading

British Association for Sexual Health and HIV. http://www.bashh.org/.

Case 180: HIV testing – needlestick injury

Candidate information

Scenario

You are the on-call medical registrar. Your SHO has been putting in a central venous catheter on a patient who presented with respiratory failure. She reports that she received a needlestick injury. She is concerned because the patient has a history of intravenous drug abuse. The local policy suggests that the SHO should be risk assessed in Accident and Emergency however the site manager has asked if you would review her due to pressures in the emergency department.

Actor information

You are the on call medical SHO. Earlier, you were asked to insert a central line into a 40-year-old man who presented with respiratory failure and is on the high-dependency unit (HDU). After you had inserted the central venous catheter, you were clearing up the sharps to dispose of them into the sharps bin. You sustained a needlestick injury on the hollow-bore needle which had been used to obtain central access. You had sterile gloves on, but the needle punctured these and the skin. You washed the wound for 10 minutes under running water. You are concerned because the patient in question has a history of intravenous drug abuse. You are worried about the risk of blood-borne virus transmission.

Approach to the case

Presume that you have not previously met the SHO and introduce yourself. 'I understand that you have sustained a needlestick injury. What I suggest we do is start with talking about exactly what happened, and then we can go on to discuss whether or not you need to consider post-exposure prophylaxis. Finally, we can talk about further testing. Is that ok?' It may be sensible to gauge the doctors understanding of the steps required following potential exposure to blood-borne viruses or make a statement such as 'I am going to work through the protocol for this assuming you have no prior knowledge, for that I apologise in advance but in my experience it is the safest way of ensuring we don't miss anything important'.

Check the exact time of the incident. Where appropriate, treatment should be instigated within 1–2 hours of exposure for the most effective reduction of risk. Furthermore, it should be ensured that practical measures have been taken, including encouraging the wound to bleed but not sucking or squeezing with excessive pressure, irrigation and washing with warm water and soap and first aid where necessary.

Clarify the details of the potential exposure. While this scenario indicates a needlestick injury, be aware of the potential for exposure resulting from a splash of fluid involving mucus membranes or broken/damaged skin.

Specifically related to needlestick injuries, establish features associated with increased risk:

- Hollow bore needle (higher risk as compared to solid bore needle). When discussing needlestick injuries during procedures in which more than one sharp implement is involved, be precise in finding out which sharp caused the injury. For example, in a central line insertion there is the hollow-bore introducer needle, the scalpel, and the solid bore suture needle
- Deep injuries and those that draw blood are both associated with increased risk of transmission of blood-borne viruses

Features associated with high risk

Mechanism:
- Deep injury
- Hollow bore needles
- Donor known to be blood-borne virus positive

Body fluid: Predominantly concern relates to blood exposure however body fluid in which virus may be present and also represent high-risk includes:
- Amniotic fluid
- Vaginal secretions
- Semen
- Breast milk
- CSF
- Peritoneal, pleural, and pericardial fluid
- Synovial

Bodily fluids including urine, faeces, sputum and vomit are generally considered low risk unless contaminated by blood.

Identify the patient, referred to as the donor. The SHO, or recipient, may have limited information on the donor's medical background or current case but attempt to establish:

- Suspected or confirmed history of blood-borne virus (HIV, HepB, HepC)
- High-risk features, including ethnic origin correlating to areas of high prevalence, intravenous drug use, sex worker status, and (increasingly less relevant) haemophilia with history of transfusion pre 1985
- What are they currently in hospital for? In this case, the donor has respiratory failure in the context of a history of intravenous drug use. It would be helpful to know what the working diagnosis is and see the plain chest radiograph to consider pneumocystis pneumonia suggestive of immunocompromised state
- Do they have capacity to consent to testing for blood-borne viruses?

High-risk situations demanding consideration of PEP:

- If the donor has confirmed HIV, the doctor should be advised to commence post-exposure prophylaxis, as soon as possible from the time of the sharps injury. A PEP consent form must be signed by the recipient
- In cases where there is a suspicion of HIV but no confirmatory evidence, discussion should take place between you and the on-call infectious disease doctor to discuss the risks of the needlestick and potential need for empirical PEP therapy until test results for HIV are available
- High risk of hepatitis B may require treatment with immunoglobulin
- The doctor who has sustained the needlestick injury will need to have blood tests for blood-borne viruses (HIV, hepatitis B and C). They will require repeat testing at time intervals up to 6 months to ensure seroconversion has not occurred
- The doctor who sustained the needlestick injury should fill in a clinical incident form

Thereafter, referral should be made to occupational health; where necessary they will facilitate immunisation such as hepatitis B booster and undertake repeat testing at 6, 12 and 24 weeks. Occupational health will also be responsible for obtaining the donor results and liaise with recipient with the outcome. Where positive, they will refer for specialist care and advice on fitness to work. Furthermore, they will also report confirmed BBV exposures to the health protection agency.

The GUM clinic will normally facilitate ongoing provision of PEP for a 4-week period and monitor for toxicity with weekly blood testing.

General considerations:
In this case, you should send the doctor home and tell the examiner you would discuss with the site manager to arrange cover for the rest of the shift.

The hospital's infection control team is responsible for monitoring implementation of sharps policy. The doctor should be offered formal training on preventing sharps injuries. Regardless of the actual scenario, be aware that the Department of Health guidance notes that 'many exposures result from a failure to follow recommended procedures, including the safe handling and disposal of needles and syringes'.

Part of the discussion with the examiner may involve addressing how to consent the donor for HIV testing. Ultimately the patient is under no obligation to consent. Testing for the sake of the recipients best interests is not necessarily in the donor's best interest. Caution should be used to avoid placing pressure or coercing the donor into testing for blood-borne viruses. The concept of informed consent is paramount. Pre- and post-test counselling should be in place. Where the patient is incapacitated and unable to consent, the physician responsible for their care should be consulted and evidence that it is in the patient's best interest sought. Blood testing should be performed either by you, as the registrar on call, or by the doctor responsible for the care of the patient provided it is not the recipient.

Further reading

Department of Health. Guidance for clinical health care workers: protection against infection with blood-borne viruses. London; Department of Health, 1998.

Case 181: Dealing with complaints – medical errors

Candidate information

Scenario

As the medical registrar covering the acute ward a patient has requested a meeting with you to discuss concerns in relation to the care that he has received.

Actor information

You are a 60-year-old man who has been in hospital for 2 days with a chest infection. Your condition has improved and you are due to be sent home to complete a course of oral antibiotics. Despite telling the doctor who saw you in casualty that you are allergic to penicillin (when you had penicillin before your 'throat closed over') you have been given amoxicillin as your oral treatment to go home with. You are extremely upset as you think your life may have been put in danger. You wish to make a complaint and have asked to see the doctor.

Approach to the case

Introduce yourself and clarify your role. Explain that you understand the patient has expressed a wish to make a complaint and that you would like to deal with any concerns he may have. Give the patient the opportunity to explain the nature of their complaint, listening attentively and resisting the temptation to interrupt, become defensive, or challenge the information outright.

Summarise the issues raised and repeat them back to the patient to ensure a shared understanding of the areas for discussion. Make efforts to understand the situation from the patients perspective, acknowledge distress if caused and empathise where possible.

Apologise for any distress caused. If appropriate apologise for the consequences of an action but you are often not in a position to apologise for the act itself, unless you were personally responsible. This may seem like avoiding the issue, but you should recognise your limitations in this situation and be clear on the concept of apologising on behalf of the team not the individual.

Discussing obvious errors made by colleagues is an extremely difficult topic. Cliché tells us that we 'all make mistakes' so it is tempting to defend colleagues and attempt to justify their actions. That, however, would not be the right and proper action. If faced with such a situation avoid commenting on colleagues' actions but rather seek to resolve the matter. You must neither try to cover up actions made by colleagues nor convict them in the court of public opinion.

Explain how you wish to resolve the situation and explain the actions you intend to take to ensure that similar does not occur. In this scenario, consider:

- Practical measures to ensure completion of a course of appropriate antibiotics. Change the prescription and ensure no delay to discharge by involving the sister in charge of the ward or alerting pharmacy
- Completion of an incident form
- Feedback to the colleague and their supervising consultant, with training or teaching where necessary
- Furthermore, a review of the ward process for such things as the ordering of discharge medication that should involve check points for allergy status including nursing staff and the dispensing pharmacist

Where an apology is deemed insufficient direct the patient to the Patient Advice and Liaison Service to support further options open to the patient in line with the complaints procedure.

Complaints procedures

Where a patient is not satisfied with a verbal apology, it is important to have an appreciation of the complaints procedure.

All patients have the right to complain about any aspect of their care. Furthermore, individuals may complain on behalf of a patient where consent to do so has been obtained. Complaints should be received as soon as possible after the event, or from the time when they were aware of a reason to complain, generally within a 12-month window.

- In the first instance patients should be encouraged to complain at a local level to the provider of the service from which they received their care and to whom the complaint refers.
- Alternatively, complaints can be made to the commissioner of the service – Clinical Commissioning Group or NHS England.
- Every service should make available, on request, a copy of their complaints procedure.

Often there will be a named individual who deals with all complaints.

It is good practice to ensure a dated response within 3 working days of receipt of a written complaint. This should include an outline the actions initiated, offer a meeting to discuss/ negotiate a plan to deal with the issues raised, and outline a timeline for a formal response (no fixed time scale).

Where the outcome or response is unsatisfactory, patients have a right to appeal to the Parliamentary and Health Service Ombudsman. In exceptional circumstances a judicial review may be required.

Support for complaints:
- Patient Advice and Liaison Service
- Complaints Advocacy Service
- Citizens Advice Bureau

Complaints cannot be directed to the Care Quality Commission however the commission can be informed of concerns with services.

Patients can make complaints about doctors directly to the General Medical Council. The GMC will review the complaint and if deemed appropriate proceed with an investigation, or alternatively it may be referred back for local resolution. In such instances, doctors should contact their defence union or British Medical Association for advice and consider the need for legal representation.

Additional themes worth consideration:

- Patients demanding financial compensation from a complaint. Be clear that financial compensation cannot be obtained from the standard complaints procedure in the NHS. Legal action is required to secure the possibility of financial compensation, where clinical negligence can be demonstrated

Definition of clinical negligence and the Bolam test

- The doctor must be proven to owe a duty of care to a patient
- A breech of that duty of care must be demonstrated, often demanding application of the Bolam test to reveal liability. Comparing the treatment or management implemented to that which would be considered reasonable or applicable by the wider medical community
- The breech of duty of care should be shown to have caused harm, referred to as causation. That is to say, harm that has resulted which would not otherwise have occurred

Common scenarios for complaints relate to:

- The patient in whom a test result has been misinterpreted with either distress resulting from misdiagnosis or inappropriate implementation of management/treatment options
- The lost test result with the need for repeated testings and delay to diagnosis or treatment
- Access to treatment issues. Often complaints relate to novel treatments for conditions with poor prognosis, where NHS availability is limited or ruled out by high cost and poor evidence of benefit. Answering this sort of complaint requires a detailed understanding of the relevant NICE guideline(s) and of the way NHS care is funded
- Delays to definitive management, with the need to apply principles of waiting lists and supply versus demand on the basis of prioritisation

Case 182: The trainee in difficulty

Candidate information

Scenario

As the medical registrar you have been working with the new intake of junior doctors for over 3 months. Concerns have been raised by the nursing staff about the performance and behaviour of one of the junior doctors with whom you have also experienced problems. There is a general feeling that the doctor is having difficulty coping with the demands of the job and you have been asked to discuss the situation with them.

Actor information

You are a 24-year-old foundation year doctor having graduated 6 months previously and moved to the city to start your training. Throughout medical school you avoided spending time on the wards during clinical attachments, instead, prioritising time in the library. The exposure to clinical medicine has been a shock and you have struggled to adapt but have felt unable to discuss the problem with your peers who seem more confident and able. Your reaction to the situation has been to isolate yourself and minimise contact with your team members. Increasingly irritable, low in mood, de-motivated and lacking in confidence you are frustrated by the downward spiral in which you find yourself and discussing the issues comes as a welcome relief.

Approach to the case

Be clear on the reasoning and evidence for any concerns raised particularly if others have raised them. Avoid conjecture and be wary of fuelling gossip or rumours. It is important to focus upon observable behaviours rather than personal characteristics or traits.

Recognising the trainee in difficulty

Difficulties may relate to:

- Lack of reliability. Persistent lateness, frequent sick leave, issues with not replying to bleeps, and disappearing during clinical duties such as extended breaks or unaccounted periods between ward and clinic work

- Slowness and inefficient use of time. Often paradoxically, the doctor who appears hyper-vigilant in arriving early and leaving late from work may in fact be attempting to compensate for problems coping
- Difficulty prioritising work, and an inability to compromise or accept constructive criticism
- Teamwork dynamics. Members of the team, including nurses and other doctors, seek to bypass the need for involving the individual in question. This is a coping strategy that fails to deal with the root cause of the problem
- Temper or behavioural outbursts on the ward often with a lack of insight and defensive responses to criticism with counter-challenges relating to the performance of others

Why is it important?

GMC guidance states: 'The safety of patients must come first at all times. If you have concerns that a colleague may not be fit to practise, you must take appropriate steps without delay, so that the concerns are investigated and patients protected where necessary. This means you must give an honest explanation of your concerns to an appropriate person.'

Understanding the process of raising concerns

Distinguishing between the trainee with difficulties versus the difficult trainee is an important concept. The former represents a failure to make satisfactory progress with training, for whatever reason, with resultant difficulties relating to their standard of clinical practice or ability to perform their role. The difficult trainee poses a problem as a result of attitudes or behaviours impacting upon professionalism and conduct. Both have a potential impact upon patient safety but practical solutions to the problems are likely to be markedly different.

Aim to deal directly with the individual. Sharing your concerns with an early conversation may rapidly identify the causes of any difficulty. Attempt to discuss the situation in a non-judgmental way, encouraging an open and honest discussion. Where the individual is reluctant to discuss the perceived problems, attempt to explain the responsibilities you have in dealing with the matter now that you have been made aware of it. This may offer a degree of separation, in that you are helping to discuss the concerns of others, not necessarily your own. Avoid a punitive or threatening tone but explain the potential for escalation if no progress can be made.

Common causes of difficulties include:

- Educational problems, balancing work pressures with revision and exams
- Career progression and anxiety in relation to lack of support in making career choices
- Perceived lack of team support, difficult team dynamics, or understaffing
- Personal or family health issues including substance misuse or dependency
- Personal relationship difficulties
- Domestic responsibilities or pressures. Inability to strike a life-work balance

Interventions and solutions

Formulating a plan of action, which is in the best interests of patients.

Understanding the reasons for difficulty should better allow you to identify avenues for help. Where legitimate problems are identified, doctors should be encouraged to share the information with their consultant who is often the clinical supervisor, or alternatively, educational supervisor. If met with a refusal to such a suggestion, a tactful explanation of your duty to do so on their behalf should follow. By escalating to seniors, the challenge of deciding the need for wider involvement including occupational health, human resources, the deanery, and the GMC is somewhat deferred. That said you should understand your responsibility to protecting the best interests of patients and the potential need to personally contact the GMC should you believe that there are issues relating to fitness to practice.

Where possible be seen to link the use of the trainee's e-portfolio and work-based assessments, both as a way of identifying trainees in difficulty, but also as a means of setting goals and monitoring improvement. Where assessments have been used honestly and openly they may be used to identify areas of weakness, such as communication skills, practical procedures, clinical reasoning, or team working. Multi-source feedback can be utilised to offer context to any complaints or concerns.

In addition to identifying areas of support, and need for specialist input or management, trainees may also be able to consider flexible training or an extension their training period.